NUTRITION AND BONE DEVELOPMENT

Nutrition and Bone Development

EDITED BY

DAVID JASON SIMMONS
Department of Surgery
University of Texas Medical Branch
Galveston, Texas

New York   Oxford
OXFORD UNIVERSITY PRESS
1990

Oxford University Press

Oxford   New York   Toronto
Delhi   Bombay   Calcutta   Madras   Karachi
Petaling Jaya   Singapore   Hong Kong   Tokyo
Nairobi   Dar es Salaam   Cape Town
Melbourne   Auckland

and associated companies in
Berlin   Ibadan

QP
88.2
.N87
1990

Library of Congress Cataloging-in-Publication Data
Nutrition and bone development/edited by David Jason Simmons.
p.   cm.   Includes index.   ISBN 0-19-504376-6
1. Bones—Growth.   2. Nutrition.
3. Bones—Metabolism—Disorders—Nutritional aspects.
I. Simmons, David Jason.
QP88.2.N87   1990   612.7'6—dc20   89-32566   CIP

9 8 7 6 5 4 3 2 1

Printed in the United States of America

TO NATALIE

Preface

Metabolic disorders of nutritional origin speak eloquently to current problems in connective tissue and skeletal biology. Well-established laboratory animal models make it possible to seek answers to basic questions about the specific influences of vitamins and trace elements on the proliferative potential of "bone cells." The authors who have contributed to this book have reviewed these issues as they pertain to the regulation of hard tissue matrix production and mineralization—how they may interact and, if known, how the cellular responses may vary across the age span. For nutrients other than calcium, phosphorus, and vitamin D, the answers to the problem across the age span are perhaps the most elusive.

The book contents have been divided somewhat artificially into five sections: (1) Development of the Musculoskeletal System; (2) Nutritional Problems in Mineral Metabolism over the Life-Span; (3) Protein, Carbohydrates, and Lipids; (4) Trace Elements and Metabolic Bone Disease; and (5) Archaeological Dietary Considerations. Such constraints beg overlap in the nature of the materials covered, but we have endeavored to keep this to a minimum. The breadth of the authors' subject matter, conjectures, and substantive conclusions cannot be adequately summarized in a preface. However, it is worthwhile to present something of the flavor of the book.

In Development of the Musculoskeletal System, John A. Ogden systematically describes the embryologic histogenesis and postnatal development of the human skeleton, with attention to specializations and patterns of growth of the physes as well as the spectrum of "normality" within the developing skeleton. He highlights the problems attendant to the use of small laboratory, primate and, wild-captive animal models to understand issues of skeletal growth and mineral metabolism in man. Subrata Saha reviews the consequences of aging and nutrition on the biomechanics of cortical and cancellous bone—issues that are central to the debilitating consequences of nutritional osteoporosis and the osteopenias. He develops and explores the thesis that agewise geometric changes in long bones (microstructure and cortical involution), their mass, and quality do not always accurately predict their loading carrying characteristics. A need is cited for data to quantify the relationships between microstructure, chemical composition, and mechanical properties in human populations.

In the section on mineral metabolism, Laura S. Hillman speaks to the clinical management of the term and preterm infant, and especially the challenges of prepared infant formulations. She emphasizes the need for constant monitoring of current neonatal practices, since, with the immaturity of the GI tract and liver in premature infants particularly, homeostatic mechanisms for mineral metabolism are often severely challenged by their dietary formulas. Phosphorus and vitamin D deficiencies are not uncommon.

Two papers follow that deal with the problem of undernutrition. Allen W. Root addresses the issue in the human, focusing on the consequences for malnutrition on the endocrine system and production of systemic and local skeletal "growth factors" that mediate skeletal growth, maturation, and mineralization. Issues of adequate supplies of calcium, phosphorus, and trace elements (Cu, Zn) are highlighted. Dike N. Kalu and Edward J. Masoro review these issues in the laboratory rat. Data are presented that argue strongly that although this animal may be an inexact model for man, it is not always an inappropriate model. It is emphasized that rat skeletons do not continue to grow throughout life and that its skeletal history (cortical involution) can make it a useful model to study certain aspects of osteoporosis/osteopenia. This chapter also focuses on the outcomes of studies that explore the skeletal consequences of undernutrition versus malnutrition. Charles W. Slemenda and C. Conrad Johnston Jr. then provide a status report on the important relationship between human bone mass, osteoporosis, and the incidence of fractures. They review the scientific bases for current concepts about the etiology of osteoporosis (activity, steroids, etc.) and its prevention via nutrition (Ca, F) and therapy—with particular emphasis on the role of inhibitors of bone resorption (estrogen, progesterone, and calciotropic hormones).

This subject matter is illuminated by two contributions about the metabolism of vitamin D and magnesium. Harriet S. Tenenhouse focuses on the elements of vitamin D metabolism, emphasizing issues pertaining to the formation and biological actions of the major metabolites. She brings into sharp focus how the metabolism of vitamin D is regulated by calcium and phosphorus and steroidal and nonsteroidal hormones, clarifying how biochemistry relates to the clinical picture of metabolic bone diseases such as D-deficient/D-resistant rickets and hypophosphatemia. Ruth Schwartz discusses the broad spectrum of action of magnesium on the endocrine–bone axis, emphasizing its centrality to the parathyroid skeletal and renal cell cell reactions, in PTH secretion, in the formation and maturation of hydroxyapatite, and its interactions with calcium, kidney, and bone cells. The skeletons of uremic–hypermagnesemia patients and magnesium-deficient rodents present some parallels with the osteoporotic skeleton, indicating that magnesium may have a life of its own apart from its interactions with the parathyroid. G. C. Chatterjee completes this section with a discussion of the role of vitamin C on the production and maturation of connective tissues, noting its action in the immunological mechanisms that effect mediators of bone resorption and its capacity to influence the metabolism of other drugs and chemical toxic to mechanisms of hard tissue maturation and calcification.

In Proteins, Carbohydrates, and Lipids, the discussions bear on how these dietary factors influence hard tissue cell function and play a role in the optimal absorption/utilization of calcium and phosphorus for skeletal mineralization. In evaluating the human and animal model data on proteins, Thomas A. Einhorn evaluates the hypercalciuric–osteopenic/osteoporotic outcome of diets that contain either suboptimal or high total protein, concluding that the mechanisms are likely to be different. Both levels impair osteoblastic function, but only low intakes reduce osteoprogenitor cell proliferation. Moreover, there appears to be an important endogenous component to the hypercalciuria at high protein levels, and the associated bone disease can be ameliorated by calcium supplementation. H. J. Armbrecht reviews the human and animal data that indicate that carbohydrates, and lactose in particular, stimulate then gastrointestinal absorption of calcium and phosphorus and enhance bone mineralization. The mechanism is in part vitamin D independent. H. Gilder and A. L. Boskey discuss the vital role of dietary lipids to bone tooth development/metabolism, with particularly valuable insights on the role membrane-rich calcium–acidic phospholipid complexes in cartilage/bone mineralization, their role in prostaglandin synthesis (bone modeling/remodeling), and the benefit of lipid-supplemented TPN solutions.

Within the context of nutritional problems that lead to osteomalacia-osteoporosis, we have not tried to deal exhaustively with the influences and interactions of the trace elements. That would be an impossibility within the confines of this book. Compromise was sought by focusing on four elements. William G. Goodman addresses aluminum toxicity which is a serious complication in the management of the dialyzed uremic patient. The paper highlights controversy about the consequences of aluminum loading for vitamin D-mediated gut calcium transport, renal aluminum excretion–tissue levels and parathyroid function, and the significance of distinctions in the expression of bone disease in renal osteomalacia where the rates of formation-resorption and mineralization may vary or grade with age and severity of disease (high turnover/osteitis fibrosa, low turnover/osteomalacia). M. R. Mariano-Meniz and his collaborators review the promising role of fluoride therapy in the long-term treatment of osteoporosis. At the "bone level," the benefits involve indices related to increased positive skeletal balance (mass and density), reduced fracture incidence, and normocalcemia-normophophatemia. Risks involve matters of bone quality and capacity for mineralization. Janet L. Greger speaks to the role of tin, which accumulates in the skeleton but appears to have no known function in the growth and maintenance of bone at the usually small dietary levels. Attention is owed tin, since dietary excesses produce toxic effects at the levels of the gut in terms of interactions with skeletally important copper, zinc, and selenium and may interfere with bone turnover and mineralization. The significance of zinc in skeletal formation-mineralization and its relationship to specific characterization of zinc nutriture is described by James C. Wallwork and Harold H. Sandstead. Their report emphasizes the teratology of zinc deficiency, the impairment of cell and tissue skeletal metabolism at suboptimal or unphysiologically high dietary levels, the interactions of zinc with vitamin D and calcium, and the benefit of vitamin D and calcium supplements to ameliorate Zn-deficient bone disease.

In the final section, Stephen Molnar provides "clues to the present" in a critical review of the literature on paleodiets, showing that much detective work still needs

to be done before the subsistence base(s) of ancient populations can be fully determined. The paleopathology and chemical composition of skeletal remains at-
tests to the significance of major and some "minor" dietary constituents for skeletal integrity.

There is a broad scientific base to the issues presented in this volume. The
contributors hope that their constructs will provide the stimulus for new hypotheses, concepts and interpretations.

Galveston   D. J. S.
September 1988

Contents

Contributors

H. J. ARMBRECHT
Departments of Medicine
   & Biochemistry
St. Louis University School
   of Medicine
St. Louis, Missouri

D. J. BAYLINK
Jerry L. Pettis Memorial
   Veterans Hospital
Loma Linda, California

A. L. BOSKEY
Department of Biochemistry
Cornell University Medical College
New York, New York

G. C. CHATTERJEE
Department of Biochemistry
College of Science
University of Calcutta
India

THOMAS A. EINHORN
Mt. Sinai Hospital
Department of Orthopedic Surgery
New York, New York

S. M. FARLEY
Department of Medicine
   & Orthopedic Surgery
Loma Linda University
Loma Linda, California

H. GILDER
Departments of Biochemistry
   & Pediatrics
Cornell University Medical College
New York, New York

WILLIAM G. GOODMAN
Department of Medicine
UCLA School of Medicine
Sepulveda, California

JANET L. GREGER
Nutritional Sciences Department
University of Wisconsin
   Medical School
Madison, Wisconsin

LAURA H. HILLMAN
University of Missouri-Columbia
School of Medicine
Department of Child Health
Columbia, Missouri

C. CONRAD JOHNSTON JR.
Department of Medicine
Indiana University School
   of Medicine
Indianapolis, Indiana

DIKE N. KALU
Department of Physiology
University of Texas
Health Science Center at San Antonio
San Antonio, Texas

M. R. MARIANO-MENEZ
Jerry L. Pettis Memorial
   Veterans Hospital
Loma Linda, California

EDWARD J. MASORO
Department of Physiology
University of Texas
Health Science Center at San Antonio
San Antonio, Texas

STEPHEN MOLNAR
Department of Anthropology
Washington University
St. Louis, Missouri

JOHN A. OGDEN
Shriner's Hospital for Crippled Children
Tampa, Florida

ALLEN W. ROOT
Department of Pediatrics
University of South Florida
College of Medicine
Tampa, Florida

SUBRATA SAHA
Department of Orthopaedic Surgery
Louisiana State University
School of Medicine in Shreveport
Shreveport, Louisiana

RUTH SCHWARTZ
Division of Nutritional Sciences
Cornell University
Ithaca, New York

CHARLES W. SLEMENDA
Indiana University School
   of Medicine
Indianapolis, Indiana

I
DEVELOPMENT OF THE MUSCULOSKELETAL SYSTEM

1

Histogenesis of the Musculoskeletal System

JOHN A. OGDEN

Evaluation of the skeleton, especially when dealing with the manifestations of congenital or acquired metabolic problems, requires an adequate understanding of developmental and maintenance chondro-osseous biology and accepted common terminology. The terms used to refer to different regions and aspects of a given bone are derived from the developing skeleton but apply readily to the adult skeleton which, while relatively static, still undergoes significant metabolic change and structural remodeling throughout the patient's life. The emphasis will be on basic development and biologic parameters of the skeleton up to the stage of skeletal maturation. However, when this occurs during adolescence (appendicular skeleton) and young adult years (axial skeleton), the skeletal components enter a phase of continual remodeling of the cortical and trabecular microanatomy. Disease and nutritional states may affect these processes throughout the adult years (e.g., loss of proximal femoral trabecular patterns in osteoporosis). Even in the senile individual the skeleton remains a relatively active organ system that is responsive to biologic demands (or lack of) and that reflects the overall health of the individual.

All skeletal elements initially form as genetically programmed mesenchymal condensations (1, 2). Some cellular groupings modulate to fibrocellular tissue and ossify directly (membranous ossification), a mechanism that characterizes cranial bones, most facial bones, and the initial formation of the clavicle. In contrast, the appendicular and axial skeletal components are derived from the initial transformation of the mesenchymal model into a cartilaginous model and the subsequent transformation to a progressively ossified structure. This integrated replacement of the pre-existent, biologically plastic cartilage by osseous tissue is termed endochondral ossification. These two basic types of bone formation—membranous and endochondral—refer *only* to the primary prenatal development of each individual structural unit, whether maxilla, femur, or phalanx. Subsequent growth of any particular unit after its initial differentiation may involve areas of each basic pattern within the same bone. Endochondral-derived bones have concomitant membranous ossification by appositional bone growth from the periosteum

(Fig. 1-1). Similarly, membrane-derived bones may undergo subsequent growth and elongation by an endochondral process, as in the clavicle or mandible.

BASIC BONE FORMATION PATTERNS

Membranous Ossification

Primary membranous bone formation occurs in the cranial and facial bones and in the clavicle. The membranous bones are formed from mesenchymal condensations that are morphological analogues of the eventual bone, similar to the cartilaginous precursor of an endochondral bone. At the site of presumptive primary ossification, small groups of cells elaborate a fibrous matrix that is calcified and ossified to form primary bone trabecula. Ossification then spreads rapidly outward from this primary ossification center to cover relatively large areas. The trabecular orientation within the expanding centers is relatively random when first formed

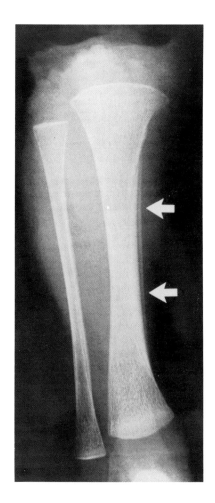

Fig. 1-1   Disarticulated tibia and fibula from a 7-week old baby victimized by child abuse. The antecedent violence had caused subperiosteal hemorrhage followed by new subperiosteal bone formation (arrows). Similar processes occur in fracture callus, tumor-responsive bone, and osteomyelitis.

but becomes progressively responsive to mechanical stresses internal and external to the developing fetus, factors that initiate early remodeling. The internal and external surfaces of the cranial and facial bones form plates through selective trabecular orientation and thickening. The clavicle is the first fetal bone to undergo membranous ossification, followed rapidly by the mandible. The clavicle and mandible subsequently form hyaline epiphyseal cartilage, but only after primary ossification is well under way. This cartilage, sometimes referred to as secondary cartilage, forms a modified growth apparatus (physis) to modulate further growth. Histologically, such cartilaginous areas either resemble the nonepiphyseal ends of the small longitudinal bones (distal end of the clavicle and mandible) or form an epiphysis capable of secondary ossification (proximal clavicle).

The axial and appendicular skeletal elements are involved in secondary membranous ossification (3–5). The diaphyseal cortex of each developing tubular bone is progressively formed (modeled) by the periosteum and modified (remodeled) by changing the woven trabecular bone to more dense cortical bone which, in turn, is further refined (remodeled) by formation of osteon systems. This peripheral periosteal process of membrane-derived ossification is extensive and rapid in some types of fracture healing, although the rate declines with increasing skeletal age. This replacement process may also be seen when portions of the developing metaphysis or diaphysis are removed for use as bone grafts, or in certain malnutrition states such as vitamin C or K deficiencies in which subperiosteal bleeding is followed by rapid neo-osteogenesis.

Endochondral Ossification

Endochondral ossification is the primary formation process of the axial and appendicular skeletal components and may recur in selected areas of established bone as part of fracture repair through the formation and maturation of callus. Put succinctly, this type of bone formation is the staged, synchronous replacement of mesenchymal tissue by cartilaginous tissue and the subsequent replacement of the cartilaginous model by osseous tissue. While the overall process is a continuum, it may be divided arbitrarily into a number of steps:

1. Formation of a mesenchymal condensation representing the basic anlage of each bone.
2. Increased extracellular matrix formation to create the precartilaginous model.
3. Extensive ground substance elaboration to form the distinct chondral anlage.
4. Further intracellular and extracellular enlargement of the entire chondral anlage, increasing hypertrophy of the central chondrocytes, formation of a trabeculated primary bone collar, associated periosteum and rudimentary vascular supply at the presumptive diaphysis, and increased intracellular and extracellular biochemical activity, especially in the hypertrophied central chondrocytes, leading to calcification within this section of the cartilaginous anlage.
5. Penetration of the primary osseous collar by the fibrovascular tissue, part of which will become the nutrient artery.

6. Progressive central replacement of cartilage by bone, initially around the area of vascular invasion, followed by extension of the process (including the bone collar) longitudinally toward each end of the anlage, thereby forming the primary ossification center (which eventually will become the diaphysis and metaphysis), the establishment of an orderly arrangement to the growth mechanism (physis), and an actively remodeling metaphysis.
7. Progressive vascularization of most of the chondroepiphyses by cartilage canal systems.
8. Appearance of secondary ossification centers within the chondroepiphyses, which is primarily a postnatal process.

Once the initial ossification center has formed and the nutrient artery has been established, expansile ossification progresses rapidly toward each end. The bone first formed is a loose trabecular network contained within a multilayered (laminated) periosteal shell (the latter being membranous bone surrounding the presumptive diaphysis). Initially, the endochondral ossification process extends at approximately equal rates toward each end of the bone. Postnatally, however, there are significant differences in the rates of physeal growth at each end of a given bone (e.g., 80% of longitudinal growth in the humerus occurs from the proximal physis).

As the primary ossification center approaches each cartilaginous end, selected areas of the cartilaginous cells increasingly resemble a physis. This process usually occurs during the third to fourth months. Concomitant with the ossification center progressing toward the cartilaginous ends, the primary periosteal collar extends toward these regions, but slightly ahead of the more central endochondral ossification process. Once the physis is morphologically established (usually after 70–80% of the initial cartilaginous anlage has been replaced by primary ossification), the periosteal ring stops further extension toward the epiphysis and remains level with the zone of hypertrophic cartilage (with which it continues growth in an integrated fashion), although it may extend further as osteoid tissue to reach the germinal zone. This periphyseal bone collar is referred to as the fibro-osseous ring of Lacroix. The cellular association of periosteal ring, bone collar peripheral physis, and fibrovascular tissue is referred to as the zone of Ranvier, which is an important area of diametric (latitudinal) expansion of the physis.

As the individual bone elongates and widens in the metaphysis by the normal process of endochondral ossification, extensive remodeling begins. When the endochondral trabecular bone and the membranous bone collar initially unite, they form a shaft of relatively uniform diameter. However, the metaphysis must progressively widen to accommodate the diametrically expanding physis and epiphysis. Active remodeling occurs in two areas of the metaphysis—central and peripheral. Bone modeling and remodeling are so active that the metaphyseal cortex is relatively porous. This porous bone is a factor in susceptibility of the immature skeleton to torus fracture and also allows spontaneous "decompression" of a metaphyseal focus of osteomyelitis into the subperiosteal space (4). As the skeleton matures, especially around and after the stage of physeal closure, the metaphyseal cortex progressively "solidifies" with osteon bone (6, 7).

SKELETAL REGIONS

The major long bones are divided into distinct anatomical areas—the epiphysis, physis, metaphysis, and diaphysis (Fig. 1-2). Each region is prone to certain patterns of injury and disease responses, with the intrinsic susceptibility changing as physiologic and biomechanical capacities change in accord with postnatal developmental modifications at both microscopic and macroscopic levels. The four regions originate and become modified as a result of the basic endochondral ossification process. Subsequently, they are supplemented by membranous bone formation along the metaphyseal and diaphyseal shafts. Finally, the regions are modeled and remodeled to create mature cortical (osteon) bone.

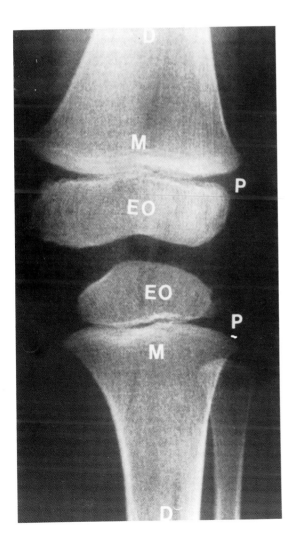

Fig. 1-2 Knee joint of a 5-year-old showing the characteristic regions of developing bone. EO, epiphyseal ossification center; P, physis; M, metaphysis; D, diaphysis. Note, in the tibia, how the thin metaphyseal cortex progressively thickens to become the diaphyseal cortex.

Diaphysis

The diaphysis comprises the major portion of each long bone. It is a product of periosteal, membranous osseous tissue apposition on the original endochondral model. This leads to the gradual replacement of the endochondrally derived primary ossification center and primary spongiosa, the latter being replaced by secondary spongiosa in the metaphyseal region. At birth, the diaphysis comprises laminar (fetal, woven) bone characteristically lacking in haversian systems. The neonatal diaphysis appears to be the only area exhibiting any significant change from the fetal osseous state to more mature bone with osteon systems (lamellar bone). Periosteal-mediated, membranous, appositional bone formation with concomitant endosteal remodeling leads to enlargement of the overall diameter of the shaft, variably increased width of the diaphyseal cortices, and formation of the marrow cavity (Fig. 1-3). Mature lamellar bone with intrinsic but constantly remodeling osteonal patterns progressively becomes the dominant feature (7–14). The active remodeling osteon is referred to as a bone metabolic unit or bone modeling unit (BMU) and is the mechanism of response within the cortex to physiologic, nutritional, and biomechanical conditions throughout life.

The developing bone in a neonate or young child is extremely vascular and appears much less dense than the maturing bone of older children, adolescents, and adults. Subsequent growth leads to increased complexity of the haversian (osteonal) systems and the elaboration of increasing amounts of extracellular matrix, causing a relative decrease in cross-sectional porosity and an increase in hardness, factors that constantly change susceptibility to fracture patterns and responses to metabolic conditions.

The inner surface of the cortex (endosteum) is the site of continual remodeling throughout life and is relatively irregular owing to the variable trabecular bone and continual remodeling. The outer cortical surface is usually smooth and covered with periosteum. This latter tissue, prior to skeletal maturation in adolescence, is highly osteogenic, progressively enlarging the bone diametrically, concomitant with endosteal removal to maintain cortical thickness. The periosteum is relatively loosely attached to the bone and may be stripped away during trauma or elevated by pathologic processes. When this occurs the normal biologic response is new bone formation external to the cortical surface.

Metaphysis

The metaphysis is a variably contoured flare at each end of the diaphysis. The major characteristics are decreased thickness of the cortical bone and increased trabecular bone in the secondary spongiosa. Extensive endochondral modeling centrally and peripherally initially forms the primary spongiosa, which is then transformed (remodeled) into more mature secondary spongiosa, a process that involves osteolytic, osteoclastic, and osteoblastic activity. The metaphyses exhibit considerable bone turnover compared to other regions of the bone, a factor undoubtedly responsible for the increased uptake of radionuclides during bone scans. The metaphysis, because of the high rate of bone modeling and remodeling, appears most susceptible to the development of lesions such as fibrous cortical defects and unicameral bone cysts.

Like the diaphysis, the metaphyseal cortex changes with time. Relative to the confluent diaphysis, the metaphyseal cortex is thinner and has greater porosity (trabecular fenestration). These cortical fenestrations contain fibrovascular soft tissue elements interconnecting the metaphyseal marrow spaces with the subperiosteal region (Fig. 1-4). The metaphyseal cortex exhibits greater fenestration near the physis than the diaphysis, with which it gradually blends as an increasingly thicker, dense bone. As longitudinal growth continues, cortical fenestration becomes a less dominant feature, and the overall width of the cortex increases, creating a greater morphologic transition between the juxtaphyseal and juxtadiaphyseal cortices. The metaphyseal region does not develop secondary haversian systems until the late stages of skeletal maturation. The microscopic anatomical changes appear to be directly correlated with changing patterns of fracture occurrence and undoubtedly influence the probability of torus (buckle) fractures, as apposed to complete metaphyseal or epiphyseal/physeal fractures. In diseases such as rickets, this porous, relatively weak bone may gradually deform, adding to the morphologic changes caused by the physis. Although the periosteum is attached relatively loosely to the diaphysis, it becomes more firmly fixed to the metaphysis owing to the increasingly complex continuity of fibrous tissue through the metaphyseal fenestrations. Such intermingling of endosteal and interosseous fibrous tissues with periosteal tissue imparts additional biomechanical strength to the region. The periosteum subsequently attaches densely into the peripheral physis, blending into the zone of Ranvier as well as the epiphyseal periochondrium. The fenestrated metaphyseal cortex extends to the physis as the osseous ring of Lacroix.

The metaphysis is the site of extensive osseous modeling and remodeling, both peripherally and centrally. The metaphyseal cortex is fenestrated, modified trabecular bone on which the periosteum elaborates membranous bone to progressively thicken the cortex. Similar endosteal bone formation occurs. As this metaphyseal region thickens, the trabecular bone is progressively replaced by diaphyseal osteon systems, not unlike osteons traversing the fracture site in primary bone healing. This converts peripheral trabecular (woven) bone to lamellar (osteon) bone, which has different biomechanical capacities, and thus progressively transforms metaphyseal cortex into diaphyseal cortex as longitudinal growth continues.

Another microscopic anatomical variation in the metaphysis occurs at the juxtaposition of primary spongiosa and the hypertrophic region of the physis. In most rapidly growing bones the trabeculae tend to be longitudinally oriented. However, in shorter growing bones, such as the metacarpals and phalanges, trabecular formation is predominantly horizontal. As growth decelerates in adolescence, a similar horizontal orientation may be seen on both sides of the physis in the major long bones.

Many bones exhibit transversely oriented, dense trabecular patterns in the metaphysis, with these lines usually duplicating the appropriate contiguous physeal contour (Fig. 1-5). They may appear after trauma, generalized illnesses, malnutrition or localized processes within the bone (e.g., osteomyelitis). They rep-

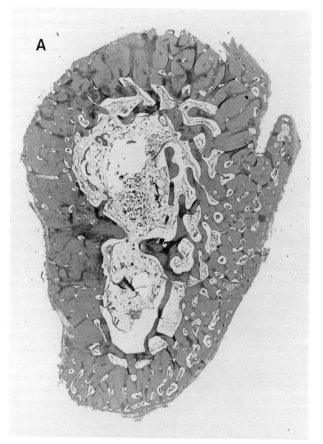

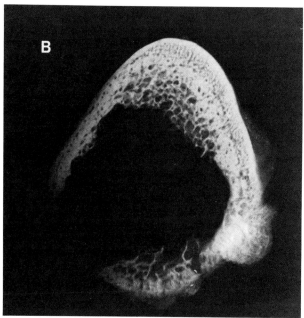

Fig. 1-3 A and B. *See legend on facing page.*

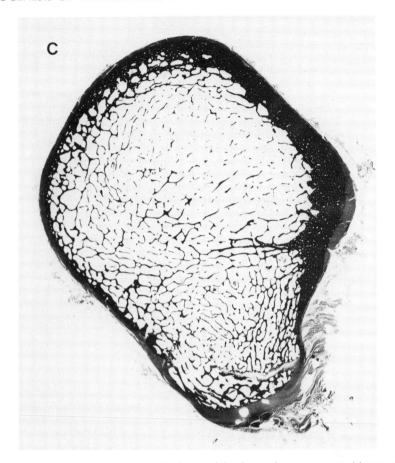

Fig. 1-3   (A). Transverse section of diaphysis of the femur from a 2-year-old. (B). Radiograph of transverse section of tibia from a 5-year-old. (C). Histologic transverse section of femur from a 15-year-old. Note the changing patterns of cortical density and osteon formation.

resent a temporary slowdown of normal longitudinal growth rates during the postinjury period or illness, and are often referred to as Harris growth arrest lines. Because of the slowdown, the trabeculae of the primary spongiosa become more transversely than longitudinally oriented as they are initially formed, creating a *temporary* thickening in the primary spongiosa adjacent to the physis. Once normal longitudinal growth rate resumes, longitudinal trabecular orientation is restored. The thickened, transverse osseous plate is "left behind" as the bone continues to elongate and is gradually remodeled as primary spongiosa becomes secondary spongiosa.

If one observes the normal, constantly changing morphology of the different bones, the more rapidly growing ones are associated with longitudinally oriented trabeculae in the juxtaphyseal region, whereas the slower-growing bones, particularly the proximal radius, the metacarpals, metatarsals, and phalanges, normally have a greater amount of transversely oriented primary spongiosa. Because this

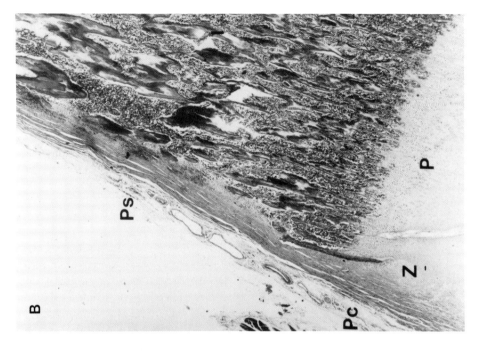

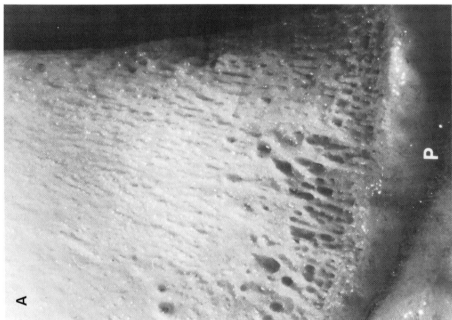

is the standard pattern of orientation in many smaller bones, transverse septae and their slower rates of growth are normal. Therefore, these particular bones will not have a sufficient difference in the orientation of trabeculae to radiographically manifest transverse lines (15).

However, when growth slows down in the rapidly growing areas normally characterized by longitudinal orientation of trabecula (e.g., distal femur), the primary spongiosa forms in a transverse orientation. Once normal rates of growth and longitudinal trabecular orientation are reestablished, the transversely oriented juxtaphyseal plate contrasts to the pre- and post-trauma or disease longitudinally oriented trabeculae and appears as a specific transverse line radiographically. As remodeling occurs with migration of the epiphysis away from this region, and with conversion of primary spongiosa to secondary spongiosa, there is a gradual breakup of this transverse trabecular orientation.

Epiphysis

At birth, with the exception of the distal femur, each epiphysis is a completely cartilaginous structure at the end of each long bone (Fig. 1-6). This includes the small longitudinal bones of the hands and the feet. Such a cartilaginous structure is referred to as the chondroepiphysis, while the corresponding ossifying structure is termed the chondro-osseous epiphysis. At a time characteristic for each chondroepiphysis, a secondary center of ossification forms and enlarges (Fig. 1-7) until the cartilaginous model has been virtually completely replaced by bone at skeletal maturity; only articular cartilage will remain (16, 17). With the exception of the distal femur, all secondary (epiphyseal) ossification is a postnatal phenomenon. The epiphyseal cartilage enlarges by both cellular multiplication, particularly at the periphery through the perichondrium, and the elaboration of increasing amounts of extracellular matrix. Eventually a portion or portions of this cartilage hypertrophies and undergoes chemical changes that eventuate in the formation of a secondary ossification center. Most centers appear as a single, expanding focus. However, certain regions such as the distal humerus (trochlea) are characterized by initial multifocal ossification. Such a center may be unifocal, as in the case of the distal femur, radius, or ulna, or it may be multifocal, as in the case of the distal humerus, where separate secondary centers develop in the capitellum, medial epicondyle, trochlea, and lateral epicondyle.

As the ossification center expands, it undergoes structural modifications (Fig. 1-8). Particularly, the region adjacent to the physis forms a distinct subchondral plate parallel to the metaphysis, creating the roentgenographically characteristic

---

Fig. 1-4   (A). Osseous preparation of distal femur from a 7-year-old human showing the physis (P) and the extensive porosity of the metaphyseal cortex. In contrast, the diaphyseal cortex is relatively smooth. (B). Histologic section of metaphyseal cortex from the distal femur of a 2-year-old human showing the physis (P), zone of Ranvier with the fibro-osseous ring of Lacroix, (Z), and the porous (fenestrated) cortex allowing fibrous communication between the periosteum (Ps) and the intertrabecular tissue. Also note how the periosteum (Ps) is continuous with the perichondrium (Pc).

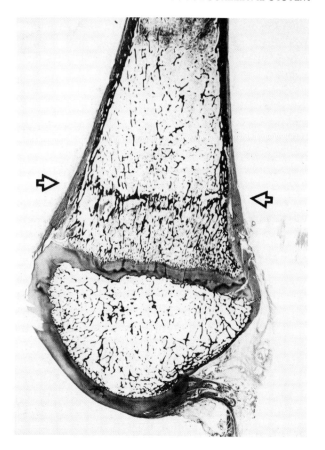

Fig. 1-5 Distal femur exhibiting a growth slow-down line (arrows). This child had been on cyclical chemotherapy for leukemia.

lucent physeal line. Certain chondroepiphyses exhibit variations in the appearance and enlargement of the ossification centers, factors that must be considered in the appropriate diagnosis of biologic variation rather than disease within these regions. The appearance and progressive development of the secondary center of ossification within a chondroepiphysis is undoubtedly affected by nutrition status. The ossification center imparts increasing rigidity to the more resilient epiphyseal cartilage as the secondary osseous tissue expands. The secondary ossification center progressively enlarges in a pattern reasonably characteristic for each epiphysis. The appearances of the secondary ossification centers are often variable when comparing one side of the skeleton to the other, and one must be very careful in the evaluation of symmetry versus asymmetry. This process is related to biomechanics, and there is often increased maturation (i.e., ossification) in the epiphyses of the dominant side compared to the nondominant side. The external surfaces of an epiphysis are covered either by articular cartilage or by perichondrium. Muscle fibers, tendons, and ligaments attach directly into the perichondrium, which is densely contiguous with the underlying hyaline cartilage. The perichondrium contributes to continued centrifugal enlargement of the epiphysis. It also blends imperceptibly into the periosteum. This perichondrial–periosteal tissue continuity contributes to the biomechanical strength of the region.

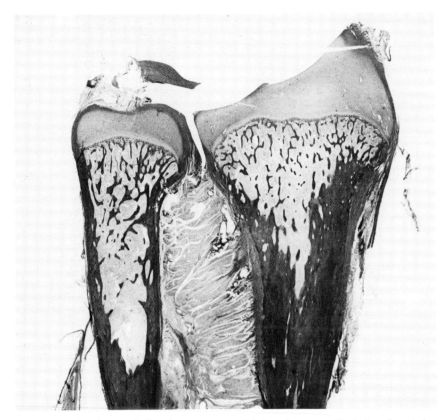

Fig. 1-6 Distal radius and ulna from a 2-year-old showing unossified chondroepiphyses and relatively transverse physes.

Physis

The growth plate, or physis, is the essential mechanism of endochondral ossification. The primary function of the physis is rapid, integrated longitudinal and latitudinal growth.

Since the physeal cartilage remains radiolucent, except for the final stages of physiologic epiphysiodesis, its appearance must often be inferred from radiographic metaphyseal, and physeal contours. The changing size of the secondary ossification center more effectively demarcates the physeal contour on the epiphyseal (germinal layer) side. As this center of ossification enlarges centrifugally to approach the physis, the originally spherical shape of the ossification center flattens and gradually develops a contour paralleling the metaphyseal contour. Similar contouring also occurs as the ossification center approaches the lateral and subarticular regions of the epiphysis. The region of the ossification center juxtaposed to the physis forms a discrete subchondral bone plate through which the epiphyseal blood vessels penetrate to reach the physeal germinal zone.

From a macroscopic viewpoint, there are two basic types of growth plates—discoid and spherical (Fig. 1-9). Primary growth plates of the major long bones

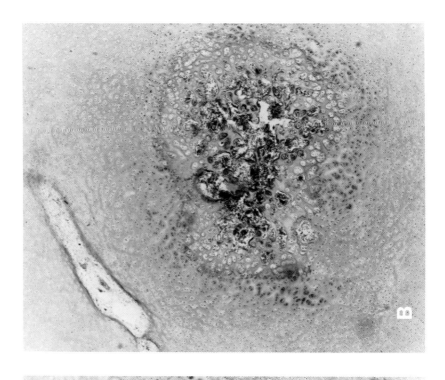

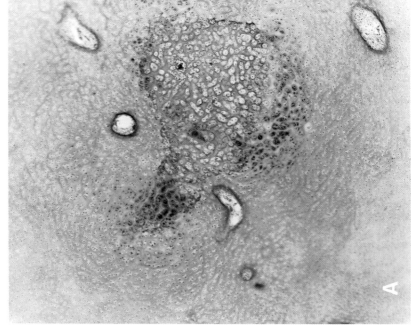

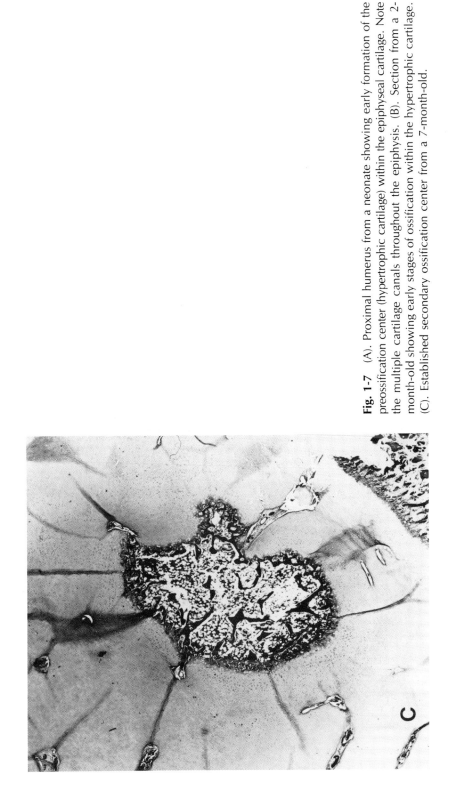

Fig. 1-7 (A). Proximal humerus from a neonate showing early formation of the preossification center (hypertrophic cartilage) within the epiphyseal cartilage. Note the multiple cartilage canals throughout the epiphysis. (B). Section from a 2-month-old showing early stages of ossification within the hypertrophic cartilage. (C). Established secondary ossification center from a 7-month-old.

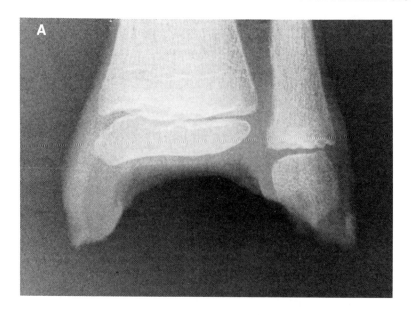

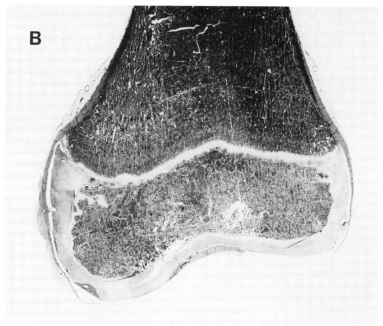

Fig. 1-8 (A). Radiograph of distal tibia and fibula from a 10-year-old showing the secondary ossification center within the epiphyses. The medial malleolus remains unossified. The contour of both physes is relatively transverse. (B). Section of distal femur from a 9-year-old. Note the irregularity of ossification at the medial and lateral margins of the ossification center. Also note the binodal contour of the physis, with the central "peak." (C). Osseous preparation of the knee from a 10-year-old. Note that the secondary center has a cortical shell with multiple fenestrations for blood vessels.

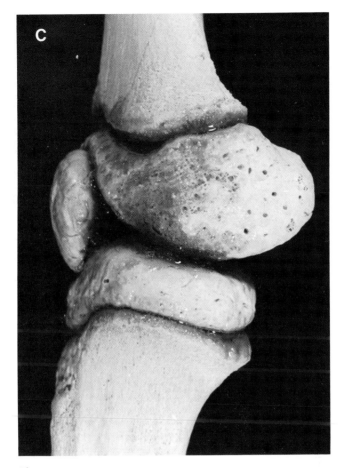

Fig. 1-8   (C).

are discoid. They are characterized by a relatively planar area of rapidly differentiating and maturing cartilage that grades imperceptibly from the epiphyseal
hyaline cartilage. Initially, most discoid physes are transversely planar, but with
subsequent response to growth and biomechanical stresses, each physis assumes
variable degrees of three-dimensional contouring while retaining the basic planar
nature. Additionally, small interdigitations of cartilage extend into the metaphyseal bone. These are termed mammillary processes. Contouring and mammillary
processes appear to contribute to the intrinsic stability of the physis, particularly
to shearing forces.

Discoid (planar) growth plates may also be found between the metaphysis and
an apophysis, which has been defined as an epiphysis subjected primarily to tensile rather than compressive forces. The tibial tuberosity is such a structure (Fig.
1-10). However, instead of the normal columnar cytoarchitecture, such a tension-
responsive structure is characterized by variable amounts of fibrocartilage that
represent a microscopic structural adaption of the physis to the high tensile forces
imparted by the quadriceps mechanism.

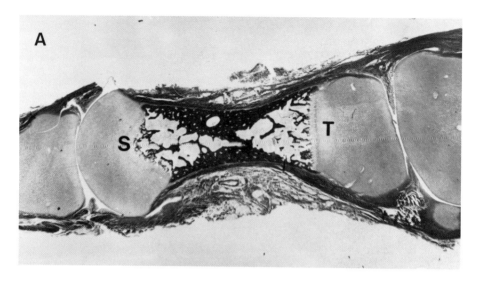

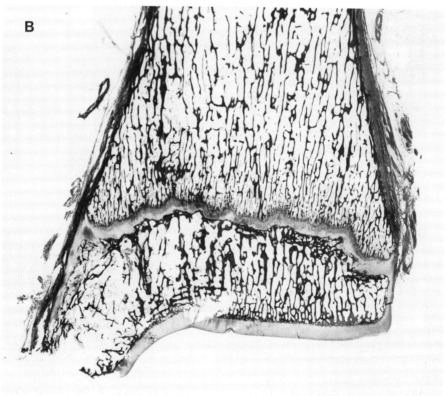

Fig. 1-9 (A). Section of a digit showing discoid transverse (T) and spherical (S) physes within a plalanx. Note also the thickened cortical bone derived primarily from membranous ossification. (B). Undulated physis of the distal tibia from a 12-year-old.

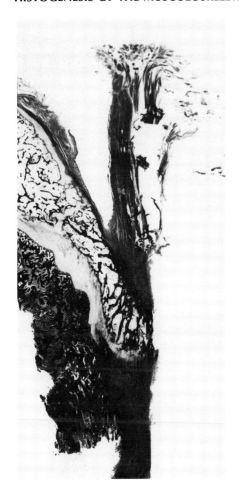

Fig. 1-10 Apophysis associated with tibial tuberosity.

In the short tubular bones (metacarpals, metatarsals, and phalanges), two discoid physes and contiguous chondroepiphyses initially form, but with subsequent skeletal growth only one end maintains a true chondroepiphysis and physis which will become the primary mechanism for longitudinal growth of each bone. In contrast, the epiphyseal hyaline cartilage of the opposite end is replaced relatively rapidly, until only a small amount remains between the articular surface and metaphysis. The associated physis assumes a spherical contour with decreased cell column length underneath the articular cartilage. This spherical physis contributes minimally to longitudinal growth but does allow contoured expansion of the metacarpal head.

An epiphyseal ossification center rarely appears in the epiphysis associated with such a spherical growth plate, although a structural variation is sometimes encountered, the pseudoepiphysis. This commonly occurs in the distal end of the thumb metacarpal, where it should be considered a normal variant. However, when found in multiple small bones, it may be indicative of a pathologic situation such as hypothyroidism. The pseudoepiphysis is not a true ossification center but

rather an upward, and subsequently expansile, enlargement of metaphyseal ossification.

The physis has a characteristic and essentially unchanging basic cytoarchitecture from early fetal life until skeletal maturation (3, 7, 18, 19). Histologic differences among the various physes are a reflection of growth rates and biomechanical stresses (20). These variations include the relative numbers of cells in
each zone, the overall height of the physis, peripheral differences in the zone of
Ranvier and specific cellular modifications, such as replacement of the zone
of hypertrophic cartilage by a zone of fibrocartilage. The basic patterns may be
analyzed as either functional or morphologic zones (Fig. 1-11).

The zone of growth is involved in both longitudinal and latitudinal (diametric)
expansion of the bone. It is the area of most concern in any fracture involving
the growth plate, for direct damage from trauma, or indirect damage by temporary
or permanent vascular injury, in contradistinction to other zones of the physis,
may have long-term ramifications for normal growth patterns. This is the cellular

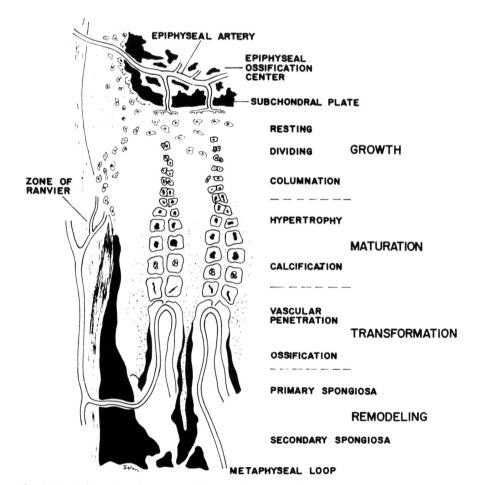

Fig. 1-11   Schematic of regions of the growth plate (physis).

zone in which mitoses and new cell formation occur. The resting and dividing cells are intimately associated with blood vessels of the epiphysis.

Adjacent to the resting cell layer is the layer of active cell division. Mitoses appear in both longitudinal and transverse directions, although principally in the former, leading to the earliest evidence of cell column formation. In an active growth plate, such as the distal femur, cell columns may comprise half the overall height of the physis. The randomly dispersed collagen of the resting and dividing regions becomes more longitudinally oriented between the cell columns.

Additional cells may also be added peripherally through a specialized region surrounding the physis—the zone of Ranvier. This zone contains fibrovascular tissue, undifferentiated mesenchymal tissue, differentiating epiphyseal and physeal cartilage, and the osseous ring of Lacroix.

The next functional area is the zone of cartilage maturation. The amount of intercellular matrix formed increases, particularly between cell columns, rather than between successive cells in a given column. The cells remain separated by a thin, transverse septum. This is composed of a distinct type of collagen that appears specifically related to endochondral ossification. The matrix exhibits cell-mediated biochemical changes, becoming metachromatic and subsequently calcifying, a necessary prelude for ossification. The chondrocytes hypertrophy.

The final functional zone is cartilage transformation. The cartilage matrix must be sufficiently calcified to allow vascular invasion by the metaphyseal vessels which break down the transverse cartilaginous septa to invade the cell columns. Osteoblasts then lay down bone collagen (primary spongiosa) on the surfaces of the performed intercolumnar cartilage matrix. This initial cartilage/bone composite will be remodeled and removed, to be replaced by a more mature secondary spongiosa, which no longer contains remnants of the cartilaginous precursor.

The regions of the cellular hypertrophy and transformation appear to be structurally weak zones most likely to be involved in pathological conditions. In certain diseases, such as rickets, the hypertrophic zone may be widened significantly because of failure to calcify the matrix. This prevents capillary invasion from the metaphysis, such that the hypertrophic zone cannot be replaced by osseous tissue. Addition to the hypertrophic cartilage zone continues, resulting in a progressively wider region that becomes mechanically unstable, and may eventually result in epiphyseal displacement.

Zone of Ranvier

The zone of Ranvier is an anatomical structure bordered outwardly by a continuation of the fibrous periosteum and inwardly by the epiphyseal and physeal cartilage. The cells and matrix within the groove are organized into three anatomic groups. It has an outer zone of fibroblasts and a region is formed over the groove by fibroblasts and collagen bundles which are continuous with the fibrous layer of the periosteum. It acts as a mechanical support for the growth plate and as an anchor for the periosteum. The innermost zone contains a region of densely packed cells high in alkaline phosphatase that function as osteoblast precursors that form the osseous ring. There is also a region of loosely packed cells characterized by increased production of glycosaminoglycans that functions as a source for cartilage progenitor cells, allowing increased diametric (latitudinal) expansion of the epiphysis and physis by appositional growth.

GROWTH

Patterns of Physeal Growth

Characteristically, the growth of bones is considered a longitudinal phenomenon. However, expansion must occur in other significant ways. Appositional growth for the diaphysis through the combined mechanisms of periosteal osteogenesis and endosteal remodeling has been described. The physis similarly expands in a diametric, or latitudinal, fashion, a process that occurs by cell division and intercellular matrix expansion within the physis (interstitial growth), and by cellular addition (appositional growth) peripherally at the zone of Ranvier (Fig. 1-12).

Interstitial growth within the physis appears directly related to enlargement of the secondary center of ossification. When the epiphysis is completely cartilaginous, or contains only a small, spherical ossification center, the biologically plastic cartilage does not present a total mechanical barrier to interstitial expansion of the juxtaposed physis. With increasing development of the epiphyseal ossification center, a discrete subchondral (cribiform) bone plate forms. Subsequent interstitial expansion of the physis is effectively precluded in the areas directly apposed to the subchondral plate. Latitudinal expansion thus becomes progressively limited to appositional growth from the peripheral zone of Ranvier, which remains peripheral to the enlarging cribiform plate.

Mechanical Control of Growth

Besides the intrinsic nature of cell division, which is a genetically controlled factor, there appears to be an anatomic restraint to rapid, uncontrolled elongation. This control factor is the periosteal sleeve. This sleeve, which is densely adherent at each end of a bone to the zone of Ranvier and the perichondrium of the epiphyses, is only loosely attached to the underlying metaphyses and diaphysis. The sleeve has an intrinsic elasticity affected by the varying collagenous composition and biochemical milieu (e.g., hormones, nutritional status). When this intrinsic tension is disrupted, overgrowth of the bone, compared to the contralateral one, is a recognized clinical phenomenon. Crilly identified this pattern of overgrowth in chicken bone by the circumferential resection of portions of periosteum. Other investigators have since added to this concept of the periosteum as a mechanical control to longitudinal growth.

Physiology of Growth

Growth within the physis and its eventual closure are also regulated by various hormones. Thyroxine is extremely important in early cartilaginous (physeal and epiphyseal) development. Lack of this hormone may cause (1) loss of integrity of the articular cartilage; (2) erosion of the hyaline chondroepiphysis by bone and

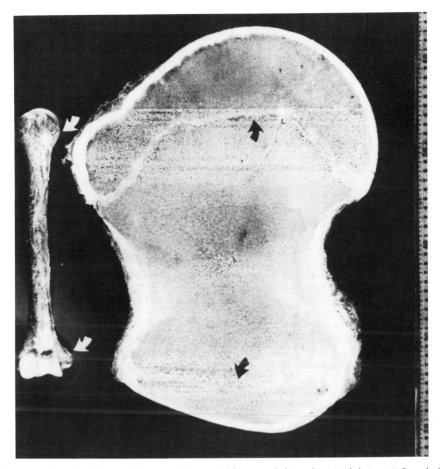

Fig. 1-12 Proximal humeri from a 16-year-old human (left) and an "adolescent" fin whale (right). The physes (arrows) of the human humerus are approximately the same distance apart as those in the whale. However, there is a massive difference in the amount of *latitudinal* growth in the whale.

fibrous tissue; (3) increased vascularization of the chondroepiphysis (there may be twice as many cartilage canal systems, without the normal canal demarcation); (4) abnormal distribution of the matrical glycosaminoglycans; and (5) decreased physeal width, particularly affecting the zone of hypertrophy. Thyroxine (or its absence) appears to have little direct effect on ossification. The most severe form of hypothyroidism is cretinism, in which overall skeletal development is retarded and pseudoepiphyses may develop. The effect of thyroxine on skeletal growth appears to be synergistic with growth hormone. Growth hormone appears to affect the cells of the resting germinal zones to induce cell division and widen the physis. The mode action is not completely understood but probably occurs through a second hormone called somatomedin (sulfation factor) and now recognized as insulin.

Sex hormones also affect physeal growth. Testosterone initially stimulates the physis to undergo rapid cell division and widening during the growth spurt (anabolic effect), but eventually manifests an androgenic effect that slows down growth and leads to consolidation of the cartilage. Estrogens suppress growth plate activity by two mechanisms: (1) an apparent indirect effect through suppression of sulfation factor (by peripheral antagonism), and (2) a direct effect to increase calcification of the matrix, which is a prerequisite to physeal closure. An additional indirect effect of estrogen may be increased collagen cross-linkage in the periosteum, increasing intrinsic tension (stiffness) within the periosteum and thereby increasing restraint to longitudinal growth. Alteration of physeal microstructure by hormonal imbalance may be a factor in susceptibility to epiphysiolysis (21–23).

SKELETAL MAINTENANCE

Cartilage and bone are dynamic, mechanically responsive tissues that constantly model and remodel, no matter what the degree of skeletal maturation. Initial responses to metabolic conditions occur at a microstructural level and represent either a direct cellular response, as in trabecular bone, or a combined cellular and vascular response, as in cortical bone. The ability to model and remodel requires active physiologic mechanisms. For joint cartilage the physiologic status is maintained through joint motion and fluid dynamics. For the osseous tissues, as well as hyaline epiphyseal cartilage, maintenance is extremely dependent upon vascularity (3, 7, 24–26).

The developing osseous and cartilaginous components are both extremely vascular. The periosteum contains multiple, small vessels that play a role in cortical osteogenesis and contribute to the increasingly complex haversian systems of the immature and mature diaphyseal cortices. The endosteal surfaces of the diaphysis and metaphyses receive blood through the nutrient artery, a major vessel whose branches also supply the intercortical canals. The epiphysis receives its blood from vessels that penetrate into and ramify through the cartilage and bone. The two major circulatory patterns—epiphyseal and metaphyseal vessels—appear to be functionally and anatomically separate, even after skeletal maturity is attained.

The epiphyseal circulation varies relative to the development and enlargement of the secondary center of ossification. Vessels initially enter the chondroepiphysis within specialized structures termed cartilage canals. These canals ramify throughout the chondroepiphysis and send branches to the resting/germinal zones of the physis. These canals have several important functional and morphologic characteristics: (1) they supply discrete regions of the epiphysis and physis, with no significant intraepiphyseal anastomoses; (2) the mesenchymal tissue within and around the canals may serve as a source of chondroblastic cells for continued interstitial enlargement of the chondroepiphysis; and (3) the canals play an integral role in the formation of the secondary center of ossification.

The vascular supply to the metaphysis comprises terminal ramifications of the nutrient artery, which constitutes about four-fifths of the vessels reaching the growth plate. The other one-fifth of the vasculature comes into the periphery through metaphyseal fenestrations. This supply is also integral to the functioning of the physeal periphery (especially the zone of Ranvier) in the skeletally immature individual. The periosteal vessels create an essentially bipartite circulation to the metaphysis, the central portion being derived from the nutrient artery, and the periphery from the periosteal vessels.

There are three functionally separate systems of circulation to the physis. One system supplies the epiphyseal surface of the physis, one supplies the peripheral portion (zone of Ranvier), and the other supplies the metaphyseal surface, with each system being essentially end-arterial. The vascular supply includes numerous branches of the epiphyseal arteries that reach the germinal and resting layers of the contiguous physis. These initially approach the physis directly through the chondroepiphysis. But with skeletal maturation and the appearance of a large ossification center, these branches eventually come through the maturing subchondral plate. The epiphyseal supply is quite abundant and necessary to normal development of the physis.

The degree of vascularity to the skeleton changes significantly over time (Fig. 1-13). In recent studies major changes in flow distribution patterns were found in the developing canine tibia and femur (27, 28). In particular, there was a dramatic quantitative decrease in tibial circulation commensurate with increasing skeletal maturation. If this occurs in humans, which is quite likely, it would explain the increasing delay in fracture healing and the high incidence of nonunion characteristic of the tibia of an adult. A poor vascular response would impair the early, crucial stages of callus formation. Adequate vascularity is a major factor in healing. These chronobiologic circulatory changes in distribution patterns also affect diagnostic tests such as radionuclide scans.

METABOLISM

The importance of an adequate calcium dietary intake and subsequent absorption for normal endochondral and membranous mineralization, ossification, and growth is reasonably well recognized. However, the specific dietary requirements of calcium and phosphate are difficult to define for any particular mammalian species or the specific stages of chondro-osseous development during or after completion of normal skeletal growth.

One of the major problems in extrapolating disease caused from one species to another is the species-specific skeletal response, as well as the species-specific nutritional demands. Fiennes felt that the so-called rickets or osteomalacia of monkeys might not be comparable to human rachitic osteodystrophies, primarily due to different metabolic pathways (29). For example, in capuchin monkeys the transporting protein for vitamin D is albumin, not α-globulin, as it is in the human. In fact, if one surveys a wide variety of species including fish, insects, amphibians, reptiles, birds, and many species of mammals, the transporting proteins are very variable—α and β globulins, albumins, and lipoproteins (30).

The aspects of vitamin D metabolism and the various types of rickets and osteodystrophy in small laboratory animals such as mice and rats have received considerable attention; however, very little information is available in larger mammals (29–44). Certainly such data would be helpful in furthering the understanding of the different manifestations of these diseases, especially when compared

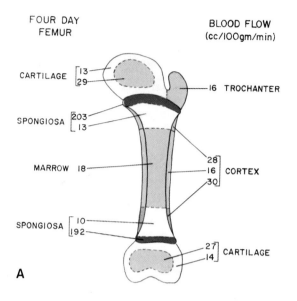

FOUR DAY
FEMUR

BLOOD FLOW
(cc/100gm/min)

CARTILAGE [13
29

16 TROCHANTER

SPONGIOSA [203
13

MARROW 18

28
16 CORTEX
30

SPONGIOSA [10
192

27 CARTILAGE
14

A

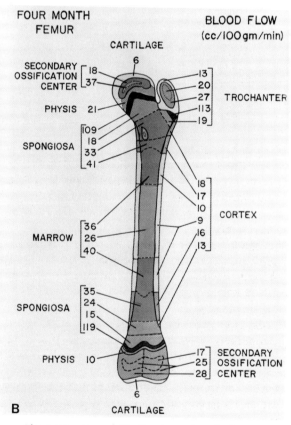

FOUR MONTH
FEMUR

BLOOD FLOW
(cc/100gm/min)

CARTILAGE
6

SECONDARY
OSSIFICATION
CENTER [18
37

13
20
27 TROCHANTER
113
19

PHYSIS 21

SPONGIOSA [109
18
33
41

18
17
10
9 CORTEX
16
13

MARROW [36
26
40

SPONGIOSA [35
24
15
119

PHYSIS 10

17
25 SECONDARY
28 OSSIFICATION
CENTER

6

B

CARTILAGE

Fig. 1-13 (A and B). *See legend on facing page.*

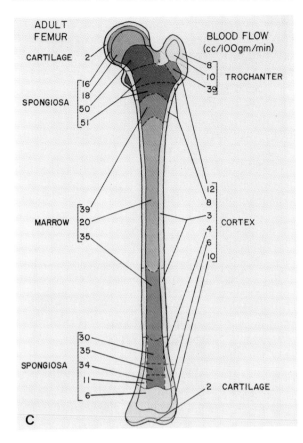

Fig. 1-13 Schematics of circulation to the canine femur in animals aged 4 days (A), 4 months (B), and 2 years (C). The white–gray–black colorations represent relative concentrations of radioactively labeled microspheres within discrete regions of bone and cartilage (black represents the highest concentration per volume). The numbers represent calculated blood flow (in cc) per 100 g osseous or cartilaginous tissue.

to the different patterns of human rachitic disorders (21, 45–51). Normal and abnormal patterns of bone growth by endochondral and membranous formation differ in smaller, faster-maturing species and may be misleading compared to the slower maturation rates and different calcification, ossification, and remodeling patterns in large-boned mammals.

The physes of any tubular bone contribute certain percentages of growth to the length of a given bone. However, the rates of endochondral growth are not linear but rather change with time. In particular, certain areas grow extremely rapidly in the adolescent human. Other mammals undoubtedly do the same during their juvenile maturation. Even within a given physis, to develop the characteristic contours, specific areas must grow more rapidly than others. For instance, in the proximal humerus an initially transverse physis must become conical, necessitating more rapid growth centrally. Similarly, in the proximal femur the capital femoral and trochanteric physes must grow at separate rates and become seemingly disparate growth units. The greater the physeal cartilaginous growth rates in a specific region of the physis as well as the overall physis, the more elongated will be the calcium-deficient cell columns that cannot be invaded by the metaphyseal blood vessels. The metaphyseal neovascularity will *not* invade cell columns that have not been prepared by adequate calcification.

Mankin suggested that excessive columnar hypertrophy and cellularity cause the mechanical disruption of the tissue that eventually leads to deformity and bowing (48). In deformed animals reported by Conlogue and Ogden (Fig. 1-14), there were variable columnar hypertrophy and propagation of tissue at the periphery of the physis, but there also was marked latitudinal disruption with the formation of intercolumnar clefts (32, 40). These clefts have not been described in human disease or in the small-animal model (e.g., rat, mouse), which may be a factor of species-specific or age-specific response patterns. The clefts, especially in the more severely involved areas, were grossly evident when the bones were split at necropsy. They undoubtedly represented loss of intercolumnar structural (matriceal) integrity, rather than postmortem change or tissue preparation artifact. It is quite possible that there is a limit to the ability of the intercellular tissue to maintain the relationship between areas, leading to this cleft disruption. Certainly the observation of these clefts offers a plausible additional reason for the epiphyseal deformity and slipping (epiphysiolysis) seen in human rachitic disease. These areas did separate quite easily from the underlying metaphyseal bone in the most severely involved areas, although the less involved areas did not exhibit the same degree of disruption between hypertrophic, elongated cell columns and metaphyseal bone.

Histopathologic studies of human slipped epiphyses in the various types of rachitic syndromes are minimal. Perhaps the most comprehensive works have been described by Krempien and Mehls (21, 22). They studied various bones removed at autopsy from seven uremic children and found that epiphysiolysis resulted from three different processes: (1) growth arrest, (2) excessive erosion of the growth cartilage and of the trabeculae of the metaphyseal spongiosa, and (3) disturbance of vascularization of the hypertrophic cartilage. By resorptive destruction, secondary hyperparathyroidism caused loss of chondro-osseous continuity. The ordered trabecular pattern of primary spongiosa was transformed into a mechanically inferior set of trabeculae consisting of woven bone and fibrous tissue. Impairment of primary mineralization, per se, could not be demonstrated. Intensive subperiosteal osteoclastic resorption led to a reduction of metaphyseal width and to fractures of the unsupported lateral parts of the growth cartilage. They also noted significant differences of involvement of physes in different localizations, which was also evident in our cases. In growth plates subjected to axial compression, signs of growth arrest prevailed (reduction of hypertrophic cartilage occlusion of the growth plate by transverse bone plate). In the growth plates subjected to shearing forces, such as the upper femur, radius, and ulna, the epiphyses slipped sideways and did not exhibit the same pattern of growth arrest.

Another very important finding was that the overall width of the epiphyseal growth plates was not systematically increased. However, at the peripheral margins near the zone of Ranvier, there was disorder to the proliferating cartilage, and this area did not appear to be making as much primary spongiosa, such that there was overlap of the lateral border of the physis in the metaphyseal bone. Within the physis the proliferating cartilage, rather than being widened, tended to be arranged in clusters (clones). Thus, these changes reported by Krempien and Mehls differ from what was described by Conlogue and Ogden in that the primary pathology appeared to be not in the physis but in the junction between

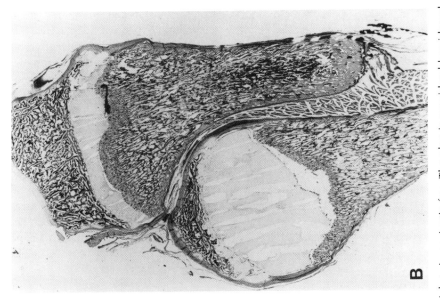

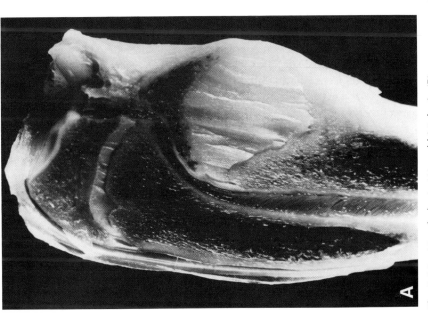

Fig. 1-14 Morphologic (A) and histologic (B) appearance of dietary rickets in an Arctic fox. The ulna is considerably widened and has developed longitudinal separations between the cell columns.

physis and metaphysis, where the normal sequence of vascular invasion, chondroclastic erosion of calcified chondroid, and osteoblastic deposition of bone matrix on the primary spongiosa were seriously disturbed.

Krempien's histologic studies failed to show any traumatic separation in the metaphyseal region or any evidence of microfractures within the metaphysis, which is where the failure has been postulated previously on the basis of roentgenologic studies. In contrast, epiphyseal slipping was shown to be the result of a coordinated lateral movement of the epiphyseal structure commensurate with intensive destructive and reparative processes at the physeal/metaphyseal juncture, most likely due to secondary hyperparathyroidism. The primary fault that ultimately led to the lateral movement of the entire physis and epiphysis appeared to be the failure of the trabeculae of the primary spongiosa to form a tight, stable interlocking complex with the growth cartilage. In advanced cases, no connection was observed between the cartilage and the metaphyseal trabeculae. Similar separations appeared to be occurring in many of the epiphyses of the animals reported by Conlogue and Ogden (32). However, the physeal widening and cleft formation also probably allowed shear deformation within the physis itself, rather than at the chondro-osseous junction of the primary spongiosa.

Recent case reports have suggested that children may develop rickets solely through a deficient intake and/or absorption of calcium without any vitamin D metabolic abnormalities (46, 47, 49). Maltz et al. described an infant with rickets presumably due to insufficient calcium intake but did not ascertain whether vitamin D intake was normal (47). More recently, Kooh et al. described infant-onset rickets definitely caused by insufficient calcium intake, with normal vitamin D levels (46). They felt that the critical factor in the development of rickets in their case was rapid growth and metabolic demand for calcium in the fifth to twelfth months. A similar mechanism probably occurred in the fox kits reported by Conlogue and Ogden (32, 40).

Although it has been established that adequate intake of calcium is necessary for normal skeletal growth and mineralization, absolute dietary requirements, whether for the human or for other animals, are hard to define (49–51). The case reported by Kooh is certainly the first human example definitely supporting the concept that an inadequate calcium intake may cause osteoporosis or rickets. The following mechanism has been postulated: protracted calcium deficiency > hypocalcemia > secondary hyperparathyroidism > hyperphosphaturia > generalized aminoaciduria hypophosphatemia. Whether the initiating event is vitamin D or calcium deficiency, the eventual biochemical manifestations and effects on the developing skeletal components are similar.

Deficiencies of calcium also have been implicated in captive, previously wild young animals subsequently raised with various artificial or high-protein diets (29, 31, 34–36, 42–44, 47). The aforementioned references have all described the development of rachitic changes after attempts to raise or maintain a previously wild animal in captivity. None of the diets totally duplicated the natural diet of the animal, and, in many cases, the captive animal only ate selected foods rather than the total diet that was presented.

The lack of exposure to sunlight may play a role in the development of rickets. Cholecalciferol (vitamin D) either must be ingested in small amounts in the diet or must be synthesized via ultraviolet radiation in the epidermis from circulating precursor molecules. The exact amount of exposure to sunlight to allow normal vitamin D metabolism in any particular animal species is unknown. In most animals, natural environmental radiation and synthesis of cholecalciferol are adequate. But in captivity, without ultraviolet radiation of these precursors and with minimal or no dietary cholecalciferol, a deficiency may develop.

Vitamin A toxicity may result in severe osseous changes that are roentgenographically similar to vitamin D malabsorption (52). This is particularly likely if excessive dietary intake of liver occurs.

EPIPHYSIODESIS

Physiologic epiphysiodesis refers to the normal, gradual replacement of the physis during adolescence. The process commences with the formation of small osseous bridges between the epiphyseal ossification center and metaphysis, and ends with the complete replacement of the cartilaginous physis by osseous tissue. This transversely oriented replacement may still be radiographically evident during adulthood, although it is usually progressively remodeled until no longer radiographically evident. Each physis appears to have its own pattern of closure, a factor that predisposes to certain types of fractures.

Several significant changes occur during normal epiphysiodesis. The epiphyseal cribiform bone plate thickens. A similar thickening of the metaphyseal bone also occurs, with formation of the transverse osseous septa instead of the more characteristic longitudinal trabeculae. The basic cellular arrangement of the physis does not change significantly while these osseous plates are initially forming. However, there is a distinct cessation of cellular proliferation and altered biochemistry, with progressive calcification and mineralization extending into the germinal and resting zones to form multiple tide lines. The cell columns are rapidly replaced as they are progressively calcified. The extension of the ossification from both sides leads to eventual perforation of the physis in several areas by small osseous bridges. Ossification then progresses outward from these perforations, replacing the cartilage and leaving a thick, physeal ghost composed of coalesced, thickened osseous plates of the metaphysis and epiphysis, which is evident on roentgenograms. The process usually starts centrally and proceeds centrifugally, so that small remnants of the physis may be found peripherally. However, certain physes show altered patterns. In particular, the distal tibial physis initially closes in the middle and medial regions, and subsequently in the lateral region.

NORMAL VARIATIONS

The developing skeleton is subject to considerable variation in the ossification patterns, many of which are retained in the mature adult skeleton (53). This is particularly prevalent in the secondary ossification centers and the carpal and tarsal bones. Such variation in either the pattern or degree of ossification may even vary from side to side and should make one cautious about the interpretation of symmetry when taking comparison radiographic views. Ossification centers do not become completely smooth until the late states of chondro-osseous maturation. Regions such as the distal femur can be very irregular, an appearance that probably reflects rapidity of chondro-osseous transformation rather than any discrete response to altered disease or nutritional states (4, 13, 54).

Care must also be taken in the arbitrary assignment of the term "variation." There is increasing acceptance, particularly in the orthopedic community, that many of the lesions defined as osteochondroses actually may be chronic, stress-related, responses (i.e., the residual of microfractures). Osgood-Schlatter's disease certainly fits such a category (4, 13). Furthermore, disorders such as bipartite patella (Fig. 1-15) and accessory navicular, while usually being interpreted as

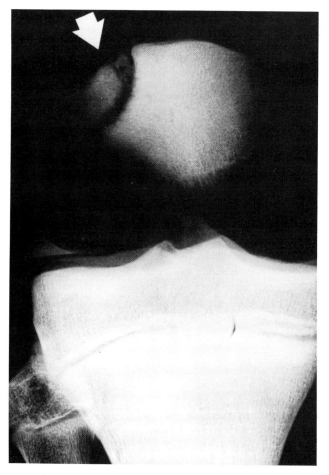

Fig. 1-15 Radiograph of a specimen of bipartite patella. Note the multiple centers and the irregular ossification margins. There was *complete* continuity of hyaline (epiphyseal) and articular cartilage. Thus, the "bipartite" nature may be osseous only, rather than involve contiguous cartilaginous separation.

radiographic "variation," may be subject to injury, and when patients with such diagnostic findings happen to be acutely symptomatic in that region, the diagnosis of superimposed acute injury must be considered (55, 56). Bone scans showing increased radionuclide uptake can help distinguish the radiologic variation from the injured variation.

The differentiation of an injury or disease process is difficult and necessitates that the physician be aware of the array of physiologic variants that can be extremely misleading in the assessment of radiographs of the skeleton, no matter what the age of the patient. These radiologic variations may represent developmental or positional artifacts. All are potentially confusing and misleading.

REFERENCES

1. Sissons, H. (1971) In: Bourne, G. H. (ed). *The Biochemistry and Physiology of Bone*, Vol. III, New York: Academic Press, p. 145.

2. Thompson, D. W. (1942) *On Growth and Form*. Cambridge University Press.

3. Ogden, J. A. (1981) In: Urist, M. R. (ed). *Fundamental and Clinical Bone Physiology*. Philadelphia: J. B. Lippincott.

4. Ogden, J. A. (1982) *Skeletal Injury in the Child*. Philadelphia: Lea and Febriger.

5. Rhodin, A. G. J., Ogden, J. A., Conlogue, G. J. (1981) Nature (London)290:244.

6. Black, J., Mattson, R., Korotsoff, E. (1974) J. Biomed. Mater. Res. 8:299.

7. Ogden, J. A. (1979) In: Albright, J. A., Brand, R. (eds). *The Scientific Basis of Orthopaedics*. New York: Appleton–Century–Crofts (2nd Edition).

8. Carter, D. R., Spengler, D. M. (1978) Clin. Orthop. Rel. Res. 135:192.

9. Cohen, J., Harris, W. H. (1958) J. Bone Joint Surg. 40A:419.

10. Enlow, D. H. (1962) Anat. Rec. 142:230.

11. Evans, F. G., Vincentelli, R. (1974) J. Biomech. 7:1.

12. Hert, J., Kucera, P., Vavra, M., Volenik, V. (1965) Acta Anat. (Basel) 61:412.

13. Ogden, J. A. (1984) In: Rockwood CA, Wilkins, K. E. and King, R. E. (eds). *Fractures*, Vol. 3, Children. Philadelphia: J. B. Lippincott.

14. Simkin, A., Robin G. (1974) J. Biomech. 7:183.

15. Ogden, J. A. (1984) J. Pediatr. Orthop. 4:409.

16. Ogden, J. A. (1983) Skelet. Radiol. 10:209.

17. Ogden, J. A., Conlogue, G. J., Jensen, P. (1978) Skelet. Radiol. 2:153.

18. Dodds, G. (1930) Anat. Rec. 46:385.

19. Dodds, G. (1932) Am. J. Anat. 50:97.

20. Ogden, J. A., Hempton, R. F., Southwick, W. O. (1975) Anat. Rec. 182:431.

21. Krempien, B., Mehls, O., Ritz, E. (1974) Virchows Arch. Pathol. Anat. 362:129.

22. Mehls, O., Ritz, E., Krempien, B., Gilli, G., Link, K., Willich, E., Scharer, K. (1972) Arch. Dis. Child 50:545.

23. Ogden, J. A., Southwick, W. O. (1977) Yale J. Biol. Med. 50:1.

24. Brookes, M. (1971) *The Blood Supply of Bone: An Approach to Bone Biology*. New York: Appleton–Century–Crofts.

25. Light, T. R., McKinstry, M. P., Schnitzer, J., Ogden, J. A. (1984) In: Arlet, J., Ficat, R. P., Hungerford, D. S. (eds). *Bone Circulation*. Baltimore: Williams and Wilkins.

26. Trueta, J. (1968) *Studies of the Development and Decay of the Human Frame*. Philadelphia: W. B. Saunders.

27. McKinstry, R., Schnitzer, J. E., Light, T. R., Ogden, J. A., Hoffer, P. (1982) Skelet. Radiol. 8:115.

28. Schnitzer, J. E., McKinstry, P., Light, T. R., Ogden, J. A. (1982) Am. J. Physiol. 242:H365.

29. Fiennes, R. N. T. W. (1972) Proc. Roy. Soc. Med. 67:309.

30. Capen, C. (1975) In: McDonald, C. E. (ed). *Veterinary Endocrinology and Reproduction.* Philadelphia: Lea and Febriger, p. 62.

31. Bullock, B. C., Bowen, J. A. (1966) Fed. Proc. 25:533.

32. Conlogue, G. J., Foreyt, W. J., Hanson, A. L., Ogden, J. A. (1979) J. Wildlife Dis. 15:563.

33. Dammrich, K. (1967) Zentralbl. Vet. Phys. Endo. Biochem. 24:597.

34. Dietrich, R. A., Vanpelt, R. W. (1972) J. Wildl. Dis. 8:146.

35. Freedman, M. T., Bush, M., Novak, G. R., Heller, R. M., James, A. E., Jr. (1976) Skeletal Radiol. 1:87.

36. Gorham, J. R., Peckham, J. C., Alexander, J. (1971) J. Am. Vet. Med. Assoc. 156:1331.

37. Graham, D. L. (1976) In: Page, L. A. (ed). *Wildlife Diseases.* New York: Plenum, p. 89.

38. Hunt, R. D., Garcia, G., Hegsted, D. M. (1966) Fed. Proc. 25:545.

39. Lehner, N. D. M., Bullock, B. C., Clarkson, T. B., Lofland, H. G. (1966) Fed. Proc. 25:533.

40. Ogden, J. A., Conlogue, G. J. (1981) Skelet. Radiol. 7:43.

41. Siegel, I. M. (1973) J. Am. Vet. Med. Assoc. 163:544.

42. Tomson, F. N., Lotshaw, R. R. (1978) J. Am. Vet. Med. Assoc. 173:1103.

43. Wallach, J. D. (1970) J. Am. Vet. Med. Assoc. 157:583.

44. Wallach, J. D. (1971) J. Am. Vet. Med. Assoc. 159:1632.

45. Dodds, G., Cameron, H. (1934) Am. J. Anat. 55:135.

46. Kooh, S. W., Fraser, D., Reilly, B. J., Hamilton, Jr., Gall, D. G., Bell, L. (1977) New Engl. J. Med. 297:1264.

47. Maltz, W. E., Fish, M. D., Holliday, M. A. (1979). Pediat. 46:865.

48. Mankin, H. J. (1974) J. Bone Joint Surg. 56A:101.

49. Tsang, R. C., Donovan, E. F., Steichen, J. J. (1976) Pediatr. Clin. N. Amer. 23:611.

50. Walker, A. R. P. (1955) Am. J. Clin Nutr. 3:114.

51. Walker, A. R. P. (1972) Am. J. Clin. Nutr. 25:518.

52. Breshau, R. C. (1957) Arch. Pediatr. 74:139 & 178.

53. Keats, T. E. (1979) *Atlas of Normal Roentgen Variants* (3rd Edition). Chicago: Year Book Medical Publishers.

54. Resnick, D., Greenway, G. (1982) Radiol. 143:345.

55. Lawson, J., Ogden, J. A., Sella, E., Barwick, K. (1984) Skeletal Radiol. 12:250.

56. Ogden, J. A., McCarthy, S., Jokl, P. (1982) J. Pediatr. Orthop. 2:263.

2
Skeletal Biomechanics and Aging

SUBRATA SAHA

The human skeleton undergoes a continuous physiologic decrease in bone mass with advancing age. The rate of loss varies from bone to bone and also with race, sex, and nutritional condition (1–5). Although several researchers have measured such age-related changes in appendicular and axial skeletons (6, 7), as well as for other bones, e.g., mandible (8), controversy exists regarding the exact nature of morphometric changes in the bone material. For instance, it is not well established that the porosity in compact bone also increases with age. Similarly, although it is generally assumed that the load-carrying capacity of the skeleton decreases after age 50 (an assumption based on the fact that the rate of long bone and vertebral crush fractures increases with age among the elderly) (9, 10), quantitative information on the actual load-carrying capacity of bones as a function of age is often lacking in the literature.

In this chapter we will focus our attention on how the biomechanical properties of the skeleton change with age.

OSTEOPOROSIS

Musculoskeletal disability ranks highest among disease groups that limit normal activity and thus affect the quality of life. Among musculoskeletal disabilities, arthritis and osteoporosis are those most commonly affecting a large percentage of our population.

Osteoporosis is the pathological condition associating diminution of bone mass that renders the skeleton vulnerable to fracture, which may occur spontaneously or by minimal trauma (11, 12). Osteoporosis is not to be confused with osteopenia, which is a condition of decreased bone density due to lower than normal/abnormal mineralization.

Osteoporosis is the most common bone disorder in the United States and is a major risk factor in fractures among the elderly (Fig. 2-1). Twenty-five to 30 percent of white women develop symptomatic osteoporosis. Of the more than one million fractures occurring annually in women 45 years or older, 70 percent are sustained by those with osteoporosis. By age 90, hip fractures occur in 33 percent of women and 17 percent of men, with a mortality rate of 12 to 15 percent; they

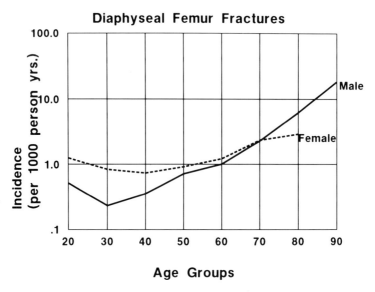

Fig. 2-1 Incidence of diaphyseal femur fractures in males and females for the age range of 20 to 90 years. [Adopted from Hedlund (9).]

are the second leading cause of death among individuals 47 to 74 years of age (13). Figure 2-2 shows the incidence of femoral neck and trochanteric fractures in Stockholm County, Sweden, from 1972 through 1981. The rapid increase in the incidence of such fractures with advancing age may not be evident due to the use of a logarithmic scale used in the vertical axis. However, the number of hip

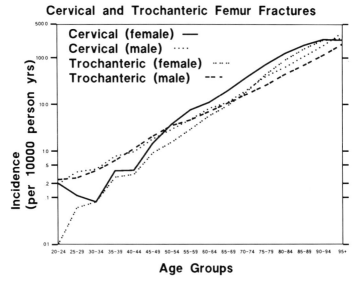

Fig. 2-2 Incidence of cervical and trochanteric femur fractures for various age groups from 20 to 95+ years. [Adopted from Hedlund (9).]

fractures occurring per 10,000 person years is impressive and has large medical and socioeconomic implications.

Of the estimated 190,000 hip fractures that occur each year, two-thirds are due to osteoporosis. Acute care for these fractures costs $1.4 billion annually. More important, hip fractures often result in a diminished quality of life. Half of the patients who survive hip fractures are unable to live independently after the fracture and must enter a nursing home (13).

Quantitative morphometric and radiographic measurements of age-related changes in normal skeletons demonstrate a progressive decrease in the cortical thickness of long bones beyond age 40 to 50 in females and beyond 50 to 60 in males. This decrease is due to an increased resorption at the endosteal surface and a decreased rate of apposition of new bone at the periosteal surface.

Clinically, it is often assumed that decreased cortical thickness with aging is indicative of decreased bone mass and associated onset of osteoporosis. This is because the degree of osteoporosis is often quantified by the cortical thickness index, which is the ratio of combined cortical thickness of long bone diaphysis $(t_1 + t_2)$ divided by the total width of the diaphysis (D) (Fig. 2-3). With decreased cortical thickness and increased diameter of long bones, the cortical thickness index, $(t_1 + t_2)/D$, will obviously decrease at a higher rate than the cortical thickness alone. However, this does not necessarily mean a decreased cross sectional area of the long bone. For a circular bone cross-section, the net cross sectional area of bone (A) is given by

$$A = \frac{\pi}{4}(D^2 - D_i)^2 \qquad (2-1)$$

where D and D_i are the outer and inner diameters of the bone (Fig. 2-4). For a thin cylinder with average diameter d, i.e., the diameter up to the middle of the cortex, and cortical thickness, t, the cross-sectional area (A) is approximately equal to (Fig. 2-4):

$$A = \pi d\, t \qquad (2-2)$$

Thus, for instance, if the cortical thickness, t, of a long bone decreases by one

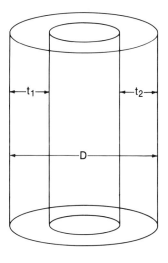

Fig. 2-3

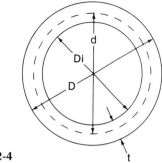

Fig. 2-4

percent per year and the average diameter, d, increases by more than one percent per year, then the net change in the cross-sectional area, A, could be positive, i.e., the cross sectional area of bone (A) may increase per year, although the cortical thickness index will show a decrease with age. It is evident, therefore, that change in cortical index may not always correctly portray the change in the cross sectional area of bone.

The amount of bone mass is controlled primarily by genetic factors. For example, blacks have greater bone mass than whites and rarely suffer from osteoporotic fractures (4, 14, 15). This may be due to the facts that: (1) aging related bone loss in black males and females are slower than that for whites; and (2) the density and mean weight of skeletons from black males and females generally exceed those of skeletons from whites (Figs. 2-5 and 2-6) (4). However, genetic factors are modified by nutrition, exercise, hormones, and exposure to environmental agents that may be toxic or protective. The exact mechanism of osteoporosis at the cellular level is unknown, but it is believed to be the uncoupling of osteoclastic-osteoblastic activity, with osteoclastic activity predominating (16).

Although it is universally accepted that osteoporosis is characterized by a decrease in bone mass and a reduced density and loss of bony trabeculae, it is unclear whether or not the cortical bone undergoes microstructural changes in the early stages of osteoporosis, nor is there enough information regarding the biomechanical properties of osteoporotic bones compared to normal ones (17). This problem becomes more complex as no definite criterion exists to divide normal skeletons from osteoporotic ones, particularly as age increases. Some authors have developed qualitative criteria to describe bones at various stages of osteoporosis. For instance the Singh Index is widely used to define the degree of osteoporosis in the proximal femur (18). However, how different degrees of osteoporosis relate to the load-carrying capacity of the bones is not known. Further research is necessary to develop the relationship between the clinical signs of osteoporosis and the resistance to fracture of whole bones. In the subsequent sections, the available data on the mechanical properties of bones and the aging process are discussed.

MECHANICAL PROPERTIES OF BONE TISSUE

Even a cursory review of the literature on the mechanical properties of bone will make it evident that a wide scatter exists in published data on various mechanical

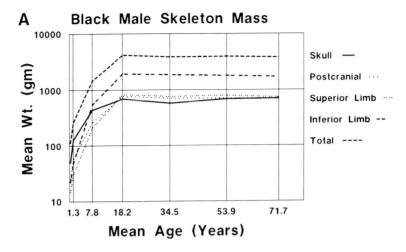

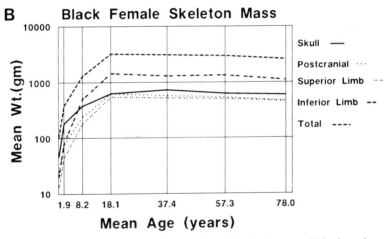

Fig. 2-5 Change with age in the mean weight of skeletal mass of black males and females. [Data adopted from Trotter and Hixon (4).]

parameters (e.g., maximum stress, ultimate strain, modulus of elasticity, and energy absorption capacity) characterizing bone. This is not surprising as many biological, physical, and experimental factors affect the measurement of mechanical properties.

These factors can be divided into two main groups and are described below:

A. Biological Factors
   1. Age
   2. Sex
   3. Race
   4. Nutrition
   5. Physiological condition (normal or diseased)
   6. Microstructure

   7. Type and region of bone
   8. Chemical composition (e.g., mineral content)
B. Experimental Conditions
   1. Type of storage (fresh, frozen, or embalmed)
   2. Specimen dimension and geometry
   3. Moisture content (e.g., wet or dry)
   4. Loading mode (tensile, compressive, shear, or bending)
   5. Strain rate
   6. Presence of stress concentrations (e.g., notches)

In this section, we will mainly focus attention on the data on variation in the mechanical properties of bone tissue according to age.

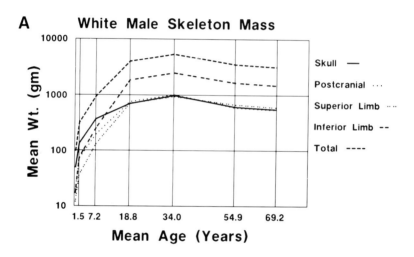

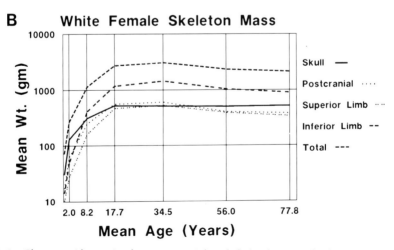

Fig. 2-6 Change with age in the mean weight of skeletal mass of white males and females. [Data adopted from Trotter and Hixon (4).]

Compact Bone

Wertheim (19) in 1847, was perhaps the first author to study the effect of age on the mechanical properties of bone. He found that the average tensile strength of four specimens from the femur and fibula of individuals less than 60 years of age was 104.6 MN/m^2 compared with an average of 52.4 MN/m^2 for four similar specimens from individuals over sixty. Rauber (20), in a similar, but more extensive study done in 1876, reported an average tensile strength of 98.9 MN/m^2 for 37 fresh specimens from the femur, tibia, and fibula of individuals less than 60 years of age compared with an average tensile strength of 76.0 MN/m^2 for a single specimen from the femur of a 70-year old man.

In contrast with these studies, Evans and Lebow (21) found no correlation between tensile or shear properties and age. Ko (22), however, found that the maximum tensile stress decreased after age 40; for the age group 60–79 years, the failure stress was approximately 70% of that for the age group 20–29. The maximum strain at fracture also decreased with age, but by a smaller amount.

During the last twenty years, several authors have investigated how aging may affect the mechanical properties of bone. Melick and Miller (23) studied age variation in the ultimate tensile strength of human compact bone and found it to decrease linearly beyond age 20. The mean strength of bone from fresh tibial cortex of adult patients under 60 was 138.2 MN/m^2 compared with a significantly lower mean strength of 118.6 MN/m^2 from patients over 60. Melick and Miller did not find significant changes in the amounts of calcium, organic tissue, or ash between these two samples. Thus, they concluded that some change in the internal bone architecture or the properties of bone fibers was responsible for the age-related decrease in tensile strength. Lindahl and Lindgren (24, 25) investigated the age and sexual variation in the tensile and compressive properties of fresh humeral and femoral cortical bone specimens from 64 autopsy subjects of various ages (ranging from 15 to 89 years). The data from the mechanical tests showed that both tensile and compressive strength decreased significantly with age from 20 years upwards in both men and women and in both femur and humerus. The decrease was approximately 10% in tension and 15% in compression. The maximum deformation also decreased, in general, with age beyond age 20 and below age 80. No significant age differences were found in the proportional limit and modulus of elasticity of specimens from both sexes.

Currey (26) investigated the effect of aging on the impact energy absorption capacity of human femoral cortical bone. Machined compact bone specimens were tested in four-point bending in a Hounsfield plastics impact tester. The impact energy absorption capacity (in kJ/m^2) was 28 for the youngest bones compared with 10 for the 90-year-olds, showing a decrease by a factor of about three between the ages of three and ninety. This decrease was associated with, and partially caused by, increased mineralization of bone. Currey hypothesized that the increased mineralization with aging probably produced decreased plastic deformation before fracture, thus making the process of crack propagation easier.

Burstein et al. (27) tested the mechanical properties of machined cortical bone specimens from human femur and tibia in tension, compression, and torsion for a population ranging from 21 to 86 years. They found consistent decreases with age for all mechanical properties except plastic modulus for the femoral specimens, but none for the tibial samples.

Recently we (28) investigated how the tensile strength of human compact bone varies along the radius and how this variation is affected by aging. Rectangular compact bone specimens were machined from the diaphysial cortex of fresh human tibia; and with the help of a diamond saw, were carefully divided into three segments along its thickness: endosteal, central, and periosteal. Dog bone shaped compact bone specimens were then prepared from these segments and these were tested in tension. The results, as shown in Fig. 2-7, suggests that the tensile strength of bone, in general, reduced with advanced age. This was not always true, perhaps due to the fact that bones from only one person was tested in each group. Figure 2-7 also shows that, in most cases, the endosteal bone was the weakest and the decrease in strength of the endosteal bone samples with age was more rapid than that for the central and the periosteal groups. This is because osteoclastic activity predominates at the endosteal surface, making it highly porous at advanced ages, thus diminishing the biomechanical strength of endosteal bone.

Trabecular Bone

The compressive strength and mineral content of cancellous bone and their relationship to age was investigated by Weaver and Chalmers (29). Cubes of cancellous bone were obtained from the third lumbar vertebrae and from the calcaneal

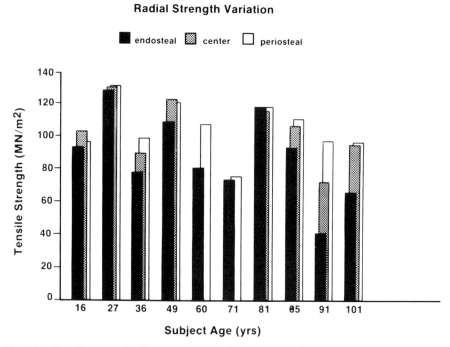

Fig. 2-7 Tensile strength of human compact bone from endosteal, central, and periosteal regions and its variation with age.

tuberosity of 137 normal cadaver (72 males and 65 females). Their study showed that:

1. The mineral content of the cancellous bone in the vertebra or the calcaneous was a reliable function of the compressive failure strength, irrespective of age or sex.
2. There was a definite and progressive trend toward decreasing bone strength and mineral content with advancing age. This decrease in bone mineral and strength developed earlier in the vertebra than in the calcaneous.
3. There was no significant difference between the strength or mineral content of cancellous bone of male and female cadaver below the age of 50. Over the age of 50, the strength and mineral content was significantly lower in the female cadaver.

Lindahl (30) tested the compressive strength of dried, defatted, spongy bone for various groups from 14 to 89 year old subjects. There was a rapid decrease in the compressive strength of trabecular bone, both from vertebra and tibia, for samples from the 14-to-60 age range, the average rate of decrease in strength being slightly higher for vertebral bone. Beyond age 60, the compressive strength still decreased for most groups, although at a diminishing rate. However, by this time, the strength had reduced to approximately 20% of the maximum strength (that is, for the age group 14–19 years). Thus, it is not surprising that, even with minimum trauma, elderly people often suffer from vertebral crush fractures.

Nokso-Koivisto et al. (31) measured the strength of cancellous bone specimens taken at autopsy from the anterior iliac crests of 28 women and 66 men. The bone strength showed a negative correlation with age. Decrease in the average bone strength was observed after the third decade of life. The trabecular bone strength was on average 15% higher in the men than in women. In females with chronic disease, the bone strength was significantly lower ($p < 0.001$) than it was in the cases of sudden death victims. The authors suggested that this is perhaps due to the lack of physical activity in patients with chronic diseases which may have produced a lower bone mineral content. They also found highly significant ($p < 0.001$) positive correlation between the bone strength and the mineral density in both males and females. Such correlations are almost universally accepted and have been reported by many other authors as mentioned before (32–34).

In a recent study, Mosekilde and Mosekilde (35) investigated how aging affects the compressive strengths of whole vertebral body and vertebral and iliac trabecular bone. The maximum compressive stress value (σ) of the whole vertebral bodies and of the vertical vertebral trabecular bone decreased with age with almost parallel linear regression lines. At any age the σ for whole vertebral bodies was about 1.6 MPa (1 MPa = 100 N/cm^2) higher than for the trabecular bone. The average cross-sectional area of the vertebral bodies increased by 25–30% from the age of 20 to 80 years. The anisotropic properties of the vertebral trabecular bone (expressed as the ratio between the vertical and horizontal σ) increased markedly with age. A highly significant positive correlation was observed between the vertical vertebral trabecular bone σ (x) and the total vertebral body

σ (y) $(y = 0.90x + 1.75$, $r = 0.88$, $P < 0.01)$. The average total vertebral body σ (range 1.5–7.8 MPa) could be predicted from mechanical tests on horizontal iliac crest bone biopsies with standard error of estimate (SEE) of 0.92 MPa. This study showed that the compressive strength of whole vertebral bodies depends mainly on the trabecular bone compressive strength, which decreases with age. The increase in vertebral trabecular bone anisotropy with age and the continuous periosteal growth will to some extent compensate for the obligatory age-related loss of vertebral trabecular bone mass. In normal individuals the average vertebral body compressive strength can be estimated from mechanical tests on horizontal iliac crest bone biopsies in spite of these age-related changes in internal and external architecture.

The mean wall thickness of packets of trabecular bone from undecalcified iliac crest bone samples was measured by Lips et al. (36). The bone specimens were obtained from 36 normal subjects (22 males with age ranging from 18 to 82 years and 14 females with an age range of 19 to 90 years). They found a significant ($p < 0.01$) decrease in the mean wall thickness with advancing age, both for males and females. This decrease in mean wall thickness corresponded to a decrease in bone formation rate at the basic multicellular unit level. This may partly explain the reduction in biomechanical strength of trabecular bone with aging (27–29, 33, 35, 36). Further details of such age-related structural changes in trabecular and cortical bone and their biomechanical implications has been discussed recently by Parfitt (39).

RESISTANCE TO FRACTURE

The load-carrying capacity of a whole bone is directly dependent on the total bone mass and the quality of the bone material itself. For instance, when the diaphysis of a long bone is loaded in pure tension, compression, or shear, the maximum load (P) that this bone can support is given by

$$P = A\sigma \qquad (2\text{--}3)$$

where A is the cross-sectional area of the bone and σ is the maximum stress of the bone material in that particular loading mode. The similar relationship for the metaphysis, containing both compact (A_c) and trabecular (A_t) bone areas, will be,

$$P = A_c\sigma_c + A_t\sigma_t \qquad (2\text{--}4)$$

assuming that both compact and trabecular bone can undergo plastic deformation. Here σ_c and σ_t represent the maximum stresses of compact and trabecular bone materials, respectively.

However, when a bone is loaded in bending or torsion, calculation of load-carrying capacity becomes more complicated. The maximum bending moment (M) a bone can support is given by (40),

$$M = \frac{I}{Y}\sigma = S\sigma \qquad (2\text{--}5)$$

where I is the moment of inertia of the bone cross section, y is the maximum distance from the neutral axis of any point in the cross section of the bone, S is the section modulus of bone cross section and σ is the ultimate bending stress of bone. If we assume that a long bone is a thin cylinder of average diameter d (up to the middle of the cortex) and cortical thickness, t, then the area (A) is given by Eq. (2–2). The moment of inertia, I, for such a bony cylinder can be shown to be (40)

$$I = \frac{\pi d^3 t}{8} = \frac{Ad^2}{8} \qquad (2\text{--}6)$$

Similarly, we can also calculate the maximum torque (T) that a bone can support (40),

$$T = \frac{J}{r} \tau \qquad (2\text{--}7)$$

where J is the polar moment of inertia, τ is the maximum shear stress of the bone material, and r is the maximum distance of any point in the bone cross section from its center. For a thin cylinder,

$$J = 2\pi r^3 t = \frac{\pi d^3 t}{4} = \frac{Ad^2}{4} \qquad (2\text{--}8)$$

Thus, we note that the bending or torsional resistance of a circular bone is not only related to its cross-sectional area (A), but it is also dependent on the shape of the bone. For instance, if d is doubled and t is reduced by half, the total cross-sectional area, A, will remain the same. But the new moment of inertia (I') will be

$$I' = \frac{\pi}{8} (2d)^3 \frac{t}{2} = \frac{\pi d^3 t}{2} = 4I \qquad (2\text{--}9)$$

Thus, the bending moment that this thinner bone with enlarged diameter can support will also be much larger (approximately double) than that of the bone of the previous example (Eq. 2–5). This will also be true for torsion.

Although the skeleton does not undergo such dramatic changes in bone size during aging, bone apposition on the periosteal surface generally continues throughout life. Consistently, the total width of a bone is larger in the last decades than in the third decade (1). However, the endosteal surface often erodes at a greater rate during advanced age, thus effectively reducing the cortical thickness.

It is evident from the previous analysis of long bones that the resistance to bending or torsional fracture may not be reduced even with a decreased cross-sectional area of the bone. However, this will only be true if there has not been a proportional decrease in its material strength (maximum stress, σ). In the previous section on mechanical properties, we have shown that results from most studies suggest that a significant decrease in the ultimate stress (σ) occurs, both for compact and for trabecular bone, beyond the ages of 30 to 40 (Fig. 2-8). Even with a small increase in section modulus (I), a drastic reduction in the load-car-

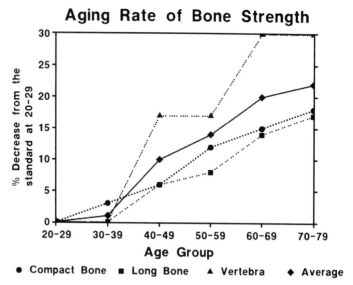

Fig. 2-8   Percentage decrease in the bone strength with aging, with respect to the standard for the age group 20–29 years. [Adopted from Yamada (38).]

rying capacity of the whole bone results, thus precipitating the likelihood of frequent fractures.

MECHANICAL STRENGTH OF WHOLE BONES

The load carrying capacities of whole bones have been investigated by many authors (38, 41). Similarly a number of researchers have also investigated the age-related structural and density changes in whole bones (1–4, 14, 15, 17). In his classic book "The Earlier Gain and Later Loss of Cortical Bone," Garn (1) documented how the total subperiosteal diameter and the medullary cavity width change with age. He also discussed the relationship between the dietary intake and maintenance of cortical bone. With the recent widespread use of non-invasive imaging techniques such as computed tomography (CT), ultrasound, and magnetic resonance imaging (MRI), and single and dual photon absorptiometery (6), it is possible to follow up accurately the structural and chemical changes in our appendicular and axial skeletons that occur from our childhood to old age. However, few have attempted to translate such age related changes in bone morphology, density and mineral content in terms of the overall load carrying capacity of the whole bone. This is partly because the clinicians studying the osteoporotic changes in bones often lack the detailed biomechanical knowledge necessary to calculate how cross-sectional and density variations may affect the mechanical strength of whole bones. Only a few authors have attempted to bridge this gap from clinical data (cortical thickness and bone density) to the prediction of mechanical behavior of whole bones.

   In order to quantify age-related changes in the mechanical integrity of the human femur, Martin and Atkinson (42) measured the cross-sectional dimensions and density at four sites in each of 37 left femoral shafts of normal human subjects aged 2-1/2 to 82 years. From the cross-sectional moment of inertia (I), and converting the density data to estimate the material strength of bone tissue (σ), and then using a formula similar to Eq. 2–5, the authors calculated the structural strength of whole bones in bending. Their results indicated that the material strength of femoral bone decreased with age equally in males and females. In males this decrease was compensated by increases in section modulus (S), so that overall load carrying capacity of the shaft remained constant. In females, the section modulus (S) decreased with age; this, combined with the effects of reduced tissue strength, resulted in greatly reduced load carrying capacity of femurs in old age.

Since the distal shaft of the radius is commonly used to monitor the bone mineral content (BMC) of aging individuals by photon absorptiometry and since this is also a common site for fractures, it is important to know if BMC is a good indicator of the mechanical integrity of the whole bone. In a more recent paper, Burr and Martin (43) investigated the effects of composition, structure and age on the torsional properties of the human radius. Similar to their previous study, they found that the bone mineral content of the scan site in the distal radius declined signifcantly ($p < 0.005$) with age in women, but in men showed no change to age 90. In spite of the loss of BMC, there was no decrease in the torsional rigidity in women. In men, torsional rigidity increased significantly ($p < 0.05$) with age, even though BMC did not change. Based on these results, the authors suggested that BMC alone may not adequately reflect the mechanical integrity of our skeleton.

Increases with aging in subperiosteal dimensions and second moments of inertia (I and J) in femoral and tibial cross sections in an archeological sample of 119 individuals were documented by Russ and Hayes (44, 45). In the femoral midshaft, the increases in the subperiosteal area with age were similar in males and females (averaging 7% in males and 11% in females), but the percentage increases in the medullary area were much greater in females (39%) than in males (19%). Thus, because of a greater endosteal resorption of bone with aging, females showed a significant decline in the compact cortical bone area (approximately 10%) whereas males showed only a small (1%) decrease in the compact cortical bone area.

In a subsequent paper by using photon absorptiometry, Ruff and Hayes (46) also measured the bone mineral content and the bone mineral width at eleven locations in forty excised femora and tibiae from the same archaelogical samples. The results indicated that locational, sex, and age-related differences in bone-mineral content were largely determined by variation in cortical area. The authors suggested that due to differences in bone geometry, variation in bone width does not reflect variation in cortical area, and as a consequence the use of bone width to standardize for volumetric or bone "size" differences produces misleading results in sex and age comparisons. In this study, decreases with age in the bone-mineral content and bone-mineral content: bone width ratio were similar to those observed in living populations. However, the bone-mineral content: cortical area ratio showed no significant decline with age for any cross section. Thus, the age-related changes in compact cortical bone appeared to be mainly volumetric, not densitometric.

SUMMARY

This chapter is a brief introduction to the topic of biomechanical changes that occur in our skeleton with age. We have mainly focused attention on the bone tissue, as relatively less is known about the effect of aging on the biomechanical properties of cartilage, tendon, and ligaments.

It has been shown by many authors that bone undergoes constant remodeling of its microstructure, as well as change in its shape (modeling) by apposition on the periosteal surface and resorption at the endosteal surface. The nature and the rate of such changes not only depend on the age of the organism, but are also highly dependent on genetic factors, nutrition, exercise, and environmental conditions. Therefore, the results of most studies cannot be universally applied.

Although many investigators have tested the load-carrying capacities of whole bones and the mechanical properties of bone tissue, only few have focused their attention on how these properties change with age. Similarly, only a limited number of authors have attempted to quantify the relationship between the changes in the microstructure and chemical composition of bone tissue and its mechanical properties. Also, little is known about how changes in the shape of a whole bone (either in diameter or cortical thickness) affect load-carrying capacity. A complete picture of the simultaneous changes in the biomechanical, structural, and microstructural variables is almost never available because authors who test whole bones often do not examine the microstructural or chemical changes in the bone tissue.

Similarly, investigators who test small, machined bone specimens often do not consider the overall size or shape of the whole bone. Therefore, a wide gap exists between our understanding of the macroscopic and microscopic aspects of bone fracture and how these relate to aging. Fracture of bone depends simultaneously on many parameters (e.g., strain rate, loading mode, chemical composition, microstructure, etc.), and a comprehensive understanding of the dynamic strength of bone requires a knowledge not only of these separate effects but also of their interaction (47). Some studies have been conducted describing how aging affects the mineral content, microstructure, mechanical properties, and size of bones (48). We need to synthesize these experimental results into a cohesive theory so that we understand how the aging process affects the structure and chemical composition of bones and how these changes are manifested in the decreased load-carrying capacity of the skeleton.

REFERENCES

1. Garn, S. M. (1970) *The Earlier Gain and Later Loss of Cortical Bone*. Springfield, Ill: Charles C. Thomas.

2. Mazess, R. B. (1982) Clin. Orthop. Rel. Res. 165:239.

3. Gordan, G. S., Genant, H. K. (1985) Clin. Geriat. Med. 1:95.

4. Trotter, M., Hixon, B. B. (1974) Anat. Rec. 179:1.

5. Notelovitz, M. (1986) In: *Current Concepts in Nutrition*. New York: John Wiley and Sons, p. 203.

6. Cohn, S. H. (1981) *Non-Invasive Measurements of Bone Mass*. Boca Raton, Fl: CRC Press.

7. Behari, J., Saha, S. (1989) CRC Crit. Rev. Bioeng. (In press).

8. Wowern, N. V., Stoltze, K. (1980) Scand. J. Dent. Res. 88:134.

9. Hedlund, R. (1985) *Incidence and Cause of Femur Fracture*. Stockholm.

10. Aitken, M. (1984) *Osteoporosis in Clinical Practice*. Bristol: Wright.

11. Sanders, M., Albright, J. A. (1987) In: Albright, J. A., Brand, R. A. (eds). *The Scientific Basis of Orthopaedics*. Norwalk, Conn: Appleton & Lange, p. 267.

12. Davies, R., Saha, S. (1985) Am. Fam. Phys. 32(5):107.

13. Grazier, K. L., Holbrook, T. L., Kelsey, J. L., Stauffer, R. N. (1984) *The Frequency of Occurrence, Impact and Cost of Selected Musculoskeletal Conditions in the United States*. Chicago: Am. Acad. Orthop. Surg.

14. Cohn, S. H., Abesamis, C., Yasumura, S., Aloia, J. F., Zanzi, I. (1977) Metabolism 26:171.

15. Melton, L. J., Riggs, B. L. (1983) In: Avioli, L. V. (eds) The Osteoportic Syndrome. New York: Grune & Stratton, p. 45.

16. Frost, H. M. (1980) In: Urist, M. R. (eds.) *Fundamental and Clinical Bone Physiology*. Philadelphia: JB Lippincott, p. 208.

17. Avioli, L. V. (1983) *The Osteoporotic Syndrome*. New York: Grune & Stratton.

18. Singh, M. (1970) J. Bone Joint Surg. 52A:457.

19. Werthium, M. G. (1847) Ann. Clin. Phys. 21:385.

20. Rauber, A. A. (1876) Elasticitat und festigkeit der knochen. Leipzig: Wilhelm Engelmann.

21. Evans, F. G., Lebow, M. (1951) J. Appl. Physiol. 3:563.

22. Ko, R. (1953) J. Kyoto Pref. Med. Univ. 53:503.

23. Melick, R. A., Miller, D. R. (1966) Clin. Sci. 30:243.

24. Lindahl, O., Lindgren, A. G. H. (1967) Acta. Orthop. Scand. 38:141.

25. Lindahl, O., Lindgren, A. G. H. (1968) Acta. Orthop. Scand. 39:129.

26. Currey, J. D. (1979) J. Biomech. 12:459.

27. Burstein, A. H., Reilly, D. T., Martens, M. (1976) J. Bone Joint Surg. 58A:82.

28. Saha, S., Engelhart, J., Lipka, J., Albright, J. A. (1989) J. Biomech. (In press).

29. Weaver, J. K., Chalmers, J. (1966) J. Bone Joint. Surg. 48A:289.

30. Lindahl, O. (1976) Acta. Orthop. Scand. 47:11.

31. Nokso-Koivisto V.-M., Alhava, E. M., Olkkonen, H. (1976) Ann. Clin. Res. 8:399.

32. Carter, D. R., Hayes, W. C. (1976) Science 194:1174.

33. Saha, S., Gorman, P. H. (1981) Orthop. Trans. 5(2):323.

34. Albright, J. A. (1987) In: Albright, J. A., Brnad, R. A. (eds) *The Scientific Basis of Orthopaedics*. Norwalk, Conn: Appleton and Lange, p. 213.

35. Mosekilde, L., Mosekilde, L. (1986) Bone 7:207.

36. Lips, P., Courpron, P., Meunier, P. J. (1978) Calcif. Tiss. Res. 26:13.

37. Evans, F. G. (1973) Mechanical Properties of Bone. Springfield, Ill.: Charles C Thomas, p. 239.

38. Yamada, H. (1973) *Strength of Biological Materials*. Huntington, NY: RE Krieger Publishing Co., p. 272.

39. Parfitt, A. M. (1984) Calcif. Tissue Int. 36:S123.

40. Timoshenko, S. P., Gere, J. M. (1972) *Mechanics of Materials*. New York: D. Van Nostrand.

41. Evans, F. G. (1957) Stress and Strain in Bones. Springfield, Ill.: Charles C Thomas.

42. Martin, R. B., Atkinson, P. J. (1977) J. Biomech. 10:223.

43. Burr, D. B., Martin, R. B. (1983) J. Biomech. 16(8):603.

44. Ruff, C. B., Hayes, W. C. (1982) Science. 217:945.

45. Ruff, C. B., Hayes, W. C. (1983) Am. J. Physical Anthrop. 60:383.

46. Ruff, C. B., Hayes, W. C. (1984) J. Bone Joint Surg. 66A:1024.

47. Saha, S. (1982) In: Ghista, D. N. (eds) *Osteoarthromechanics*. New York: McGraw Hill, p. 1.

48. Riggs, B. L., Melton III, L. J. (1988) *Osteoporosis, Etiology, Diagnosis and Management*. New York: Raven Press.

II
NUTRITIONAL PROBLEMS
IN MINERAL METABOLISM
OVER THE LIFE-SPAN

3

Nutritional Factors Affecting Mineral Homeostasis and Mineralization in the Term and Preterm Infant

LAURA S. HILLMAN

As the field of neonatology has grown in both size and complexity, one area that has required additional study is nutrition, especially related to bone mineralization. The population of women at highest risk for delivering infants with prematurity, growth retardation, or multiple neonatal problems is a population also at risk for many nutritional disorders. The effect of maternal nutrition on *in utero* nutrition is only beginning to be studied. Even if maternal nutrition is adequate, premature birth or compromised uteran blood flow may limit the infant's development of *in utero* stores. Current neonatal practices have survival rates greater than 95 percent for the 1,000- to 1,500-g infant and about 70 percent for the 750- to 1,000-g infant. The survival rates for the 600- to 750-g infants may reach 25–50 percent. In these very low birth weight infants (<1,000 g), attempts to do the enormous job usually done by the human placenta, particularly supporting bone formation, are compromised by immaturity of many organ systems necessary to nutritional adequacy—the gastrointestinal tract, liver, and kidney. In both the extremely ill term infant and the extremely premature infant, the problems are further complicated by secondary illness and complications of prolonged intensive care. Most instances of severe bone mineralization problems in the neonate are related to multiple factors and may often involve multiple nutritional deficiencies.

Thus, it is important first to define what is normal *in utero* and during the first year of life for the infant who goes to term. Once we define the capacities for mineral homeostasis and the nutritional requirements of the term infant, we will better be able to define any limitations or additional requirements found in the premature infant. Once we have defined maximal capacities and minimal requirements found of the healthy premature fed normal enteral feeding regimens, we can deal with the complicated problems that face most neonatologists.

IN UTERO MINERALIZATION

Placental Transport of Minerals and Vitamin D

Mineralization of the cartilaginous fetal bones occurs primarily during the third trimester, a time when enormous amounts of mineral are supplied across the placenta. During the second trimester poorly understood changes occur in the mother that allow her to increase mineral absorption and retention, increase bone stores, and supply the fetus without obvious strain on classical mineral homeostatic mechanisms (i.e., PTH and $1,25(OH)_2D$ within normal limits) (1). The amount of minerals crossing the placenta and being deposited in bone (additional minerals undoubtedly cross and are excreted in the fetal urine) at different gestational ages has been calculated from body composition studies of stillborn fetuses, but the data are rather limited in terms of both the number of infants and the ability to assign a gestational age accurately. These older compositional data have been combined and reworked by three separate investigators to generate estimates of fetal calcium and phosphorus accretion versus gestational age (2–4). Three different equations have been generated to describe the accretion process. (Clinicians or investigators attempting to "match *in utero* accretion" have chosen different curves. Clearly it is easier to match the curve of Ziegler et al. than that of either Forbes or Shaw). Greer has recently summarized these data in Tables 3-1 and 3-2 (5). Accomplishment of this large daily transfer of minerals appears to require active transport by the placenta of calcium, magnesium, and phosphorus. At all gestations, fetal cord blood concentrations exceed maternal serum concentrations

Table 3-1   Fetal Calcium Accretion (mg/kg day) from 25 to 36 Weeks' Gestational Age

Gestational age (weeks)	Forbes (3)	Shaw (4)	Ziegler et al. (2)	Mean
25	129	121	92	114
26	125	123	104	118
27	128	126.5[a]	108.5	121
28	126	129	107	121
29	130	131[b]	101.5	121
30	130	133	98	120
31	135	136.5[c]	97	123
32	135	140	99	125
33	143	142.5[d]	103.2	130
34	141	145	108.5	132
35	134	148[e]	113.5	132
36	119	151	119	13

Source: Greer and Tsand (5).
[a]Mean value of 26 and 28 weeks.
[b]Mean value of 28 and 30 weeks.
[c]Mean value of 30 and 32 weeks.
[d]Mean value of 32 and 34 weeks.
[e]Mean value of 34 and 36 weeks.

Table 3-2 Fetal Phosphorus Accretion (mg/kg day)

Gestational age (weeks)	Shaw (4)	Ziegler et al. (2)	Mean
25	71.5	59	65.4
26	73	67	70
27	74.5[a]	69.5	72
28	76	68.5	71
29	77[b]	65.5	71
30	78	63	71
31	79[c]	62.5	71
32	80	63.5	72
33	82[d]	66	76
34	84	68.5	76
35	85[e]	71	78
36	86	74	80
37	—	—	—
38	—	—	—

Source: Greer and Tsang (5).
[a]Mean value of 26 and 28 weeks.
[b]Mean value of 28 and 30 weeks.
[c]Mean value of 30 and 32 weeks.
[d]Mean value of 32 and 34 weeks.
[e]Mean value of 34 and 36 weeks.

in spite of lower protein binders in the fetal circulation. What regulates this transfer is currently undefined. In animal models, neither maternal parathyroidectomy nor maternal vitamin D deficiency seems to have much effect, and it has been suggested that the fetus may regulate its supply of minerals *via* fetal $1,25(OH)_2D$ or fetal PTH (6–8). However, infants with absent kidneys, Potters Syndrome, have normal bones (Glorieux, Personal communication).

The fetus also relies on the placenta for its supply of vitamin D. Although passage of the parent compound, vitamin D, has been shown using radioactive tracers in rats (9), it is unlikely that much of the parent compound is transferred to the human infant. Cord blood vitamin D levels in term infants are quite low (10). Serum vitamin D in premature infants prior to the institution of vitamin D supplementation and in infants fed 25-hydroxyvitamin D (25-OHD) instead of vitamin D were very low to undetectable (11). The major transfer across the placenta is in the form of the first metabolite, 25-OHD. The correlation of maternal and cord 25-OHD is shown in Fig. 3-1A. A similar correlation has been seen in infants delivering prematurely (Fig. 3-1B) (12). This high correlation has been replicated in over a dozen studies.

In all studies, infant 25-OHD levels are usually below maternal levels, averaging about 80 percent of maternal levels, and this has been interpreted as representing passive transfer. However, since vitamin D binding protein (DBP) is markedly elevated during pregnancy and is low in infants delivering prior to term (13, 14), one can calculate an uphill gradient for free 25-OHD which suggests facilitative or active transfer. From a practical point of view, placental transfer of 25-OHD cannot efficiently compensate for maternal 25-OHD deficiency. If the mother has a normal 25-OHD serum concentration, the infant will begin life with a normal 25-OHD serum concentration. However, if the mother has a low serum 25-OHD, the infant will be born with a low 25-OHD.

Maternal serum 25-OHD concentrations depend on sun exposure and oral intake of vitamin D. Sun exposure is a combination of season, latitude, dress, and, to a lesser degree, race. Seasonal changes are a key factor. In pregnant women in St. Louis, the August 25-OHD levels (42 ± 14 mg/ml, $N = 61$) are threefold greater than February levels (15 ± 6 ng/ml, $N = 56$) (15). In pregnant New Zealand women, Birkbeck and Scott found identical mean values with the months reversed (February 49.3 and October 17.4 ng/ml) (16). At moderate latitudes, infant 25-OHD deficiency is rare in Caucasian populations, since maternal 25-OHD levels are high. At cool latitudes (Finland, Norway, South Africa), winter 25-OHD levels <6 ng/ml are very common in women who are not supplemented with vitamin D and in their infants (17–19). Dress customs that decrease sun exposure put certain populations at additional risk for maternal and infant 25-OHD deficiency (e.g., the Asian population in Britain and the bedouins) (20).

Although Hollis has shown a lower serum vitamin D in response to ultraviolet radiation in heavily pigmented individuals (blacks) (21), the conversion of vitamin D to 25-OHD in the adult population is so efficient that it is difficult to determine the existence of racial differences in serum 25-OHD. In our experience, mothers who receive prenatal care (usually vitamin supplementation) and delivered at term did not show a racial difference in total serum 25-OHD (15). Hollis has also shown a decrease in the D_3 metabolites in black mothers and their infants, as would be expected with decreased skin synthesis (10).

In multiple clinical studies, black premature infants tend to have a lower total 25-OHD than Caucasian infants (22–23). Vitamin D intake was only weakly correlated with serum 25-OHD in pregnant women during the winter in St. Louis (15). However, maternal supplementation of 400 IU D during pregnancy has markedly improved maternal and infant 25-OHD in northern latitude populations and in populations such as the Asians in Britain (24, 25). Through mechanisms that remain unclear, such maternal vitamin D supplementation has markedly altered the incidence of late neonatal hypocalcemia seizures in the British Asian population (24, 25). Limited studies of the effect of maternal vitamin D status and calcium supplementation on infant bone mineralization and growth have shown a positive correlation (25–28).

1,25-Dihydroxyvitamin D ($1,25(OH)_2D$) probably crosses the placenta to a lesser degree than 25-OHD, and the fetus is not dependent on placental transport as its source of this metabolite. Numerous studies have compared maternal serum and cord serum $1,25(OH)_2D$. A majority of these reports cite a significant but highly variable correlation, but a (significant) minority failed to find any correlation (10, 29, 30). The discrepancies probably relate to the ability of the infant *in utero* from very early gestation to produce $1,25(OH)_2D$ in the kidney and possibly in a number of extrarenal sites (6). The placenta also produces significant quantities of $1,25(OH)_2D$, and it has been speculated that this may be important in regulating calcium transport (31). Thus, the exact contributions of maternal, placental, or infant $1,25(OH)_2D$ to total infant serum $1,25(OH)_2D$ is unknown;

however, cord $1,25(OH)_2D$ is normal, and deficient levels have not been reported.

$24,25(OH)_2D$ probably also has little transplacental passage with variable correlations of maternal and cord concentration reported (10, 29, 32). Since $24,25(OH)_2D$ levels appear less regulated and usually relate positively to 25-OHD levels, a positive maternal–cord relationship of $24,25(OH)_2D$ may reflect normal independent $24,25(OH)_2D$ production from 25-OHD levels that are correlated. Again, infant $24,25(OH)_2D$, although lower than predicted, is adequate (32). This may be important, since a possible role in chondrogenesis is one of the few postulated roles for $24,25(OH)_2D$ (33). Fetomaternal relationships of all vitamin D metabolites seem to be the same with premature birth (12, 34).

Fetal Homeostatic Mechanism

Since it is 25-OHD rather than vitamin D that crosses the placenta, the fetal liver has little need to convert vitamin D to 25-OHD. Animal (rat) studies of liver 25-hydroxylation show that onset of hydroxylation and excretion of 25-OHD are timed to gestational age but not postnatal age (35). As discussed, the synthesis of $1,25(OH)_2D$ and $24,25(OH)_2D$ by the fetal kidney appears normal.

Although PTH secretion can be demonstrated in the fetus as early as 12 weeks' gestation, factors such as the active transport of calcium across the placenta and the high serum calcium levels, as reflected in cord blood, are unlikely to provide an additional stimulus. PTH concentrations in cord blood are either low or normal depending on the study assay. PTH levels return to normal or overshoot as serum calcium levels fall postnatally, confirming the intact nature of the system (36–38). Low maintenance levels of PTH seem ideal to promote *in utero* bone growth without excessive resorption.

The fetal thyroid contains a concentration of calcitonin producing C cells that is 10 times higher than in the adult (39). It is not suprising that cord levels of calcitonin are higher than those of normal or pregnant adults (36, 40). About 2 h after birth there is a marked surge in calcitonin which peaks at 12 h in the term infant and then falls to normal within a few days (36, 40). The stimulus to this surge is unclear, but it is increased by asphyxia during delivery and may well be the primary cause of early neonatal hypercalcemia in that group (40, 41). Premature infants begin life with even higher values; their peak is higher, and the time to return to baseline is markedly prolonged (36, 42). The increase in calcitonin produced by bolus calcium given during exchange transfusion postnatally is also inversely proportional to gestational age of the infant (43). This suggests that the high concentrations of C cells seen during *in utero* life may be associated with a static high level of calcitonin secretion and that those cells are responsive to stimuli *in utero*. This would be the ideal *in utero* situation, since the bone resorption blocking effects of calcitonin could oppose any resorbing effects of the low-level PTH.

Thus, the placenta supplies all of the necessary building blocks for bone mineralization (minerals and 25-OHD), and the infant produces all the necessary regulating hormones [PTH, calcitonin, $1,25(OH)_2D$] at appropriate concentration to promote bone growth accretion. The result is a steady increase in bone growth and bone mineral content. Using a variety of photon absorption techniques, a

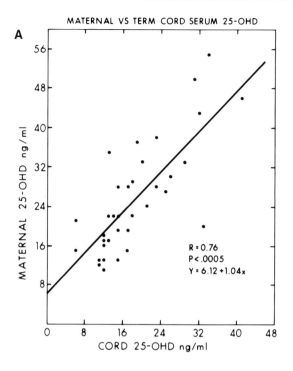

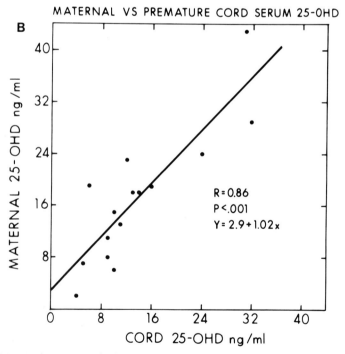

Fig. 3-1 Maternal serum 25-hydroxyvitamin D (25-OHD) compared to cord blood 25-OHD in (A) infants born at term and (B) infants born prematurely (11).

number of investigators have generated *in utero* bone mineral content curves by measuring BMC at birth in infants of varying gestations (44–46). In general the curves have shown a steady increase in BMC with increasing gestation. Careful curve fitting may suggest some concavity to the curve early on and some convexity at term. The curve generated by Dr. Greer for the radius using the radiometer machine can be seen in Fig. 3-2 (45). The curve we have generated on the midshaft of the humerus using the Norland–Cameron model 278 can be seen in Fig. 3-3. Bone width also increases during late gestation, and clearly significant remodeling accompanies this growth. It is therefore difficult on the basis of BMC measurements alone to comment about the mineral content of areas of bone or about the relative changes of growth and increased mineralization. Unfortunately, detailed histological analysis of infants dying at or shortly after birth at different gestations has yet to be done. This is an exceedingly difficult task because of the problems of defining comparable locations during growth.

POSTNATAL MINERALIZATION IN TERM INFANTS

At birth, the "reliable" supply of minerals and 25-OHD ceases. The infant now has an increased need to be able to regulate mineral absorption and retention and, if necessary, to mobilize bone mineral stores to maintain normal serum mineral concentrations. As already noted, all of the necessary calcium-regulating hormone systems are functioning at the time of birth. However, a transition must occur from the levels that support the fetal state to the levels that govern in the infant state. As serum calcium concentrations decline after removal of the placenta sup-

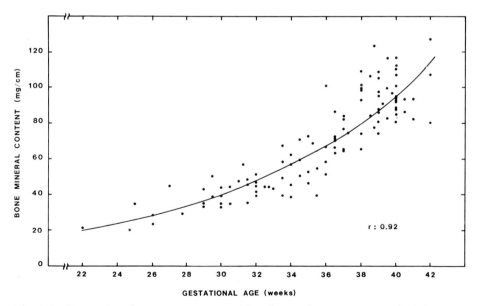

Fig. 3-2 Bone mineral content as measured by photon absorptiometry in the left radius of 114 newborn infants by gestational age (44).

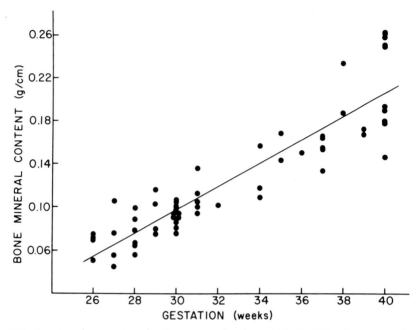

Fig. 3-3 In *utero* bone mineralization curve for the midshaft of the humerus using of Norland model 278 bone densitometer. Bone mineral content in grams per centimeter wide slice of bone after birth compared to gestational age of live-born premature and term infants.

ply, serum PTH increases (36). The exact course of these reciprocal changes depends on the assay system, but most studies agree that serum PTH achieves normal levels or overshoots by 48 h of age and then settles down to normal adult levels by a week or 2. Clearly, a subgroup of infants fail to attain or maintain normal PTH levels at 5–10 days of age, and they present as late neonatal hypocalcemia seizures (neonatal tetany) (49). In the United States, most of these infants are hypomagnesemic, and this may be the etiology of the PTH suppression (50). PTH certainly returns to normal with magnesium correction and time.

PTH remains within normal adult ranges throughout the first year of life on all usual feeding regimens when vitamin D sufficiency is assured (47). As noted, there is a surge of calcitonin postdelivery, but normal adult levels are also reached after a week or 2 (36). 1,25(OH)$_2$D production increases over the first 24–48 h, probably in response to the concomitant rise in PTH discussed (30). Our data show the highest levels of 1,25(OH)$_2$D at 2 months of age with falloff to 6-month levels only slightly above adult levels (47). There may thus be a developmental pattern superimposed on normal responsiveness to calcium and phosphorus needs. It has been speculated that these high early levels are important in inducing 1,25(OH)$_2$D receptors. Using these mechanisms, the term infant maintains a serum calcium over 10 mg/dl and a serum phosphorus between 6 and 8 for the first year of life—levels certainly designed to encourage mineralization (47).

Mineral intakes vary depending on the feeding regimen. In most areas of nutrition, human breast milk is considered the gold standard. And after several decades of predominantly formula feeding, much of the world has returned to a predominance of breast feeding. Human breast milk, however, contains relatively low levels of minerals compared to all other mammalian milks. Calcium and phosphorus exist in a 2:1 ratio. Calcium, probably for a number of reasons, is better absorbed from human milk than from formulations based on other mammalian milk such as cow's, and may reach absorption rates of over 80 percent. Phosphorus is over 90 percent absorbed from most feeding regimens and has its major regulation in renal reabsorption rather than intestinal absorption. Phosphorus not only is important for bone mineral accretion but also is a very important intracellular ion needed for soft-tissue accretion. Indeed the wisdom of the body would appear preferentially to use phosphorus for soft-tissue accretion when supplies are limited.

These factors combine to make phosphorus the more limiting element. Both Widdowson et al. (51) and Slater (52) showed that calcium and magnesium urine excretion was high in breast-fed infants whereas phosphorus excretion was low. Both groups showed further that addition of phosphorus decreased the excretion of both calcium and magnesium without altering gastrointestinal absorption, thereby increasing the retention of all three minerals (51, 52). In these older studies the vitamin D sufficiency of the infants was not documented.

We have studied breast-fed infants given an additional supplementation of 400 IU vitamin D in whom normal serum concentrations of vitamin D 25-OHD and $1,25(OH)_2D$ of 25-OHD were documented (47). Compared to infants fed standard cow's milk-based formula or soy formula, we again saw a higher urine calcium excretion (but not magnesium) and a lower phosphorus excretion until 9 months of age, when the addition of other phosphorus-containing solid foods reversed the situation. At 6 months of age serum phosphorus was significantly below the formula-fed groups and fell below 6 in the breast-fed group ($\bar{X} \pm SD$, 5.5 $\pm$ .3). At 12 months this returned to 6.2 $\pm$ .7 ($\bar{X} \pm SD$). However, urine phosphorus was higher in our studies than in the other studies, possibly reflecting a better vitamin D status. In spite of this suggestion that phosphorus content could be limiting mineral accretion, we could find no difference in bone mineral content. Serum alkaline phosphatase was only slightly higher in the breast-fed infants until 12 months, when it was significantly greater than in both other groups (47).

Cow's milk-based formulas with both higher mineral contents and calcium:phosphorus ratios of 1.5:1 or less appear to provide adequate amounts of both calcium and phosphorus (perhaps excessive phosphorus), at least as judged by urine levels of the minerals (47). Previous studies in soy formula have shown decreased phosphorus absorption because of the phytate complexing and also decreased fat and calcium absorption. Most soy formulas have attempted to compensate for this by increasing the mineral content of the formula. Manufacturers of soy formula have recently further improved their mineral suspension system. We studied infants fed ProSobee and found normal serum and urine levels as well as normal bone mineralization after 2 months of age (47).

The provision of vitamin D also varies by the feeding regimen plus a number of other factors. Of great importance is the level of 25-OHD sufficiency at birth. As noted, infant cord blood serum 25-OHD is dependent on maternal serum 25-OHD, which is dependent on the season of birth, sun exposure variables, and oral intake. Since the half-life of 25-OHD is 3 weeks, infants born with high levels may "coast" on these levels for a number of weeks before they require sun exposure or oral intake of vitamin D. Some degree of *in utero* soft-tissue stores of 25-OHD may also exist, and these are also dependent on maternal 25-OHD sufficiency. However, limited data would suggest that the infant uses primarily exogenous vitamin D supplies to maintain or increase serum 25-OHD (53). It is thus crucial that infants born to relatively vitamin D-deficient mothers be provided with sources of vitamin D either in the form of adequate sunlight exposure or as an oral intake of vitamin D.

Very early studies in term infants showed that 100 IU of vitamin D per day would result in normal calcium balance, and a recommendation for 400 IU was made to assure adequacy for all infants (54). Formula as well as cow's milk has been supplemented with about 400 IU of vitamin D per quart for many years. Our recent data confirm that this level is certainly adequate. Indeed, serum vitamin D levels in term infants were quite high at 2 months of age but fell to normal adult values by 6 months (47). That infants maintain or attain normal serum 25-OHD concentrations on this degree of supplementation has been documented by many investigators (17–19, 55–57). Although unnecessary, a large percentage of newborns in the United States may also receive additional vitamin supplements containing 400 IU vitamin D. Breast-fed infants receiving 400 IU D as a supplement have serum D and 25-OHD concentrations identical to infants receiving 400 IU D from their formula with normal 25-OHD levels being obtained even in infants starting life with very low serum 25-OHD (17–19, 55–57).

The much discussed "controversy" revolves around the need to supplement breast-fed infants. However, if one looks at all the available data, the answer appears clear, albeit complicated. Very old studies suggested that the biologically active levels of vitamin D in breast milk were very low. After a period of disbelief that "nature could have erred so," newer technologies have confirmed that levels of 25-OHD and 1,25(OH)$_2$D are indeed low in breast milk from most women. Breast milk levels are a small percentage of the maternal serum concentrations [25-OHD is 1% of serum, and 1,25(OH)$_2$D is 3% according to Hollis et al. (58)]. Recent studies have suggested that raising maternal serum 25-OHD to pharmacologic ranges can increase breast milk 25-OHD to significant levels (18, 55, 59).

Table 3-3 summarizes published maternal and infant serum 25-OHD concentrations at about 2 months of age with different levels of maternal supplementation in populations of varying degrees of maternal 25-OHD sufficiency (i.e., polar latitude and winter birth—least sufficient; and moderate latitude and mixed season of birth—most sufficient). No supplementation or even 400 IU maternal supplementation results in acceptable infant 25-OHD concentrations only in moderate latitude–mixed season of birth populations (56, 57). Data on higher levels of maternal supplementation exist only for polar latitude populations. In these populations even 1,000 IU D maternal supplementation does not result in acceptable infant levels (17, 18, 55). Supplementation at 2,000 IU D per day does result in normal infant 25-OHD levels; however, maternal levels were often excessive (over 40 ng/ml after 8 weeks' lactation), and the safety of these maternal levels might be questioned (18, 55). When infant 25-OHD sufficiency is in question, supplementation of the infant is clearly the easiest and most reliable route. Certainly

Table 3-3 Serum 25-OHD Concentrations ng/ml in Breast-Fed Infants and Their Mothers with Varying Maternal or Infant Vitamin D Supplementations (values closest to 2 months selected from available data)

	South Africa	New Zealand	Finland	Norway	USA (Utah)	USA (Ohio)	Finland	USA (Missouri)
Season	Winter	Mixed	Winter	Winter	Mixed	Mixed	Mixed	Fall
Age (weeks)	6	13	8	6	9	6	8	8
No supplementation								
Mother	10 ± 6	23 ± 7	9					
Infant	1 ± 1	19 ± 4	5					
Mother 400 IU								
Mother	14 ± 5				19 ± 7			
Infant	10 ± 6			8	17 ± 9	22 ± 12		
Mother 1,000 IU								
Mother	15 ± 4		25 ± 12[a]				41	
Infant	9 ± 2		12 ± 5[a]				15	
Mother 2,000 IU								
Mother			27 ± 10				48	
Infant			21 ± 9				30	
Infant 400								
Mother	11.0 ± 4		10 ± 5[a]		19 ± 7			
Infant	15 ± 4		24 ± 14[a]		19 ± 10	39 ± 9		23 ± 9

[a]Previous study mean: maternal 1000 IU—mother 15, infant 5; infant 400 IU—mother 7, infant 18.

vitamin D supplementation during lactation should be recommended for the mother's own mineral economy. We must remember, however, that man and even babies were meant to get vitamin D from skin production in response to sunlight.

Prevention is always preferable to treatment, and the need to provide adequate maternal vitamin D supplementation during pregnancy cannot be overly stressed. The recommended dose of 400 IU D intake for all pregnant women is reasonable; however, depending on the location, season of the third trimester, and ethnicity, higher doses may be appropriate. Studies of routine prenatal supplementation of the Asian population in Britain have shown marked improvement in maternal and infant 25-OHD concentrations (25). A very concrete benefit in this vitamin D-deficient population was a reduction in late neonatal hypocalcemia (25). Cord magnesium was significantly reduced with maternal supplementation, and serum calcium was significantly increased at 1 week of age (60). (How the vitamin D deficiency late-neonatal hypocalcemia of the Asian population in Britain relates to the magnesium and PTH deficiency late-neonatal hypocalcemia of the United States is unclear.)

Except in cases of extreme vitamin D deficiency, when $1,25(OH)_2D$ levels may decline for lack of substrate or increased utilization, $1,25(OH)_2D$ is one of the few measurements that may suggest how hard the infant's homeostatic mechanisms are having to work to meet requirements on a given feeding regimen. In our recent study, serum $1,25(OH)_2D$ was lower in breast-fed infants than either cow's milk formula or soy protein formula infants, and infant levels were similar to our adult norms (47). This observation again emphasizes the probable adequacy of breast milk minerals during the first 6 months of life, when vitamin D supplementation is assured. A further elevation of $1,25(OH)_2D$ at 2 and 4 months in infants fed soy formula is difficult to explain (47). Neither elevation of PTH nor significantly low serum phosphorus was present to act as stimulus to $1,25(OH)_2D$ production.

Having lauded the term infants' ability to adapt, but having noted his dependence on adults to supply adequate minerals and vitamin D, we must address the fortunately infrequent problem of term infants who develop problems with bone mineralization. The very old literature suggested that it was the cow's milk-fed infants who developed rickets and that breast-fed infants were relatively spared. With the advent of vitamin D supplementation of milk and formula and the practice of early introduction of solid foods, rickets became rare in all infants in the United States (61). Now as part of a general return to nature, the breast milk-fed infants are becoming at increased risk of what is undoubtedly a combination of vitamin D and phosphorus deficiency rickets (62–64). Usually a multiplicity of preventable factors combine to produce the deficiency. Factors in typical cases are seen in Table 3-4. The affected infants are usually those born to mothers who were vitamin D insufficient for the reasons discussed. No supplementation of the infant is provided, and the nursing mother maintains her vitamin D-insufficient state, providing milk that is certainly inadequate in vitamin D metabolites.

These infants are often black, inner-city dwellers whose social patterns and skin pigmentation combine to limit correction of the deficiency by sun exposure. Introduction of solid foods is markedly delayed in most cases, often to beyond a year, and when foods are introduced they have often been vegetarian diets. This delay in solid foods has two effects—limited access to other vitamin D-containing foods, and limited access to additional phosphorus. Their rickets often becomes symptomatic at about a year, when the infant is essentially experiencing the same conditions that led to the mother's initial vitamin D insufficiency (often the infants are born in winter and present symptomatic the next winter, having never sufficiently corrected the situation in between). Major educational efforts are needed and are being carried out in high-risk populations such as the Asians in Britain. However, additional education is needed for groups such as vegetarian and religious sects, the latter of which wear totally occlusive dress. These two groups are trying to do their best by their infants by prolonged breast feeding (65).

The infant who completes a normal gestation has developed a skeleton where the long bones, at least, are mineralized, and normal handling and movement are well tolerated. The newborn infant, however, is not a weight-bearing animal, and the musculoskeletal system undergoes numerous changes in the first year of life: arm weight bearing (3 months), upright trunk in sitting (6 months), four-limb

Table 3-4 Vitamin D Deficiency Rickets in Breast-Fed Term Infants

Age of onset: late in first year
Season of onset: winter
Season of birth: winter
Infant diet: exclusive breast feeding
Maternal diet: vegetarian
Maternal dress: covered
Race: black > white

weight bearing (8 months), upright two-limb weight bearing with support (10 months), and two-limb weight bearing without support (12 months). Body proportions are also changing, with a steady increase in the ratio of leg length to overall length. These changes clearly require a great deal of skeletal modeling and remodeling. As minerals continue to be deposited in the cortex and as the bone marrow cavity enlarges with the increased bone diameter, the "average density" of the bone $[BMC/\pi(BW)^2]$ actually decreases. Such changes produce a relatively lighter bone with good mechanical strength (47). Attempting to evaluate "bone density" using a "bone densitometer" is clearly an impossibility and a misnomer under these growth conditions. A symposium on the use of bone mineral content measurements in infants has been published recently (48).

However, assuming normal growth, measurements of bone mineral content (BMC = total mineral content in a cross section of bone 1 cm thick) may be useful to define group pathology and to follow individuals longitudinally. This approach would be useful to define the normal pattern as well as change of BMC over a set time period, $\Delta BMC/month$ ($\Delta BMC/M$) and would be helpful in an assessment of the mineral needs of the growing infant. Such data have been developed for the midshaft of the humerus (Fig. 3-4). Independent of the feeding regimen, BMC increases over the first 4 months, plateaus at 6 months, then slowly increases further. $\Delta BMC/M$ fell from .07 g/cm to no increase over the first 6 months then averaged out at about .04 g/cm. This pattern of need for minerals generally follows normal mineral intakes per kilogram body weight over the first year.

POSTNATAL MINERALIZATION IN PREMATURE INFANTS

Mineralization problems are more frequently met in premature infants. Again, the problems are multifactorial, and in each infant one must look at a number of factors, the most important of which are (1) mineral availability, (2) vitamin D availability and metabolism, (3) gestational effects related to increased demands and efficiency of mineral regulation, and (4) complications of prematurity and NICU care. We will, however, attempt to define these factors separately for the sake of discussion.

Mineral Availability

The *in utero* mineralization mineral needs, already reviewed, emphasize the large job to be done if ones goal is to match *in utero* accretion (2–5). Many researchers would suggest that this is an unrealistic goal, one that places unnecessary stress on immature systems. The extreme alternative would be to try to establish the minimal mineral intakes that would result in acceptable mineralization and growth. Some feeling for what can be considered tolerable limits has been gained by studying infants on the various available feeding regimens. By chance, limitations of calcium and phosphorus have occurred under different circumstances, and those effects can be assessed somewhat independently.

The effects of limiting calcium can best be seen in premature infants fed the

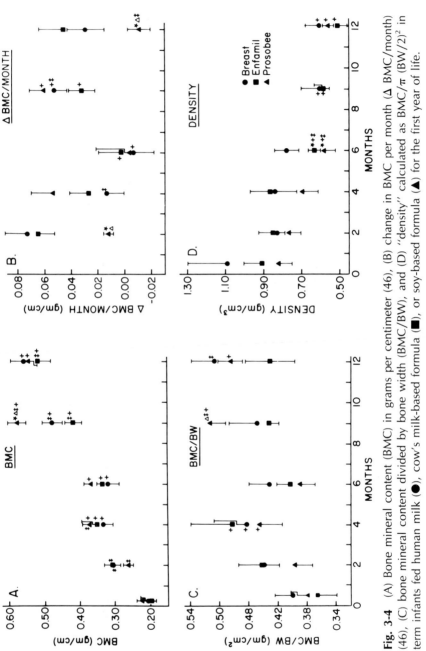

Fig. 3-4 (A) Bone mineral content (BMC) in grams per centimeter (46), (B) change in BMC per month (Δ BMC/month) (46), (C) bone mineral content divided by bone width (BMC/BW), and (D) "density" calculated as BMC/π (BW/2)² in term infants fed human milk (●), cow's milk-based formula (■), or soy-based formula (▲) for the first year of life.

standard formula designed for term infants. The calcium content of standard casein predominant formula was about 500 mg/L and mean percent absorption reported was 35–50 percent (5), so an infant taking 200 ml/kg—a generous amount—
would obtain only 35–50 mg/kg, about one-third (35/120 = 29%) of the *in utero*
accretion rate. Phosphorus content was, however, high—390 mg/day with 90
percent absorption for an intake of 70 mg/kg which matches *in utero* accretion.
We followed 69 infants <1,500 g on such a formula for 12 weeks (23). Serum
calcium was between 8.9 and 9.1 mg/dl until 12 weeks, when it increased to
9.6. Mean serum phosphorus also slowly fell over the first 9 weeks, from 6.8 to
4.8 mg/dl, and then increased at 12 weeks to 6.8. Mean serum alkaline phosphatase was between 360 and 430 IU throughout the period.

Radiographic evaluation showed moderate demineralization in over 50 percent
of infants until 12 weeks, when mineralization improved in all but 15 percent of
infants who still showed moderate demineralization. No infant who had maintained steady formula and vitamin intakes showed rachitic change or fractures.
Infants were divided on the basis of whether they were able to reach intakes of
80 mg/kg calcium by 3 weeks of age, an arbitrary level which rather equally
divided the group. As seen in Fig. 3-5, the group with the lower calcium intake
had a lower serum calcium, higher alkaline phosphatase, and worse bone mineralization. However, even in this group improvement occurred at 12 weeks. Serum
PTH was high-normal in a subset of these infants, and calcitonin also remained
elevated for the first 12 weeks.

The results of phosphorus deficiency were more impressive. In 1975 we described nine infants with classical vitamin D deficiency who were also on either
soy formula or PM 60/40, a formula with a mineral composition of breast milk.
These infants clearly displayed the consequences of both vitamin D and phosphorus deficiency (66). A larger series of soy formula-fed infants who presented
with rickets, the etiology of which was less well described, was reported by Kulkarni (67) and Callenbach (68). Kulkarni also performed a prospective study in
which the incidence of rickets was 50 percent (69). Although the phosphorus
content of soy formula was the same as standard cow milk-based formula, the
presence of phytate made a portion of the phosphorus unavailable. The complexity
of the problem, in part, generated the studies of another soy formula in term
infants previously described. Although that formula performed well in term infants, the recommendation to avoid prolonged use of soy formula in preterm infants remains appropriate because of their increased needs and potential limitations.

A much clearer example of phosphorus limitation is the use of breast milk in
preterm infants. Although the composition of breast milk varies considerably, reasonable estimates of mineral content would be 300 mg/L calcium and 150 mg/
L phosphorus. Balance studies of Senterre and Salle would suggest the percent
calcium absorption with 1,200 IU vitamin D of 70 percent (70). Thus, infants
consuming 200 cc/kg would have calcium intakes of 42 mg/kg, still less than
half of *in utero* accretion rates (42/120 = 35%) but indeed higher than standard
formula. The intake of phosphorus assuming 90 percent absorption (70), however,
would be only 27 mg/kg, or less than half of *in utero* accretion (27/71 = 38%).
Since a key factor in supporting mineralization is bone matrix fluid phosphorus,

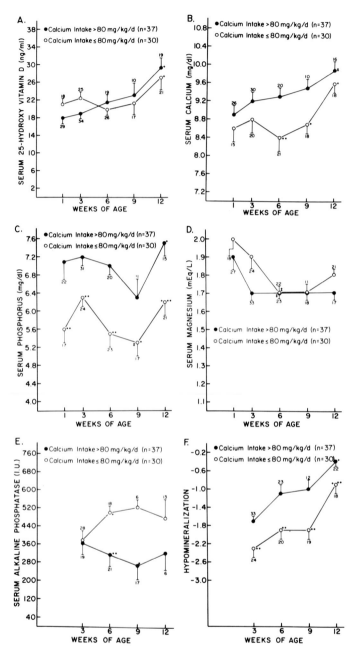

Fig. 3-5 (A) Serum 25-OHD, (B) serum calcium, (C) serum phosphorus, (D) serum magnesium, (E) serum alkaline phosphatase, and (F) hypomineralization by age in infants with calcium intakes at three weeks >80 mg/kg/day (N = 37) (●) and ≤80 mg/kg/day (N = 30) (○). *Difference between group; †change from initial value; and ‡difference from start of increase or decrease. One symbol: $p < .05$; two symbols: $p < .01$ (22).

which is in equilibrium with serum phosphorus, it is clear why such a decreased intake might have negative results. Further, as already discussed, phosphorus is important for building lean body mass, and phosphorus appears to be preferentially used for that function over bone mineralization.

Balance studies on premature infants fed human milk have shown that absorption of phosphorus and renal conservation of phosphorus are maximal, so that essentially all intake is retained (70–73). Calcium is also well absorbed, but urinary calcium losses are large, and calcium retention is limited because of the limits of phosphorus intake. Calcium cannot be incorporated into bone without phosphorus, so when phosphorus is limited, the extra calcium is excreted. Both Senterre and Salle (72) and Schandler et al. (73) have shown that provision of additional phosphorus increases calcium retention and decreases urinary calcium losses. Those studies were performed during the first 3–4 weeks of life in infants over 1,000 g. The clinical significance of this balance data becomes clear when one follows premature infants, especially those <1,100 g, over a longer period of time. We followed 14 exclusively breast-fed infants <1,300 g for 3 months (74). Six of the infants required phosphorus supplementation based on (1) falling serum phosphorus, (2) increasing urinary calcium, and (3) poorly mineralized bones.

In general, the infants who required phosphorus supplementation were those weighing <1,100 g and those whose serum 25-OHD levels failed to increase. The time course of their serum and urine minerals compared to bottle-fed infants can be seen in Fig. 3-6. Significant falloff of serum phosphorus and increase in urine calcium did not begin until 5–6 weeks of age, and those infants who reached levels initiating supplementation did so between 8 and 10 weeks of age. The dramatic response to 1 week of supplementation with 20–25 mg/kg of phosphorus as neutrophos or neutrophos K can be seen in Table 3-5. None of these infants developed rickets, perhaps because they were closely monitored and benefited from early intervention. Bone mineralization by X-ray was comparable to infants fed standard formula; over half remained moderately demineralized at 9 weeks. It is interesting that the time course is similar to that which we have seen with soy formula or PM 60/40 where rickets was diagnosed at 12 weeks of age and severe demineralization and occasionally fractures without rickets were diagnosed at about 9 weeks (66, 75). Nine to 12 weeks represents the normal time when 1,000-g infants leave the hospital and potentially remain undiagnosed at home. In Kulkarni's experience with soy formulas, many of the infants were diagnosed during the healing stages of rickets (67). Spontaneous healing appears to occur in many infants after 3 months. This time frame corresponds to changes in both vitamin D metabolism and mineral homeostasis, which occurs when term gestation is reached (to be discussed later). The point to be made here is that some of the failure to appreciate the potential problems of feeding human breast milk to extremely premature, <1,100 g infants is the failure to follow these infants long enough to detect the problem.

Thus, based on these two groups of infants, one might suggest that one can provide as little as 30 percent of *in utero* requirements of calcium (with phosphorus provided) and get by with a poorly mineralized bone which will not fracture or become rachitic and will spontaneously improve when the infant reaches term gestation. Provision of 40 percent of *in utero* phosphorus requirements re-

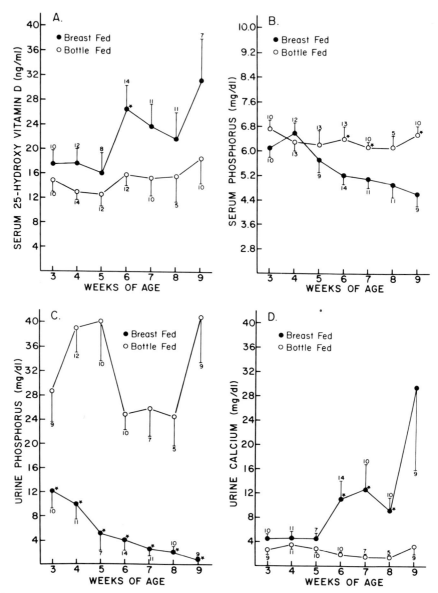

Fig. 3-6 (A) Serum 24-OHD, (B) serum phosphorus, (C) urine phosphorus, and (D) urine calcium by age in infants fed human milk (●) or standard infant formula (Similac 20 calories) (○) (72).

sulted in 43 percent (6/14) infants <1,300 g and (6/7) 86 percent of infants <1,000 g developing phosphorus deficiency as defined by serum and urine values (74). What percentage would have developed rickets if not treated? This is unknown, but based on the soy data, it could be substantial. These data again emphasized that phosphorus is the key element in bone mineralization and its need for soft-tissue accretion. Undoubtedly, part of what allowed both groups to do as

Table 3-5 Serum and Urine Minerals (mg/dl) Prior to (B) and 1 Week after (A) Supplementation with 25 mg/kg/day Phosphorus

Patient No.	Age (weeks)	Serum phosphorus B	Serum phosphorus A	Urine phosphorus B	Urine phosphorus A	Serum calcium B	Serum calcium A	Urine calcium B	Urine calcium A
1	9	4.6	7.6	.1	9.9	8.3	8.7	9.3	3.2
2	9	4.5	6.1	.1	15.6	9.7	9.1	10.3	.8
3	9	1.7	4.7	Und	.4	9.8	9.0	18.3	1.8
4	10	4.1	7.3	.3	2.4	9.8	9.4	70.0	1.9
5	8	3.9	6.5	.8	19.1	8.7	8.7	9.4	8.5[a]
6	8	3.7	5.6	.1	.7	9.0	10.6	17.5	4.8
Mean		3.8	6.0[b]	.2	8.0[b]	9.2	9.3	13.0[c]	3.8[c]
SE		±.4	±.4	±.1	±3.4	±.3	±.3	1.9	±1.3
Mean Δ ± SE		2.6 ± .3		7.8 ± 3.3		.03 ± .4		9.1 ± 2.5	

Source: Hillman et al (74)

[a]Urine calcium never decreased in this infant in spite of correction of serum and urine phosphorus.

[b]Different from before values by paired *t*-test, $p < .05$.

[c]Value excludes patient No. 4 because of extreme value of 70 mg/dl.

well as they did preserving bone mineralization was a concomitant limitation of the growth rate, particularly in the breast-fed infants. Great caution must be taken not to assume similar results if other factors are altered to increase growth rate.

It should be further noted that many factors can increase or decrease the percentage of calcium absorption, as will be discussed later. For phosphorus, absorption is less easily influenced and cannot generally be increased. The infant's major regulation of phosphorus is through renal conservation and, as noted in Fig. 3–6, even very premature infants have a remarkable ability to conserve phosphorus, with urine phosphorus being undetectable in many breast-fed prematures. Thus, although there may be alternatives to increasing calcium intake, there probably are not reliable alternatives to increasing phosphorus intake.

The approach previously taken by many nurseries has been to add either calcium or phosphorus or both in varying amounts to infants on standard formula or breast milk. Companies have now made available formulas for premature infants that have incorporated many of the changes that may alter the percent calcium absorption and have also markedly increased the content of both calcium and phosphorus. However, all companies have increased calcium out of proportion to phosphorus to achieve the 2:1 calcium:phosphorus ratio seen in breast milk. These formulations appear to be a reasonable place to start, and the calculated accretions are in line with *in utero* accretions. The major difference between the three major American premature formulas are in their calcium and phosphorus contents (Table 3-6). European formulas have been limited by law to the lowest level of 700 mg/L calcium.

Whether there is an active component to calcium absorption in the premature infant will be discussed later. Clearly there is a very large nonactive, unsaturable, non-vitamin D-dependent, calcium absorption in premature infants. The premature infant calcium intake data would suggest that the more calcium that is given,

Table 3-6 Composition of Premature Formula and Breast Milk Fortifiers per 100 ml

	Similac Special Care (24 cal) (liquid)	Similac Natural Care Breast Milk Fortifier 1:2 with straight breast milk (liquid)		Enfamil Premature Formula (24 cal) (liquid)	Enfamil Breast Milk Fortifier plus breast milk (powder)	SMA Premie (liquid)
Calcium	175	170	98	95	85–90	75
Phosphorus	92	85	60	47.5	49–53	40
Sodium	37	38	46	31.7	35–46	32
Protein	2.2	2.2	2.2	2.4	2.0–2.7	2.0
Vitamin D	123	120	61	264 IU	260	51

the more that gets across (76, 77). That is not to say that the "more" that is put into a formula, the "more" that gets into the infant. The initial formulation at the highest mineral levels was plagued by problems of sedimentation in the bottle and in the tubing used to feed the infants (78). Although calcium absorption rates were reported to be as high as 70 percent with this formulation (79), we still detected moderate demineralization in 25 percent of infants at 6 weeks, and in the group as a whole, serum and urine calcium were only moderately increased.

A lower serum phosphorus compared to standard formula suggested that the very high calcium levels could be limiting phosphorus absorption (Fig. 3-7). Bone densitometry data on this formula showed falling BMC in four of 12 infants (80). Balance studies on a new formulation of the highest mineral formula commercially available still show somewhat low serum phosphorus and only 75% phosphorus absorption, suggesting that high calcium content may interfere with phosphorus absorption (81). Feeding a higher mineral level did not alter serum 25-OHD levels. Since we wished to study increased minerals plus increased vitamin D, we switched to a more conservative formula (900 mg/L calcium) as the base formula for further studies. Both serum calcium and phosphorus normalized, and we have essentially not seen an infant with moderate demineralization on X-ray. However, commensurate with this have been a consistent increase in urinary calcium and, whether or not related, a generalized aminoaciduria in 80 percent of infants. Despite normal serum levels and increased urine levels of calcium, bone mineralization has not paralleled the *in utero* curve (Fig. 3-7).

We were concerned that the calciuria and aminoaciduria might relate to the high protein load of this formula (3.0 g/100 kcal), since calciuria secondary to protein overload has been reported in adults and animals (82, 83) and patients on total parenteral nutrition. We had prepared three identical high-mineral formulas that varied only in protein content (the two lower-protein formulas having 2.7 and 2.2 g/100 Kcal—the same content as the first high-mineral formula tested and standard formula, respectively). To our surprise, the lower protein formula resulted in greater calciuria, and the aminoaciduria persisted. Infants on the lower-protein, high-mineral formulas also developed serum proteins significantly below those previously seen at similar protein levels with standard minerals (84). The

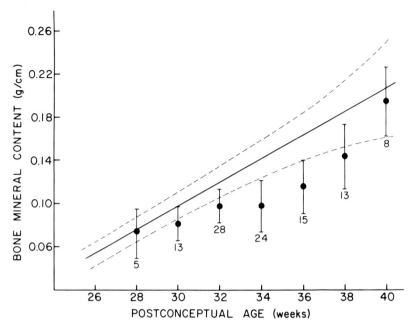

Fig. 3-7 Bone mineral content by postconceptual age in premature infants fed a high-mineral premature formula (Enfamil Premature Formula) compared to the *in utero* bone mineralization curve for the humerus using the Norland model 278 bone densitometer.

most likely explanation is that providing adequate minerals increased growth and protein needs, and, conversely, when protein was limited, absorbed calcium was not retained for growth. An alternative hypothesis would be to postulate a calcium protein interaction during absorption. This possibility requires further study.

To investigate the possibility that calcuria and aminoaciduria represented renal tubular damage, we used measurements of urinary B_2 microglobulins and N-acetylglutamate (NAG). These measures were not increased in infants on the high-mineral formula when compared to data from premature infants fed standard formula (85). This finding was somewhat reassuring, but it does not rule out a tubular effect. Attempts to alter urine calcium with vitamin D were also unsuccessful and will be discussed later. In short, the passive absorption of calcium may allow the premature to increase net absorption; however, retention of calcium and mineralization comparable to *in utero* accretion may not be easily achieved without significant calcuria.

In attempting to provide uniform supplementation for breast milk-fed premature infants, two of the formula companies have developed "breast milk fortifiers." Mead Johnson has produced a powder that, when added to breast milk, brings the protein, mineral, and vitamin concentrations of the breast milk up to the level found in their premature formula. Ross Labs has produced a liquid designed to be mixed half and half with breast milk, and this results in mineral and vitamin levels somewhat lower than that found in their premature formula, making it comparable to the Mead Johnson fortifier. (It should be noted that mixed half and half, this results in dilution in half of human milk factors not present in the fortifier and that, fed alternately, this represents the highest mineral load presented to the GI tract of any present feeding regimen).

Experience with these fortifiers is limited. How mineral supplementation affects some of the benefits of breast milk such as immunologic protection is totally unstudied. It should be cautioned that human milk is very low in protein, and spontaneous cases of clinical hypoproteinemia in extreme prematures occur (usually at about 3 months of age, after the infant has gone home). However, supplementation with minerals alone was associated with hypoproteinemia in two of our six infants. Our data on the effects of protein levels on mineral balance with premature formula would suggest that one might markedly increase the chance of clinical hypoproteinemia by providing minerals alone. Fortunately, both commercial fortifiers include generous protein supplementation.

Vitamin D

Given the clear existence of a passive calcium transport system in premature infants that can be pushed by increasing calcium intake and the excellent absorptions and retention of phosphorus in premature infants, one may ask whether there is a role for vitamin D. There remain a large group of neonatologists who are uncomfortable with feeding high-mineral intakes. With lower mineral intakes, it would be important to maximize percentage absorption by vitamin D-mediated transport. We have already noted that high-mineral intake alone does not normalize bone mineralization. Will altering vitamin D status promote renal reabsorption of calcium or influence bone mineral deposition? Before trying to address these clinical questions, it is important to review (1) the premature infant's ability to absorb and metabolize vitamin D and the implications of this for required intakes of vitamin D, and (2) the ability of the premature infants and organ targets to respond to the vitamin D metabolites.

As noted, very old balance data in term infants (54) suggested that 100 IU of vitamin D was adequate intake, and our recent measurements of vitamin D would suggest that 400 IU is more than adequate, possibly excessive (47). Old balance studies in premature infants in Germany suggested that 1,000 IU of vitamin D was necessary. Newer studies in France have shown improvements in calcium balance with up to 2,000 IU of vitamin D (70) and as high as 2,400 IU needed to normalize serum 25-OHD (86). However, in the United States, older studies in term infants suggested that 1,800 IU/day was associated with linear growth retardation (87). It is difficult to compare these studies because of the lack of measurements of vitamin D metabolites, especially 25-OHD. Clearly these populations may differ in their level of vitamin D sufficiency (the French population is clearly a more vitamin D-deficient population than the U.S. today), and thus infants may be entering studies with different levels of vitamin D sufficiency. If one assumes that the average requirement is 1,000 IU/day, this is 10-fold the requirement of the term infant. If one normalizes for weight, then the requirements per kilogram for the 1-kg premature is 30-fold that of the 3-kg term infant. This is a marked increase in requirement and would suggest a number of potential problems: (1) inefficient absorption of vitamin D; (2) inefficient hydroxylation of vitamin D to 25-OHD by the immature liver; (3) inefficient hydroxylation of 25-OHD to 1,25(OH)$_2$D; and (4) increased utilization of 1,25(OH)$_2$D. We will attempt to address each of these steps separately and would reemphasize that what is in question is not the infant's *ability* to perform each step but the *efficiency* of performing each step.

Vitamin D is a fat-soluble vitamin, and absorption is influenced by factors that influence fat absorption. Premature infants have well-documented problems with fat absorption based on both decreased bile acids and decreased pancreatic lipase, and one would thus assume some decreased efficiency of vitamin D absorption. Until recently the inability to measure serum vitamin D limited assessment of this problem. Although absorption of 25-OHD and absorption of vitamin D are not totally comparable, 25-OHD absorption tests have been used in normal adults (88) and adults with gastrointestinal disease to try to assess vitamin D absorption (89). We performed 25-OHD absorption tests in eight larger premature infants (1,704 ± 63 g BW) and found that although the time course of the peak in serum 25-OHD levels (4–8 h) was the same as seen in adults, the magnitude of the increase was only half of what would have been expected suggesting a decreased efficiency of absorption (see Fig. 3-8). More recently we have measured serum vitamin D in a small number of premature infants at 37.2 ± 4.3 days of age fed standard formula with 400 or 800 IU D, doses representing almost 400–800 IU/kg. Adults given the dose of 800 IU/kg had serum vitamin D levels of 70–90 ng/ml (90). Mean infant levels were 20.3 ± 4.8 with a range of 5–31 ng/ml (normal adult 1.1 ± 0.1, N = 10). Although these infant levels are high, they are less than a

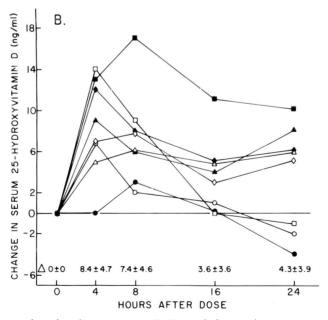

Fig. 3-8 Change from baseline serum 25-OHD (ng/ml) in eight premature infants given a single dose of 2 μg/kg 25-hydroxycholecalciferol.

third of predicted values and thus support the concept of decreased absorption of vitamin D.

Immaturity of the gastrointestinal tract may be of further importance by decreasing enterohepatic circulation of 25-OHD in the premature infant. The existence or importance of an enterhepatic 25-OHD circulation in man is unclear and still debated. However, if important, the premature infant could experience significant loss of 25-OHD through this mechanism. Of note is that at least two of the high-mineral premature formulas already discussed contain 40 or 50 percent medium-chain triglycerides which, because they bypass the need for bile salts and pancreatic lipase, result in very high levels of fat absorption in premature infants. In studies of infants eating standard formula, 2 μg/kg of 25-OHD$_3$ was established as a dose that reliably produced serum 25-OHD concentrations between 25 and 30 ng/ml, the level achieved by a vitamin D-sufficient premature at postconceptional term (47). Use of a somewhat lower dose, 2 μg without correction for birth weight, in infants eating Enfamil Premature Formula resulted in levels twice that high (54.5 $\pm$ 14 ng/ml at 4 weeks and 53.7 $\pm$ 10.3 at 6 weeks), suggesting—as one explanation—markedly improved adsorption of 25-OHD in the face of medium-chain triglycerides. In summary, it would appear that decreased absorption of vitamin D (and possibly reabsorption of 25-OHD) is one factor accounting for the increased vitamin D requirements of the premature infant.

The liver is a second organ known for its inefficiency in the premature infant. Decreased synthesis of clotting factors has been known for many years (91). More recently we have shown decreased levels which return to normal at postconceptional term for albumin (92), ceruloplasmin (92), somatomedin C (93), and vitamin D binding protein (DBP) (14). Drug metabolism, particularly metabolism that requires hydroxylation and the P-450 system, has been shown to be also decreased in premature infants (94). Studies of rat pups have shown that although the 25-hydroxylase is present in 19-day-old fetuses, increases to adult levels do not occur until 3 days of life. Delivery of rats at different days suggested that this increase was postconceptually, not postnatally, timed (35). These same authors showed that liver uptake of vitamin D was decreased until weaning, then rapidly increases (35). Since vitamin D-dependent calcium absorption is not present in the rat until weaning, this timing seems appropriate (95). Evaluation of the hydroxylating capacity of the liver of one human fetus failed to show significant hydroxylating capacity (96).

During the first week of life we were unable to see increases in serum 25-OHD with 250 IU vitamin D given intravenously (22); however, Salle et al. showed increases in 25-OHD by 5 days in infants given 2,000 IU orally (97). Koo et al (98) have shown that as little as 25 I.U./kg i.v. vitamin D will support normal 25-OHD serum levels in premature infants give TPN. It would thus appear that enzymatic activity is present and that acceptable amounts of 25-OHD can be generated if large amounts of substrates are given. We were interested in what happens over time and establishing what levels of vitamin D supplementation was needed to assure adult or term infant serum 25-OHD concentrations. Our adult serum concentrations, using the assay of Haddad and Chyu, are 21.7 $\pm$ 4.9 (SD), and values in term infants show means of between 25 and 27 ng/ml over the first year of life (47).

Both in the cord blood studies and in all subsequent studies the mean 25-OHD serum concentration that a St. Louis premature infant population (mixed season of birth and >50% black infants) begins life at is 16 ng/ml. However, there is a huge range, from 5 to 35 ng/ml. Very early limited studies giving premature infants the amount required by term infants, 100 IU/day, resulted in dangerously low levels of serum 25-OHD, even with their smaller size (22). Subsequently, infants were studied using the currently recommended dose of 400 IU/day.

Infants were grouped into four catetgories depending on the pattern of their serum 25-OHD levels from birth through 6 or 9 weeks of age (Fig. 3-9) (23): 22 percent maintained normal levels, whereas 27 percent were unable to maintain normal levels; 24 percent were able to correct low levels, whereas 26 percent were unable to correct low levels. Combination of these groups resulted in 46 percent of infants for whom 400 IU of vitamin D appeared adequate and 54 percent of infants for whom it appeared inadequate. In all groups but the group with falling 25-OHD levels, a significant further increase in serum 25-OHD occurred between 9 and 12 weeks postnatal age, the time at which postconceptual term was reached in this 30-week-gestation population. This suggested a postconceptional timing to increased efficiency of 25-hydroxylation.

In the study of infants fed 400 IU D and standard formula, those infants maintaining or achieving serum 25-OHD levels did better than those with persistent or subsequently low 25-OHD levels (i.e., higher serum calcium, lower alkaline phosphatase, more mineralized bones) (Fig. 3-10). Similarly the breast milk-fed premature infants who did not end up requiring phosphorus supplementation had higher

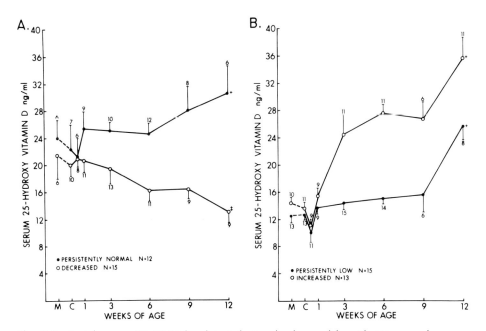

Fig. 3-9 Serial serum 25-OHD level in infants who began life with (A) normal serum 25-OHD, 15 mg/ml, or (B) low serum 25-OHD, ≤15 mg/ml, divided by success or failure in maintaining or attaining 25-OHD levels >15 ng/ml by 6 or 9 weeks of age.

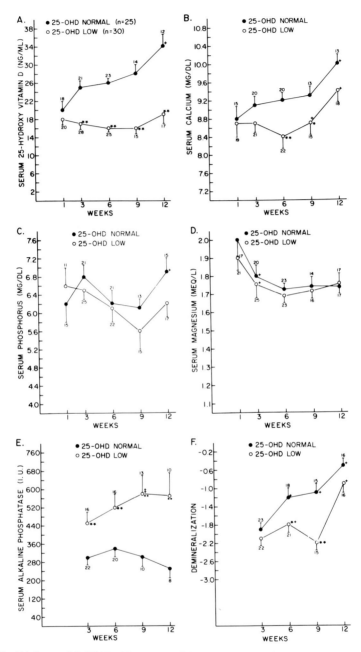

Fig. 3-10 (A) Serum 25-OHD, (B) serum calcium, (C) serum phosphorus, (D) serum magnesium, (E) serum alkaline phosphatase, and (F) demineralization by age in infants divided by infant's ability to maintain or attain normal serum 25-OHD (>15 ng/ml) over the first 6 or 9 weeks of life (●) or failure to maintain or attain normal serum 25-OHD (●). *Different between groups; †change from initial values; ‡change from start of increase or decrease. One symbol: $p < .05$, two symbols: $p < .01$ (22).

serum 25-OHD than those requiring phosphorus supplementation (74). It thus seemed important to try to normalize serum 25-OHD in all infants. Two methods were chosen: (1) to give more vitamin D with the assumption that increased substrate would result in more 25-OHD, and (2) to bypass any potential problems of absorption and/or hydroxylation by giving 25-hydroxycholecalciferol (25-OHD_3) (11). Absorption studies of 25-OHD_3 were first carried out to assess the premature infant's ability to absorb 25-OHD and give guidelines for dosage. These studies suggested that a dose of 1 μg/kg birth weight might be adequate; however, clinical trials suggested that 2 μg/kg birth weight would more reliably result in serum 25-OHD values between 20 and 30 ng/ml. The 800 IU dose of vitamin D_2 resulted in normalization of serum 25-OHD in all infants but was slower than with 25-OHD_3 in many infants. Control infants had the same 25-OHD levels as previously seen (Fig. 3-11). It also resulted in a higher serum calcium and better mineralization than 400 IU D_2; however, to our surprise neither serum calcium or mineralization was improved with 25-OHD_3. Indeed, we saw a suppression of PTH with a concomitant increase in serum phosphorus and decrease in serum magnesium. $1,25(OH)_2D$ levels were similar in all groups.

We do not have a good explanation for these findings. If these findings are confirmed, then we indeed have disparate effects of the parent compound and its first metabolite. Very early German studies using very large doses of 25-OHD, 9 or 18 μg/day, recorded decreases in alkaline phosphatase (99, 100). Since a clear benefit of 25-OHD over increased vitamin D does not exist, we would sug-

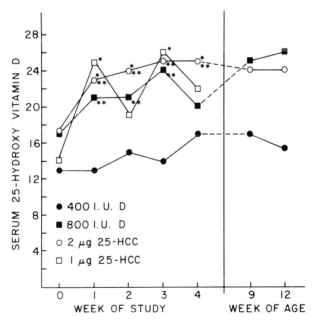

Fig. 3-11 Serial serum 25-OHD by week of study in premature infants fed 400 IU vitamin D (●), 800 IU vitamin D (■), 2 μg 25-hydroxycholecalciferol (25-HCC) (○), or 1 μg 25-HCC plus values at 9 and 12 weeks of age all on 400 IU vitamin D (□). Different from 400 IU *p < .05, **p < .01 (10).

gest that use of 25-OHD be reserved for research studies and that higher doses of vitamin D be used to attain normal serum 25-OHD. It should be noted that the vitamin D use was D_2, whereas the 25-OHD was 25-OHD$_3$.

Since 25-OHD$_3$ would not mimic the effect of vitamin D_2, it is possible that the response to increased vitamin D seen in premature infants is not the same as that in normal children and adults or adult animals. Infant rats have initially entirely a non-vitamin D-dependent calcium absorption (a passive absorption), and then at weaning they develop a vitamin D-mediated active calcium absorption in the duodenum (the ileum remains primarily passive). Eventually the passive absorption decreases, but for a period of weeks calcium absorption is a combination of active and passive transport with active transport more important at low calcium concentrations and passive transport more important at higher calcium concentrations. The development of an active calcium absorption responsive to $1,25(OH)_2D$ depends on the development of a critical number of $1,25(OH)_2D$ receptors in the duodenum.

When the human infant develops adequate numbers of $1,25(OH)_2D$ receptors in the intestine is unclear. Senterre (70) found increased calcium absorption in infants given .5 μg of $1,25(OH)_2D$ at 2–4 weeks of age; however, the levels of serum $1,25(OH)_2D$ reached are unknown. Seino (101) used 1α vitamin D with good clinical success; however, $1,25(OH)_2D$ values were near 200 pg/ml. We have shown elevated serum $1,25(OH)_2D$ levels in premature infants fed standard formula plus 400 or 800 IU vitamin D (102) (Fig. 3-12), and Markstad has shown this in breast-fed infants (103). Premature infants with rickets have even higher

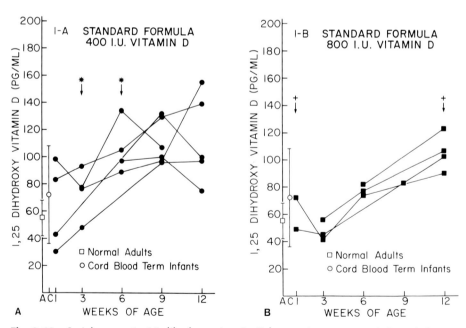

Fig. 3-12 Serial serum 1, 25-dihydroxyvitamin D by age in premature infants fed standard formula (Similac 20 caloried) plus a supplement of (A) 400 IU vitamin D or (B) 800 IU vitamin D (98).

serum 1,25(OH)$_2$D concentrations (104). Chesney noted a response to exogenous 1,25(OH)$_2$D in a premature infant whose endogenous serum 1,25(OH)$_2$D was already >150 pg/ml (105). These data suggest that 1,25(OH)$_2$D receptors may be present in amounts adequate to respond to pharmocological levels but may not have reached concentrations to respond to physiological levels or that 1,25(OH)$_2$D may have a nonreceptor effect. Studies of lower doses of 1,25(OH)$_2$D measuring both serum 1,25(OH)$_2$D levels and acute effects on calcium absorption are needed to answer the question of when the premature infant develops functional receptor numbers and a receptor-mediated active calcium transport.

If the response that we saw going from 400 to 800 IU D or that was seen by Salle comparing no supplementation with 1,000 IU D represents classical vitamin D-responsive active calcium transport, it makes sense that it was seen in feeding regimens with low mineral intakes (standard formula or breast milk) (11, 70). One might predict that vitamin D would be less important for calcium absorption if mineral intakes were increased to levels where passive absorption would predominate. Vitamin D is also felt to play a role in renal reabsorption of calcium and may be important in the mineralization process itself. We thus studied whether increasing either vitamin D or giving 25-OHD$_3$ in infants fed high-mineral formula would alter urine calcium losses or normalize bone mineral content prior to post-conceptional term.

Doses of 400 IU D$_2$, 800 IU D$_2$, and 2 μg 25-OHD$_3$ were again compared using premature formula (900 mg/L calcium, 450 mg/L phosphorus). No differences were seen among groups. The urine calcium losses persisted, and BMC did not significantly increase until after 6 weeks of age (see Table 3-7). Thus, when large mineral intakes are given, it is difficult to show an additional vitamin D effect. Doses of 400 IU D$_2$ and even 25-OHD$_3$ performed as well as 800 IU D$_2$. It must be noted that all these supplements resulted in normal or elevated levels of 25-OHD and 1,25(OH)$_2$D. There is a case report of one infant given high-mineral formula but only 100 IU D$_2$ who developed vitamin D deficiency rickets (106), and premature infants given cow's milk but no vitamin D occasionally developed rickets in the studies of VonSydow (107). Lack of an effect on urine excretion or bone mineralization again raises the question of developmental factors.

Developmental Factors

In all studies the effects of gestational age are clear. The smaller and younger the infant, the more likely that the infant will develop significant bone problems. The mean gestation of the nine infants we reported with combination vitamin D and

Table 3-7 BMC of Humerus (g/cm) by Postnatal Age (weeks)

Supplement	(N)	2W	4W	6W	9W	12W
400 IU D$_2$	(23)	.09 ± 0.2	.10 ± .02	.12 ± .03	.17 ± .03*	.14 ± .02
800 IU D$_2$	(18)	.09 ± .01	.11 ± .03	.10 ± .02	.13 ± .03*	.17 ± .03
2 μg 25-OHD$_3$	(7)	.08 ± .02	.10 ± .03	.13 ± .04	.18 ± .03*	.19 ± .03

Source: Day et al (108)

phosphorus deficiency rickets was 28 weeks and birth weight 1,000 g (66). The infants developing significant phosphorus deficiency on breast milk were all <1,100 g (74). Clearly, much of this relates to the huge mineral demands of this gestation and the difficulties consistently providing the necessary mineral intakes over a long period of time (about 8–10 weeks, to 2,000 g). However, there appear to be gestationally timed factors that further complicate the situation.

Breakdown by birth weight of the large group of infants studied on standard formula and 400 IU D showed that serum calcium and phosphorus (but not magnesium) and mineralization were lower and alkaline phosphatase higher as one went lower in gestation (Fig. 3-13) (23). However, in all groups improvement occurred without any changes in feeding regimen when postconceptional term (12-week postnatal age for the 28-week infants) was reached (23). Prior to 12 weeks, serum calcium, phosphorus, and alkaline phosphatase could be correlated with vitamin D intake but not serum 25-OHD. At 12 weeks serum calcium and phosphorus were *directly* and alkaline phosphatase *inversely* correlated with serum 25-OHD, suggesting a change to a more classical vitamin D responsiveness (23). Although serum minerals were normalized and bone mineralization improved significantly with either high-mineral formula or higher-dose vitamin D, a similar, gestationally timed delay in the normalization of bone mineralization was still apparent by either radiographic evaluation or photonabsorptiometry (11, 108).

In the low-mineral feeding regimens, we would postulate that much of the improvement in serum calcium and phosphorus seen with reaching term gestation was improved calcium and phosphorus absorption, possibly related to the same type of $1,25(OH)_2D$ receptor number maturation described in the rat, rabbit, and chick (109–111). Clearly an active transport mechanism would be more apparent at low calcium concentrations. Much of the improvement in bone might be expected from the normalization of serum minerals.

Explanation of the data on higher mineral intakes may involve more than maturation of an active transport intestinal absorption. The persistence of renal losses in the face of bones that are not fully mineralized suggests possible developmental factors at the level of either the bone or the kidney. Primary developmental delays in bone mineralization seem unlikely, since mineralization proceeds normally *in utero*. Both PTH and calcitonin levels remain such as to promote mineralization (42). Bone cells with $1,25(OH)_2D$ receptors have been shown to contain receptors very early in gestation (indeed, their main functions may be in early differentiation). More likely are developmental changes in the kidney. $1,25(OH)_2D$ receptors certainly exist in the kidney and may be important in renal conservation of urine calcium.

If receptor numbers are developmentally decreased in the intestine, until term, a similar pattern could exist in the kidney. However, even more important for calcium retention may be PTH. In term infants the renal response to PTH develops within a few days of birth (112). Data in premature infants looking at cyclic AMP responses to PTH suggest that PTH responsiveness develops at a later postnatal age than in term infants. Again, this may be a development of efficiency or number of PTH receptors (112–114). Finally, calcitonin can increase urinary calcium excretion and also produce an aminoaciduria (116). We have shown that calcitonin remains high in premature infants, even on standard mineral intakes (42). Since

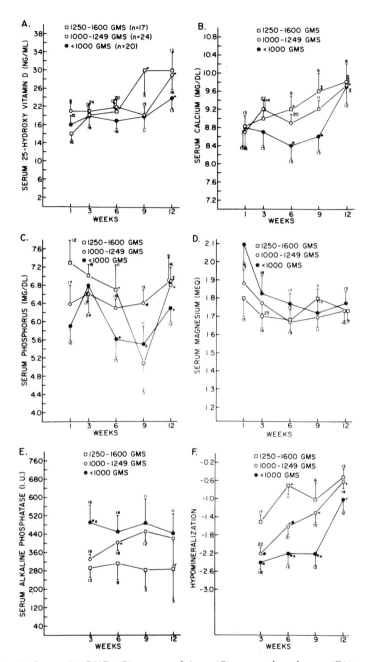

Fig. 3-13 (A) Serum 25-OHD, (B) serum calcium, (C) serum phosphorus, (D) serum magnesium, (E) serum alkaline phosphatase, and (F) hypomineralization by age in infants of birth weight 1,250–1,600 g (□), 1,000–1,249 g (○), and <1,000 g (●). *1,000 g different from 1,260–1,600 gm; #1,000–1,249 different from 1,250–1,600 g; △1,000 g different from 1,000–1,249; †different from initial values; ‡different from start of increase or decrease. One symbol: $p < .05$, two symbols: $p < .01$ (22).

calcium is the major stimulus to calcitonin production, it is possible that high-mineral formula may increase this further.

Since (a) mineral intakes, (b) vitamin D metabolites, and (c) developmental effects may all have primary effects on calcium absorption, it is important to be able to assess "percent true calcium absorption." This is now possible using stable isotopes of calcium. We have recently published a method employing [46]Ca as an intravenous isotope and [44]Ca as an oral isotope which uses primarily 24-hour urine collection to ascertain the percent true calcium absorption (115). We hope to apply this technique to examine such questions.

It should be cautioned that the previous discussion primarily applies to calcium. The mechanisms for phosphorus absorption and reabsorption appear near maximal at all gestations, and the effects of vitamin D may therefore be small. The major variable is phosphorus intake which is frequently compounded by phosphorus loss secondary to elevations in PTH secondary to problems with calcium metabolism. As a result, we are seeing increasing reports of long-term problems with mineralization in situations where phosphorus deficiency is the major problem. Simple techniques to assess the effects of multiple factors on phosphorus absorption have not been reported.

Complications of Newborn Intensive Care

Providing adequate nutrition for normal growth and bone development often becomes exceedingly difficult in the context of modern newborn intensive care because of the complexities of the disease processes and their treatment. By far the largest problem is that of chronic lung disease (bronchopulmonary dysplasia). The disease is characterized by a long-term dependence on oxygen and, frequently, mechanical ventilation. Just the logistics of providing oxygen and mechanical ventilation make providing adequate volumes of enteral feedings difficult. Many neonatologists are hesitant to feed intubated infants enternally because of the risk of chronic aspirations. Gastrointestinal reflux and decreased gastric emptying are common in these infants. The frequent presence of cor pulmonale in these infants makes fluid restriction necessary. Limitation of intake limits both calories and mineral intake. Neonatologists frequently use very concentrated formula to attain calories, 27 or 30 calories per ounce of formula, but many are hesitant to concentrate the high-mineral premature formula to that degree because of concerns of increased osmolarity.

Limitation of fluids is often not adequate to treat cor pulmonale, and diuretics are often used. The diuretic in most common use is Lasix, which causes significant urine losses and has been reported associated with nephrocalcinosis and renal stones (117–119). Studies of the use of the calcium-sparing diuretics, chlorothiazides, are just beginning in humans. We have used these drugs as first-line diuretics in BPD for many years; however, most severely affected infants will eventually also require the use of Lasix.

The severe derangements of acid–base balance in these infants (respiratory acidosis with compensating metabolic alkalosis) may also interfere with bone mineralization. Severe acidosis may even interfere with production of 1, 25 $(OH)_2D$ in the infant kidney.

Unfortunately, this results in a vicious cycle, since bone demineralization and rib fractures, plus the myopathy produced by vitamin D or phosphate deficiency, markedly reduce chest wall strength. The severely reduced lung compliance of these infants makes the need for a strong respiratory effort even greater. Failure to sustain adequate chest wall excursion results in additional atelectasis and infection. One essentially adds "rachitic lung disease" to the underlying BPD, all of which makes correction of bone mineralization and mineral homeostasis even more difficult. A close look at all of the reports of rickets in premature infants will reveal a high percentage with what would now be called BPD (120–124). A French review described a triad of liver disease, lung disease, and bone disease in many premature infants (125).

Intestinal tract problems in infants clearly limit enteral intake and thus minerals. The function of the gastrointestinal tract in extremely premature may be limited just by their extreme prematurity through a combination of volume limits, vagal predominance, and absence of lactose. Many of these infants require the use of a nonlactose, often elemental, formula to achieve enteral feedings. The problems associated with the long-term use of soy protein-based formula in premature infants has been discussed (66–69). Other nonlactose cow's milk protein hydrolysis formulas are also associated with a higher risk of bone problems. These formulas have the same mineral content as standard formula; however, it is assumed from the increased problems that absorption or retention is decreased. The reasons for this are unclear. Lactose is important for calcium absorption in animal studies; and Zeigler et al. (126) have shown that it aids calcium absorption in the human infant. Further studies of these formulas and possibly the development of a higher-mineral nonlactose formula is needed.

Neonatologists are necessarily cautious in instituting enteral feeding because of the inherent gastrointestinal limitations and also because of fear of the most common gastrointestinal complication, necrotizing enterocolitis (NEC). The etiology of NEC is unclear, with leading theories involving vascular insult to the intestine or an infectious etiology. NEC is rarely seen in the absence of enteral feeding; however, the role of feeding in the pathogenesis of NEC is unclear. NEC has been reported on any feeding regimen and occurs anywhere from the first few days to 4–6 weeks of age. Although the incidence of NEC increases with decreasing gestation, it can be seen in any size premature and even term infants. Many neonatologists delay enteral feedings in smaller premature infants in an attempt to avoid NEC. Since to avoid NEC completely would involve limiting feedings to a large number of infants for a long period of time, we have elected cautious enteral feeding, immediately stopping feeding at the first suggestion of NEC. Once a diagnosis of NEC is made, this usually means the withholding of enteral feeding for 1 or 2 weeks and in many centers the immediate institution of total parenteral nutrition. Neonatal sepsis presents with many of the gastrointestinal symptoms of NEC and also results in withholding of feedings.

Failure secondary to a patent ductus arteriosus (PDA) also leads to poor gastrointestinal function and the need to limit fluid intake and use diuretics for cardiac function. In most centers a significant PDA is closed either medically, with indomethacin, which itself may compromise intestinal blood flow, or surgically. However, the time involved in diagnosis and therapy certainly imposes an additional period of decreased mineral intake. The presence of a PDA is often one of the factors that lead to the chronic lung disease (BPD) already discussed.

With all of the above limitations, complications, or concerns, many premature infants either begin nutrient intake by the parenteral route, total parenteral nutrition (TPN), or end up receiving TPN for a portion of their neonatal course. Among the complications of TPN, the two major problems are liver disease and bone mineralization problems. The liver disease is a cholestatic jaundice, which, at least in children and adults, does not appear to alter 25-hydroxylation of vitamin D significantly (127). Its effect on serum 25-OHD in the premature infant has not been studied.

The bone disease seen with TPN both in the adult and in the infant is a multifactoral problem that remains poorly understood. However, the problem in the premature or term infant may well be somewhat different from that seen in adults. The major problem until recently has been the inability to add enough calcium and phosphorus to the solution without causing precipitation. Early on, problems of phosphorus deficiency were described, and many places have decreased calcium content to accommodate increased phosphorus content. Decreasing calcium may increase PTH and result in increased renal phosphorus losses and decreased serum phosphorus. A method of increasing both the calcium and phosphorus content of TPN solutions has recently been described (128) and has been tested in term infants (129). However, much additional work is needed to establish the appropriate amounts of calcium and phosphorus and the ratio of the one to the other. In addition to the problems of mineral intake are problems of mineral losses. Urinary excretion of both calcium and phosphorus is very high in premature infants on TPN. Whether this is the effect of a higher protein or amino acid load (82, 83), the described calcium–phosphorus imbalance, or immaturity of the premature kidney is unclear. Urine losses of trace elements are also large and may affect bone mineralization. Different TPN solutions deliver different acid loads, and systemic acidosis can occasionally interfere with mineralization as discussed. Clearly there appears to be room for improvement in most TPN solutions; however, limitation of the duration of TPN and introduction of adequate enteral mineral intakes need to continue to be stressed. A frequently seen combination in infants who develop bone disease is weaning from TPN to unfortified breast milk, compounding phosphorus deficiency.

This is just a partial list of the complications of prematurity and modern neonatal care. Providing adequate minerals and vitamin D to prevent rickets, fractures, or severe demineralization long enough for development of normal mineral homeostatic mechanism to result in normal mineralization is clearly easier said than done. However, continued concern for problems of bone mineralization and a concerted attempt to maximize mineral intake and vitamin D intake whenever possible will significantly decrease the incidence of bone mineralization problems. One nursery has reported bone problems in one of five infants (130). In our nursery cases of radiographic rickets or severe demineralization with fractures are rare, possibly due to a concerted effort to reduce the use of TPN, unfortified breast milk, and (calcium-losing) diuretics.

REFERENCES

1. Pitkin R. (1975) Am J Obstet Gynecol 121 (5):724.
2. Ziegler E. E., O'Donnell A. M., Nelson S. E., Fomon S. J. (1976) Growth 40:329.
3. Forbes G. B. (1976) Pediatrics 57:976.
4. Shaw J. C. L. (1973) Pediatr Clin North Am 20:333.
5. Greer F. R., Tsang R. C. (1985) In: Tsang R. C. (ed) *Vitamin and Mineral Requirements in Preterm Infants*. New York: Marcel Dekker.
6. Moore E. S., Langman C. B., Favus M. J., Coe F. L. (1985) Ped Res 19:566.
7. Ross R., Care A. D., Robinson J. S., Pickard D. W., Weatherley A. J. (1980) J. Endocrinol 87:17.
8. Rodda C. P., Kubota M., Heath J. A., Ebeling P. R., Moseley J. M., Care A. D., Caple I. W., Martin T. J. (1988) J Endocr 117:261.
9. Haddad J. G. Jr., Boisseau V., Avioli L. (1971) J Lab Clin Med 77:908.
10. Hollis B. W., Pittard W. B. (1984) J Clin Endo Metab 59:652.
11. Hillman L. S., Hollis B., Salmons S., Martin L., Slatopolsky E., McAlister W., Haddad J. (1985) J Pediatr 106:981.
12. Hillman L. S., Haddad J. G. (1974) J Pediatr 84:742.
13. Haddad J. G. Hillman L., Rojanasathit S. (1976) J Clin Endocrinol Metab 43:86.
14. Hillman L., Haddad J. G. (1983) J Clin Endocrinol Metab 56:189.
15. Hillman L. S., Haddad J. G. (1976) Am J Obstet Gynecol 125:196.
16. Birkbeck J. A., Scott H. F. (1980) Arch Dis Child 55:691.
17. Rothberg A. D., Pettifor J. M., Cohen D. F., Sonnendecker E. W. W., Ross F. P. (1982) J Pediatr 101:500.
18. Ala-Houhala M. (1985) J Ped Gastro Nutr 4:220.
19. Markestad T. (1983) Acta Pediatr Scand 72:817.
20. Watney P. J. M., Chance G. W., Scott P., Thompson J. M. (1971) Br Med J 2:432.
21. Hollis B. W., Jacob A. I., Sallman A., Santiz Z., Lambert P. W. (1982) In: Norman A. W., Schaefer K., Herroth D. V., Grigoleit H. G. (eds) *Vitamin D. Chemical, Biochemical and Clinical Endocrinology of Calcium Metabolism*. New York: Walter de Gruyter, p 1157.
22. Hillman L. S., Haddad J. G. (1975) J Pediatr 86:928.
23. Hillman L. S., Hoff N., Salmons S., Martin L., McAlister W., Haddad J. (1985) J Pediatr 106:970.
24. Cockburn F., Belton N., Purvis R., Giles M., Brown J., Turner T., Wilkinson E., Forfar J., Barrie W., McKay G., Pocock S. (1980) Br Med J 2:11.
25. Brooke O. G., Brown I. R. F., Bone C. D. M., Carter N. D. Cleeve H. J. W., Maxwell J. D., Robinson V. P., Winder S. M. (1980) Br Med J 280:751.
26. Finola G. C., Trump R. A., Grimson M. (1937) Am J Obstet Gynecol 34:955.
27. Krishnamachari K. A. V. R., Iyengar L. (1975) Am J Clin Nutr 28:482.
28. Raman L., Rajalakshmi K., Krishnamachari K. A. V. R., Sastry J. G. (1978) Am J Clin Nutr 31:466.
29. Markestad T., Aksnes L., Ulstein M., Aarskog D. (1984) Am J Clin Nutr 40:1057.
30. Steichen J. J., Tsang R. C., Gratton T. L., Hamstra A., DeLuca H. F. (1980) N Engl J Med 302:315.
31. Weisman Y., Harell A., Edelstein S., David M., Spirer Z., Golander A., (1979) Nature 281:317.
32. Hillman L. S., Slatopolsky E., Haddad J. G. (1978) J Clin Endocrinol Metab 47:1073.

33. Corvol M. T., Dumontier M. F., Garabedian M., Rappaport R. (1978) Endrocinology 102:1269.

34. Delvin E. E., Glorieux F. H., Salle B. L., David L., Varenne J. P. (1982) Arch Dis Child 57:754.

35. Plourde V., Haddad P., Gascon-Barre M. (1985) Pediatr. Res. 19:1206.

36. Hillman L. S., Rojanasathit S., Slatopolsky E., Haddad J. G. (1977) Pediatr Res 11:739.

37. David L., Anast C. S. (1974) J Clin Invest 54:287.

38. Noguchi A., Eren M., Tsang R. C. (1980) J Pediatr 97:112.

39. Leroyer-Alizon E., David L., Dubois P. M. (1980) J Clin Endocrinol Metab 50:316.

40. David L., Salle B. L., Putet G., Grafmeyer D. C. (1981) Pediatr Res 15:803.

41. Schedewie H. K., Odell W. D., Fisher D. A., Krutzik S. R., Dodge M., Cousins L., Fiser W. P. (1979) Pediatr Res 13:1.

42. Hillman L. S., Hoff N., Walgate J., Haddad J. G. (1982) Calcif Tissue Int 34:470.

43. Dincsoy M. Y., Tsang R. C., Laskarzewski P., Ho M., Chen I-W., Davis N. (1982) J Pediatr 100:782.

44. Minton S. D., Steichen J. J., Tsang R. C. (1979) J Pediatr 95:1037.

45. Greer F. R., Lane J., Weiner S., Mazess R. B. (1983) Pediatr Res 17:259.

46. Linkhart T. A., Ghosh B., Baylink D., Vyhmeister N. (1984) Measurement of preterm infant humerous bone mineral content with the Norland Bone Densitometer 278A. Program American Society for Bone and Mineral Research.

47. Hillman L. S., Chow W., Salmons S., Weaver E., Erickson M., Hansen J. (1986). Submitted for publication.

48. Filer L. (ed) (1988) J Pediat 113 (Suppl).

49. Fakhraee S., Bell M., Hillman L. (1980) Pediatr Res 114:571.

50. Chiswick M. L. (1971) Br Med J 3:15.

51. Widdowson E. M., McCance R. A., Harrison G. E., Sutton A. (1963) Lancet II:1250.

52. Slater J. E. (1961) Br J Nutr 15:83.

53. Kobayashi T., Okano T., Shida S., Nakao H., Kuroda E., Kodama S., Matsuo T. (1982) In: Norman A. W., Schaefer K., Herroth D. V., Grigoleit H. G. (eds) *Vitamin D Chemical, Biochemical and Clinical Endocrinology of Calcium Metabolism*. New York: Walder de Gruyter, p. 817.

54. Jeans P. C. (1936) J Am Med Assoc 106:2066.

55. Lamberg-Allardt C., Salmenpera L., Perheentupa J., Siimes M. A. (1985) In: Norman A. W., Schaefer K., Grigoleit H. G., Herroth D. V. (eds) *Vitamin D Chemical, Biochemical and Clinical Update*. New York: Walter de Gruyter, p. 665.

56. Chan G. M., Roberts C. C., Folland D., Jackson R. (1982) Am J Clin Nutr 36:438.

57. Greer F. R., Searcy J. E., Levin R. S., Steichen J. J., Steichen-Asche P. S., Tsang R. C. (1982) J Pediatr 100:912.

58. Hollis B. W., Roos B. A., Draper H. H., Lambert P. W. (1981) J Nutr 111:1240.

59. Greer F., Hollis B., Cripps D., Tsang R. (1984) J Pediatr 105:431.

60. Brown I. R. F., Brooke O. G., Haswell D. J. (1981) Clinica Chimica Acta 111:109.

61. Harrison H. E. (1966) Am J Public Health 56:734.

62. Edidin D. V., Levitsky L. L., Schey W., Dumbovic N., Campos A. (1980) Pediatrics 65:232.

63. Bachrach S., Fisher J., Parks J. S. (1979) Pediatrics 64:871.

64. Dwyer J. T., Dietz W. H., Hass G., Suskind R. (1979) Am J Dis Child 133:134.

65. Bachrach S. (1980) Pediatrics 66:332.

66. Hoff N., Haddad J., Teitelbaum S., McAlister W., Hillman L. S. (1979) J Pediatr 94:460.

67. Kulkarni P. B., Hall R. T., Rhodes P. G., Sheehan M. B., Callenbach J. C., Germann D. G., Abramson S. J. (1980) J Pediatr 96:249.

68. Callenbach J. C., Sheehan M. B., Abramson S. J., Hall R. T. (1981) J Pediatr 98:800.

69. Kulkarni P. B., Dorand R. D., Bridger W. M., Payne J. H., Montiel D. C., Hill J. G. (1981) Southern Medical Journal 7:13.

70. Senterre J., Salle B. (1982) Acta Ped Supl 296:85.

71. Atkinson S. A., Radde I. C., Anderson G. H. (1983) J Pediatr 102:99.

72. Senterre J., Putet G., Salle B., Rigo J. (1983) J Pediatr 103:305.

73. Schanler R. J., Garza C., Smith E. O. (1985) J Pediatr 107:767.

74. Hillman L. S., Salmons S. J., Slatopolsky E., McAlister W. H. (1985) J Pediat Gastro Nutr 4:762.

75. Hillman L. S. (1979) Ross Clinical Research Conference.

76. Baltrop D., Mole R. H., Sutton A. (1977) Arch Dis Child 52:41.

77. Day G. M., Chance G. W., Radde I. C., Reilly B. J., Park E., Sheepers J. (1975) Pediatr Res 9:568.

78. Steichen J. J., Gratton T. L., Tsang R. C. (1980) J Pediatr 96:528.

79. Shenai J. P., Reynolds J. W., Babson S. G. (1980) Pediatrics 66:233.

80. Greer F. R., Steichen J. J., Tsang R. C. (1982) J Pediatr 100:951.

81. Rowe J. C., Goetz C. A., Carey D. E., Hoar E. (1987) J Pediat 110:581.

82. Margen S., Chu J. Y., Kaufman N., Calloway D. (1974) Am J Clin Nutr 27:584.

83. Bengoa J., Sitrin M., Wood R., Rosenberg I. L. (1983) Am J Clin Nutr 38:264.

84. Hillman L. S., Salmons S. J., Erickson M. M., Hansen J. W., Hillman R. E. (1985) Pediatr Res 19:232A.

85. Hillan L. S., Salmons S. J., Erickson M. M., Hansen J. W., Robson A. M., Hillman R. E., Chesney R. W. (1985) Pediatr Res 19:378A.

86. Garabedian M., N'Guyen T. M., Guillozo H., Grimberg R., Balsan S. (1981) Arch Fr Pediatr 38:857.

87. Jeans P. C., Stearns G. (1938) J Pediatr 13:730.

88. Haddad J. G. Jr., Rojanasathit S. (1976) J Clin Endocrinol Metab 42:284.

89. Stamp T. C. B. (1974) Lancet II:121.

90. Clemens T. L., Adams J. S., Hollick M. F. (1982) Calcif Tissue Int 345:549.

91. VanCreveld S., Paulssen M. M. P., Ens J. C., Mey R. A. M., Versteg P., Verstegh E. T. B. (1954) Etud Neonata 3:53.

92. Hillman L. S., Martin L., Fiore B. (1981) J Pediatr 98:311.

93. Hillman L. S., Blethen S. L. (1981) Pediatr Res 15:509A.

94. Vest M. F., Rossier R. (1961) Ann NY Acad Sci 3:183.

95. Toverud S. U., Dostal L. A. (1986) J Ped Gastro and Nutr 5:688.

96. Satoh K., Fukoka H., Sakamoto S. (1983) Program and Abstracts of Workshop, Japan, p. 40.

97. Glorieux F., Salle B. L., Delvin E. E., David L. (1981) J Pediatr 99:640.

98. Koo W., Tsang R. C., Succop et al (1989) J Pediat Gastroenterol Nutr (In press).

99. Burmeister W., Kramer D., Kirsh W. (1972) Klin Padiatr 184:190.

100. Wolfe H., Kerston B., Keston J. (1975) Klin Pediatr 187:331.

101. Seino Y., Ishii T., Shimotsuji T., Ishida M., Yabuuchi H. (1981) Arch Dis Child 56:628.

102. Hillman L. S., Salmons S., Dokoh S. (1985) Calcif Tissue Int 37:223.

103. Markestad T., Aesnes L., Finne P. H., Aarskog D. (1984) Pediatr Res 18:269.

104. Steichen J. J., Tsang R. C., Greer F. R., Ho M., Hug G. (1981) J Pediatr 99:293.
105. Chesney R. W., Hamstra A. J., DeLuca H. F. (1981) Am J Dis Child 135:34.
106. Cifuentes R. F., Kooh S. W., Radde I. C. (1980) J Pediatr 96:252.
107. VonSydow G. (1946) Acta Paediatr 33:1.
108. Hillman L. S., Erickson M. M., Salmons S. J. (1985) Pediatr Res 19:223A.
109. Halloran B. P., DeLuca H. F. (1981) J Biol Chem 256:7338.
110. Duncan W., Walsh P., Kowalski M., Haddad J. G. (1983) Calcif Tissue Int 35:692.
111. Seino Y., Yamaoiki K., Ishida M., Yabuuchi H., Ichikawa M., Ishige H., Yoshino H., Calcif Tissue Int 34:265.
112. Linarelli L. G. (1972) Pediatrics 50:14.
113. Linarelli L. G., Bobik C., Bobik J. (1973) Pediatr Res 7:329A.
114. Mallet E., Basuyau J. P., Brunelle P., Devaus A-M., Fessard C. (1978) Biol Neonate 33:304.
115. Hillman L. S., Tair E., Covell G. D., Vieira N. Yergey A. (1988) Ped Res 23:589.
116. McInnes R. R., Scriver C. R. (1980) Pediatr Res 14:218.
117. Venkataraman P., Han B., Tsang R., Daughery C. (1983) Am J Dis Child 137:1157.
118. Hufnagle K. G., Khan S. N., Penn D., et al (1982) Pediatrics 70:360.
119. Koo W. W. K., Guab Z., Tsang R. C., Laskarzewski P., Neumann V. (1986) Pediatr Res 20:74.
120. Burnard E. D., Grattan-Smith P., Picton-Warlow G., Grauaug A. (1965) Aust Pediatr J 1:12.
121. Glasgow J. F. T., Thomas P. S. (1977) Arch Dis Child 52:268.
122. Chudley A. E., Brown D. R., Holzman I. R., Ho K. S. (1980) Arch Dis Child 55:687.
123. Bosley A. R. J., Verrier-Jones E. R., Campbell M. J. (1980) Arch Dis Child 55:683.
124. Oppenheimer S. J., Snodgrass G. J. A. I. (1980) Arch Dis Child 55:945.
125. Boissiere H., Cagnat R., Poissonnier M., d'Angely S. (1964) Ann de Pediatrie 40:367.
126. Zeigler E. F., Fomon S. J. (1983) J Pediat Gastroenterol Nutr 2:288.
127. Russell R. M. (1979) Med Clin North Am 63:537.
128. Vankataraman P. S., Brissie E. O. Jr., Tsang R. C. (1983) J Pediar Gastro Nutr 2:640.
129. Koo W. W. K., Hollis B. W., Horn J., Steiner P., Tsang R. C., Steichen J. J. (1986) J Pediatr 108:478.
130. Koo W. W. K., Shermon R., Succop P., Oestrich A. E., Tsang R. C., Krug-Wisse S. K., Steichen J. (1988) J Bone Min Res 3:193.

4

Undernutrition as a Modulator of General and Bone Aging in the Rat

DIKE N. KALU AND EDWARD J. MASORO

In 1934, McCay and Crowell (1) reported their now classic finding that restricting the food intake of rats markedly increases longevity. Since then much research has been done on this phenomenon which has clearly established this increase in longevity to be due to the retardation of the aging processes by food restriction.

EVIDENCE FOR RETARDATION OF THE AGING PROCESS

That a manipulation increases longevity does not necessarily mean it has retarded the aging processes. An analysis of possible survival characteristics will make this evident. Survival curves are a good tool for this analysis, and Kirkwood and Holliday (2) have presented survival curves for four hypothetical populations (Fig. 4-1). The vertical axis represents the percent of the population born in a segment of time (e.g., in the year of 1900) that is alive at the ages indicated on the horizontal axis. Curve a is an exponential decay curve in which mortality rate is not influenced by age; that is, the number of deaths per unit time per unit of population does not change with age. Exponential decay curves do not describe the survival characteristics of any known animal population. Curve b, which is similar to curve a but shifted to the right, describes the survival of small mammals living in the wild. In the case of curve b, aging has a small effect on the rate of mortality, but the hazards of the environment (e.g., predators, infectious agents), not aging, are the predominant forces responsible for death. With increasing protection from environmental hazards, the shape of the survival curve becomes progressively more rectangular in appearance (e.g., curves c and d) which gerontologists term the rectangularization of the survival curve. In the case of highly protected populations with mortality characteristics described by rectangular survival curves such as curve d, aging is a major factor underlying death. In addition to the survival curve, the following terms in regard to longevity should be defined: life expectancy, median length of life, and life-span of the species. Life expectancy is defined as the average length of life projected for individuals of a given age. It is usually projected from birth but can be and often is estimated for individuals

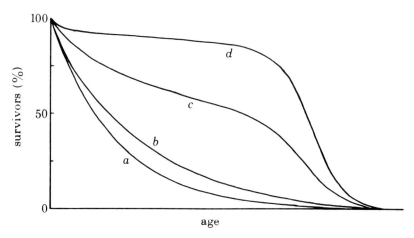

Fig. 4-1 Survival curve for four hypothetical populations. [From Kirkwood and Holliday (2).]

of any given age. The median length of life of a population is the age at which 50 percent of a population born at a given time have died. The life-span of the species refers to the length of life of the longest-lived members of the species (e.g., the 0.1 percentile survivors). Of course, to estimate the life-span of a species accurately requires that the size of the population assessed be large.

In our analysis of survival characteristics, it is instructive to discuss the changes in longevity that have occurred in the human population of the United States during the twentieth century. In 1900, life expectancy from birth was 47 years, the median length of life 58 years, and the human life-span was projected as approximately 100 years. The projections for 1940 were a life expectancy of 63 years, a median length of life of 67 years, and a life-span of approximately 100 years. The projections for 1980 were a life expectancy of 73 years, a median length of life of 78 years, and a life-span of approximately 100 years. The technological and medical advances of the twentieth century have markedly increased longevity by protecting the population from environmental hazards; that is, the survival curve has been rectangularized. These advances, however, do not appear to have influenced the aging process per se, since there has been little or no change in the human life-span (this is an example of an increase in longevity not being due to retarding the aging process).

The effects of food restriction on the survival characteristics of rats are illustrated in Fig. 4-2 from a publication of Yu et al. (3) in which a study of highly protected, barrier-maintained rats was reported. Food restriction did not rectangularize the survival curve but rather shifted the entire curve to the right, resulting in marked increase in life expectancy, median length of life, and species life-span. It is the marked increase in life-span that provides strong evidence that food restriction retards the aging processes.

Food restriction also retards most, but not all, age changes in the physiologic systems of rats (4). Examples of this action include retardation of the age-related increase in plasma cholesterol levels (5); modulation of the age-related loss in

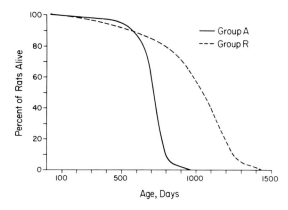

Fig. 4-2 Survival curves for male Fisher 344 rats. Group A refers to *ad libitum*-fed rats, and Group R. refers to rats fed 60 percent of the *ad libitum* intake from 6 weeks of age on. Each curve was generated from 115 rats. [From Yu et al. (3). With permission.]

response of adipocytes to insulin (6), catecholamines (7), and glucagon (8); slowing the loss of dopamine receptors in the corpus striatum (9); and delay of reproductive senescence (10). It also influences age changes in bone and in the hormones that regulate bone metabolism, and these will be discussed in depth in the sections on bone and calcium metabolism. In addition, food restriction slows the progression of and/or delays the appearance of most age-related disease processes. Indeed, so striking are its effects on age-related disease that it is important and valuable to describe some of our recent findings in this area in depth before turning to possible mechanisms by which food restriction retards the aging processes. However, it should be noted that although the retardation of age-related physiologic change and age-related disease processes is consistent with an action of food restriction on the aging processes, they do not provide as strong evidence for such an action as does the extension of species life-span.

AGE-RELATED DISEASE

Many studies (3,11–17) have shown that food restriction slows the progression or delays the occurrence or both of a broad spectrum of age-related diseases of rats. A presentation of the highlights from a recent paper from our laboratory (18) will provide the reader with an appreciation of the magnitude of this effect of food restriction. In that work, the following five dietary groups were studied: Group 1 was fed *ad libitum* a semisynthetic diet (caloric composition: 21% protein, 57% carbohydrate, and 22% fat); Group 2 was fed a similar diet but restricted to 60 percent of the intake of Group 1 rats from 6 weeks of age on; Group 3 was fed a similar diet and restricted like Group 2 rats but from 6 weeks to 6 months of age only; Group 4 was fed a similar diet and restricted to 60 percent of the intake of Group 1 rats from 6 months of age on; Group 5 was fed *ad libitum* a different semisynthetic diet (caloric composition: 12.67% protein, 65.4% carbohydrate, and 22% fat). The caloric intake of the rats in Group 1 and Group 5 was similar, and the protein intake of Groups 2 and 5 was similar.

Chronic nephropathy is a major age-related disease in rats. The severity of lesions was graded as follows: Grade 0, no lesions; Grade 1, lesions of minimal severity; Grade 2, lesions of mild severity; Grade 3, lesions of moderate severity; Grade 4, very severe lesions; Grade E (or 5), end-stage lesions. Rats with Grade 1, 2, or 3 lesions had normal serum creatinine and urea N levels, and rats with Grade 4 lesions had somewhat elevated serum levels of these compounds. However, rats with Grade E lesions not only had markedly elevated serum creatinine and urea N levels but in most cases also had osteodystrophy, metastatic calcification, and parathyroid gland hyperplasia. The effects of age and diet on the progression of chronic nephropathy in rats sacrificed at various ages are summarized in Fig. 4-3.

In the case of the Groups 1, 3, and 5 rats, there was a marked age-related progression in the severity of chronic nephropathy, but in the case of the rats in Groups 2 and 4 there was not a statistically significant progression in the severity of the lesions with age. Further insight was obtained by analysis of the rats that died spontaneously (Table 4-1). Severe lesions were observed at death in almost none of the rats in Groups 2 and 4. Severe lesions at death were observed in almost three-fourths of the rats in Group 1, in about one-half of the rats in Group 3, and in only one-third of the rats in Group 5. Clearly, food restriction started either soon after weaning or in young adult life almost abolished the progression of chronic nephropathy, whereas food restriction limited to early life was much less effective. Lifelong protein restriction in the absence of caloric restriction did retard the development of chronic nephropathy but less effectively than lifelong food restriction.

Another commonly occurring age-related disease process in these rats is cardiomyopathy. It was graded as follows: Grade 0, no lesions; Grade 1, minimal severity lesions; Grade 2, moderate severity lesions; Grade 3, very severe lesions.

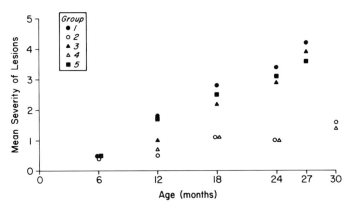

Fig. 4-3 Influence of age and diet on the severity of chronic nephropathy lesions. Group 1 refers to ad libitum-fed rats; Group 2 refers to rats fed 60 percent of the ad libitum intake from 6 weeks of age on; Group 3 refers to rats fed 60 percent of the intake of ad libitum-fed rats from 6 weeks to 6 months of age and thereafter fed ad libitum; Group 4 refers to rats fed 60 percent of the ad libitum intake from 6 months of age on; Group 5 received the protein intake of Group 2, the caloric intake of Group 1, and a somewhat greater carbohydrate intake than Group 1. Data on which illustration is based are from Maeda et al. (18), and each point refers to the findings from the analysis of the 10 rats killed from each group at the specified age.

Table 4-1 Percent of Rats Dying Spontaneously with Severe Renal Lesions

		Percent of rats with:		
Group	N	Grade 4 lesions	Grade E lesions	Grade 4 or E lesions
1	71	21	51	72
2	56	0	2	2
3	60	25	32	57
4	56	0	4	4
5	68	26	10	36

Source: Maeda et al. (18).

There was a marked age-related progression in the severity of these lesions (Fig. 4-4) in the rats of Groups 1, 3, and 5. The rats in Groups 2 and 4 did not show a statistically significant progression of the cardiomyopathic lesions. Further insight is provided by the data obtained from rats that died spontaneously (Table 4-2). These data confirm that food restriction started either soon after weaning or in young adulthood protects the rats almost completely from the occurrence of severe cardiomyopathy. They also show that protein restriction without caloric restriction is protective although less so than food restriction.

The number of tumors in the 10 rats of each dietary group sacrificed at ages 6, 12, 18, 24, 27, and 30 months is shown in Fig. 4-5. The percent of the rats dying spontaneously that had tumors is presented in Table 4-3. In all groups, rats sacrificed before 18 months of age were free of tumors. Rats in Groups 2 and 4 sacrificed at 18 and 24 months of age had significantly fewer tumors than those in Groups 1, 3, and 5. By 30 months of age the rats in Groups 2 and 4 also had many tumors. In the case of spontaneous deaths (Table 4-3), the percentage of rats that had tumors was at least as great for rats in Groups 2 and 4 as for the

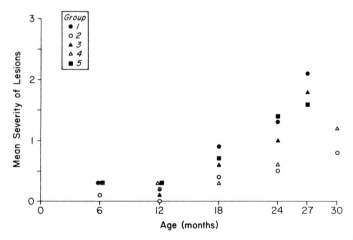

Fig. 4-4 Influence of age and diet on the severity of cardiomyopathy lesions. The dietary Groups 1, 2, 3, 4, and 5 are the same as described in Fig. 4-3. Data on which illustration is based are from Maeda et al. (18), and each point refers to the findings from the analysis of the 10 rats killed from each group at the specified age.

Table 4-2   Percent of Rats Dying Spontaneously with Severe Cardiomyopathy

Group	N	Percent of rats with Grade 3 lesions
1	71	21
2	56	0
3	60	13
4	56	2
5	68	7

Source: Maeda et al. (18).

other rat groups. The conclusion to be drawn is that food restriction started soon after weaning or in early adult life delays the occurrence of neoplastic disease but does not prevent it. Moreover, restriction of protein but not calories neither delays nor prevents the occurrence of neoplastic disease.

MECHANISMS BY WHICH FOOD RESTRICTION MODULATES AGING

The mechanisms by which food restriction retards the aging processes have been sought by many. Indeed, McCay and his colleagues executed their early studies (1, 19) in the belief that food restriction would increase longevity by slowing growth and development. The data in Table 4-4 from the study of Yu et al. (20) show that food restriction initiated in rats after most of growth and development is complete (i.e., at 6 months of age) is as effective in increasing life-span as food restriction started soon after weaning; moreover, food restriction limited to the rapid growth and development phase of life (i.e., 6 weeks to 6 months of age) did not markedly increase longevity. Such data make it unlikely that slowing growth

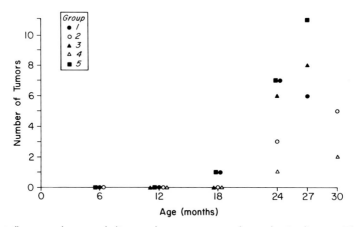

Fig. 4-5   Influence of age and diet on the occurrence of neoplastic disease. The dietary Groups 1, 2, 3, 4, and 5 are the same as described in Fig. 4-3. Data on which illustration is based are from Maeda et al. (18), and each point refers to the findings from the analysis of 10 rats killed from each group at the specified age.

Table 4-3 Neoplastic Disease in Rats That Died Spontaneously

Group	Total number examined	Percent of rats with tumors
1	71	53
2	56	68
3	60	63
4	56	68
5	68	56

Source: Maeda et al. (18).

and development plays a major role in the action of food restriction on the aging processes.

The reduction of body fat by food restriction has been proposed as the mechanism by which food restriction increases longevity (11). This view gained considerable popularity because of the widely held belief that there is a strong direct relationship between adiposity and mortality in humans (21). However, work on food restricted and *ad libitum*-fed rats by Stuchlikova et al. (24) and Bertrand et al. (23) has yielded correlative information that strongly indicates that food restriction does not act on the aging processes by reducing adiposity. A similar conclusion has been drawn by Harrison et al. (24) based on their food restriction studies with obese (ob/ob) mice and their lean littermates.

A widely held view is that food restriction retards the aging processes by decreasing the metabolic rate (25). The mechanism envisioned is that this reduction in metabolic rate decreases the rate of oxygen free-radical generation (26). However, the report of Masoro et al. (27) that food restriction does not decrease the daily caloric or other nutrient intake per gram body weight casts doubt on the validity of this metabolic rate hypothesis. Also recent work of McCarter et al. (28) showed that the metabolic rate (measured as $\dot{V}_{O_2}$) per gram body mass or per gram "metabolic mass" (i.e., body weight to the 0.67 or 0.75 power) under the usual 24-h living circumstances was not reduced by food restriction. It seems clear, therefore, that food restriction does not influence the aging process by reducing the metabolic rate.

Table 4-4 Longevity Findings

Dietary regimen[a]				Age (days)		
4–6 Weeks	6 Weeks to 6 mos	6 Months to death	N	Median length of life	Tenth percentile survivors	Death of last survivors
Ad lib[b]	*Ad lib*	*Ad lib*	40	701	822	941
Ad lib	Restricted	Restricted	40	1,057	1,226	1,295
Ad lib	Restricted[c]	*Ad lib*	40	808	918	1,040
Ad lib	*Ad lib*	Restricted	40	941	1,177	1,299

Source: Yu et al. (20).
[a]Rats were weaned at 4 weeks of age.
[b]*Ad libitum* feeding of semisynthetic diet described in Yu et al. (20)
[c]Restricting dietary intake to 60 percent of that of the *ad lib* intake.

Indeed, the findings of Masoro et al. (27) challenge the classic view that food restriction acts by reducing the intake of calories or any other nutrient per unit metabolic mass. The lean body mass of the food-restricted rats adjusts to the reduced food intake such that caloric intake as well as the intake of other nutrients is not reduced in food-restricted rats below that of the *ad libitum*-fed rats. Thus, future hypotheses of mechanism of action of food restriction must be based on total input of calories or other nutrients per rat, since the input per unit of metabolic mass is not decreased. A likely way that total input of calories or other nutrient per animal could be coupled to the aging process is by its influence on endocrine control systems or the regulation of intermediary metabolism or endocrine–metabolic interactions. Data in these areas in relation to aging and food restriction are scant and should be the subject of intensive future study.

AGING AND BONE LOSS IN RATS

While food restriction is established as an effective and reproducible technique for increasing the length of life of laboratory rodents (3, 19, 20), there is lack of complete understanding of the quality of life that accompanies the life extension. In humans a common pathology that diminishes the quality of life of aging individuals is the loss of bone that leads to osteoporosis (29), an age-related disease characterized by a decrease in bone mass below the fracture threshold. Since in rodents food restriction retards aging and maintains physiological processes near youthful levels (5–10, 30–33), it is of interest to enquire how undernutrition influences age-related changes in bone in these animals. But first, basic information on the effects of aging on the rat skeleton is in order. There has been a widespread notion that the rat skeleton is continuously growing throughout life, and there is no doubt that laboratory rats fed *ad libitum* continue to increase their body weight for a substantial part of their life-span (3). Because most early studies on rats were carried out with young growing animals, this led to the view that rat skeleton is also continuously growing. Several observations indicate that this may not be so.

For instance, Yu et al. (3) have demonstrated that in male F344 rats, increase in body weight after adulthood is due more to the deposition of fat than to an increase in lean body mass, and that at advanced age rats lose both lean body mass and adiposity. Secondly, Simpson et al. (34) observed that in rats linear bone growth increased rapidly and plateaued at about 120 days of age. Thirdly, Berg and Harmison (35) showed that in both male and female Sprague-Dawley rats linear growth of the tibia was rapid until about 170 days and then declined abruptly, and in old animals there was no longer evidence of osteogenesis in the epiphyseal growth plate, indicating that linear bone growth had stopped.

Although in every instance where rats have been studied carefully over a prolonged period, linear bone growth has been reported to slow down appreciably and eventually stop at advanced age, there is lack of agreement on the timing of the stoppage. This is due to several factors: (1) most of the studies have used animals of different strains and sexes, thereby precluding a rigorous comparison; (2) different diets were employed, and it is known that both the quality and quantity of food intake affect general body and skeletal growth; (3) in most cases the time intervals in which bone measurements were made were not short enough to determine precisely when stoppage of linear bone growth occurred; and (4) all the studies were cross-sectional and, therefore, subject to the problems of unintentional selection of animals as they age. Nevertheless, most of the available data indicate that linear bone growth plateaus at a time beyond which rats are still getting heavier (Fig. 4-6).

The data on age-related changes in bone mass in rats are even more sketchy than the information on linear bone growth. This is unfortunate, because the definition of osteoporosis is based on the size of bone mass. Weiss et al. (36) reported that in male and female Holtzman rats bone calcium content, an index of bone mass, increased quite rapidly and peaked by 7 weeks of age with little change thereafter. Since the age of the oldest rats in this study was only indicated as 104+ weeks and there was no information on the maximum length of life of the Holtzman rats studied, it is not possible to say whether these rats lose bone mass at advanced age. However, there may be strain differences in the pattern of change in bone mass with age in rats.

In contrast to the findings of Weiss et al. (36), in an ongoing study of female Wistar rats, we observed that by 18 months of age neither the length, the wet weight, the volume, the dry weight, nor the dry defatted weight of the femur had reached a plateau level. The information currently available supports the view that, following maturity, rats do not experience a progressive age-related loss of bone mass analogous to the skeletal loss that starts in humans in the fourth and fifth decades of life. However, as will be discussed later and indicated on Fig. 4-6, at very advanced age rats may suffer from terminal bone loss that may be analogous to human senile osteopenia (37). Also it appears that in rats as in humans the onset and magnitude of age-related bone loss is determined in part by whether the bone in question is cortical or cancellous. We observed recently that in female Wistar rats, 1 to 18 months old, the cortical bone area of the tibial diaphysis at the lower trochanter ridge increased with age and peaked at 6 months with no further change thereafter. In contrast, the percentage of cancellous bone

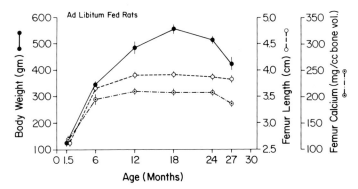

Fig. 4-6 Relationship of body weight, femur length, and femur calcium to aging in male F344 rats. Each point is mean of data from seven to 10 animals, and the vertical bars are standard errors.

area per sq mm of tissue area in the proximal metaphysis peaked at 3 months but declined progressively thereafter (38).

CALCIUM MALNUTRITION AND BONE IN RATS

Most of the information on the modulation of rat skeleton by undernutrition relates to the effects of general malnutrition or the effects of the deficiency of specific nutrients. The most studied of these nutrients are calcium and proteins.

Before we examine the effect of prolonged ingestion of suboptimal amounts of dietary calcium on the rat skeleton, it is necessary to inquire what the optimum level of dietary calcium is for rats. Bell et al. (39) have evaluated the physical characteristics of the bones of albino rats maintained on diets with calcium concentrations that ranged from 0.075 to 1.390 g calcium per 100 g dry food. The weight of the rats at the beginning of the study was 60 g, and they were maintained on their respective diets for 8 weeks. With an increase in the percent of calcium in the diet, there was a progressive rise in total body calcium retention, in the weight and calcium content of the femur, and in their bending and twisting strengths. The maximum values in these skeletal indices were observed in animals maintained on a diet containing 0.36 percent calcium, and no further increase in the skeletal parameters measured was produced by diets with higher dietary calcium content.

Bell and his colleagues concluded that in rats a dietary calcium content of 0.36 percent is optimum for maximum bone quality to be achieved. A deficit of this study is the lack of definition of the $Ca:PO_4$ ratio of the diets used in view of the notion that the magnitude of the ratio may be more important than the absolute amounts of calcium and phosphate in determining the quality of bone in rats. Differences in dietary $Ca:PO_4$ ratios might explain why a study published a year earlier arrived at the opposite conclusion to that of Bell et al. Bachmann et al. (40) studied the skeleton of three groups of female albino rats fed three diets with different calcium and phosphorus concentrations but the same $Ca:PO_4$ ratios. The calcium contents of the diets were 1, 0.6, and 0.4 percent; the phosphate contents were 0.57, 0.34, and 0.23 percent; the $Ca:PO_4$ ratios were virtually the same at 1.75, 1.76, and 1.74, respectively, and the animals were maintained on these diets from weaning for 70 days. It was observed that a progressive increase in the percentage of calcium in the diet mixture well above the 0.36 percent optimum reported by Bell et al. (39) resulted in a corresponding increase in the wet weight, dry weight, ash weight, and calcium and phosphorus contents of the rat skeleton.

The calcium-deficient diets used in most early studies were deficient in other essential nutrients as well, and it was not always clear whether the resultant bone rarefaction of dietary calcium deficiency was osteoporosis or osteomalacia. These deficits were overcome by the studies of Harrison and Fraser (41), who demonstrated with the use of well-defined calcium-deficient diet and histologic assessment of the rat bones that "pure" dietary calcium deficiency produces osteoporosis in rats, whereas vitamin D deficiency and calcium deficiency lead to osteomalacia or thin bones with wide osteoid seams. Parathyroid hormone activity, determined by subjective evaluation of parathyroid gland size, was increased by calcium malnutrition and was believed to be the cause of the bone atrophy. The latter conclusion derived from the finding that the increase in bone resorption and formation observed in calcium-malnourished animals did not occur when the animals were made hypoparathyroid by parathyroidectomy (42). These findings were later confirmed with microradiographic demonstration of increased bone resorption (43) and reports of increased immunoreactive plasma parathyroid hormone in calcium-malnourished rats (44). A major deficit of all these studies is that they were carried out only with young animals and for a short period, whereas dietary calcium requirements may differ according to the age and physiological state of the animal.

PROTEIN MALNUTRITION AND BONE

Although several observations indicate that protein malnutrition retards bone growth in rats, restriction of protein intake is often associated with reduced food intake, making it difficult to differentiate between their separate actions. In a study by Frandsen et al. (45), the confounding effects of reduced food intake in protein malnutrition were addressed by pair-feeding the rats. Young male rats were fed diets containing 24, 6, 3, and 0 percent casein ad libitum. Similar groups of rats were fed the 24 percent casein control diet in amounts corresponding to those ingested by each group of protein-malnourished animals. In both protein-malnourished and food-restricted rats, skeletal growth was retarded, and there was a decrease in the width of epiphyseal cartilage plate, diminished number and size of cartilage cells, and fewer and coarser bone trabeculae. When protein-malnourished animals were compared with pair-fed controls, the former were invariably more severely affected than the corresponding pair-fed controls, indicating that protein deficiency per se was a factor in the observed skeletal changes.

It is also necessary to consider whether the skeletal effects of protein malnutrition are secondary to dietary calcium deficiency due to the accompanying reduction in food intake and to determine whether age modifies the response of the skeleton to nutritional challenge. El-Maraghi et al. (46) carried out a series of studies to address these questions. Male and female rats varying in age from 3 weeks to $2^1/_2$ years were fed diets whose calcium concentrations varied from 0.11 to 0.44 percent and whose dietary protein content varied from 2 to 25 percent casein. The caloric contents of the diets were equalized by replacing (w/w) casein with starch. It was observed that at all ages a decrease in dietary protein resulted in low radiographic bone density and low bone ash weights. Improving the protein content of the diet increased bone ash when dietary calcium was adequate (0.44%) but caused a slight fall in bone ash when dietary calcium was suboptimal (0.11%). Reducing the dietary calcium reduced bone ash content more when dietary protein was high than when it was low, and low dietary calcium (0.11%) resulted in severe osteoporosis in young rats but caused insignificant changes in the bones of aged animals. These findings indicate that a complex interaction exists between dietary calcium, protein, aging, and the regulation of bone mass in rats.

UNDERNUTRITION WITHOUT MALNUTRITION AND BONE

The final type of nutrient undernutrition we shall consider involves the restriction of calories without malnourishing the animals by denying them essential nutrients. The effects of food restriction without malnutrition on bone is poorly defined, and the experimental paradigms that have been employed by different investigators vary, precluding rigorous comparisons.

Shires et al. (47) semistarved rats such that they lost 25–30 percent of their initial body weight at the end of 7-week experimental period. This semistarvation regimen decreased the rate of bone turnover as evidenced by paucity of osteoid, decrease in the number of osteoclasts, failure of bone to take up tetracycline label, and reduced urinary hydroxyproline excretion. In contrast, neither the bone weight, the percentage of ash per bone, nor the concentration of calcium and phosphorus per gram bone ash was altered by food restriction. Shires et al. (47) concluded that in rats food restriction causes osteopenia in spite of the paradoxical finding that the tibial weights of their rats were not decreased by the restricted food intake.

Saville and Lieber (48) arrived at an exactly opposite conclusion from their studies on the effects of undernutrition on skeletal mass and density. They fed two groups of weanling rats *ad libitum* or restricted them to two-thirds of the *ad libitum* food intake, and two rats were killed biweekly from each group, and the femur and humerus were removed and analyzed (48). It was observed that at any given age, the *ad libitum*-fed rats were bigger and had more body calcium than the restricted animals. However, when total body calcium was expressed as a function of body weight, the restricted rats had significantly more body calcium. Similarly, femur calcium, density, and the diaphyseal cortex of the femurs were greater in the restricted than in the control rats when considered on the basis of body weight. From these findings Saville and Lieber (48) suggested that maximal growth rate is incompatible with optimal skeletal characteristics. The main difficulty in assessing the significance of this study is the use of body weight to normalized femur characteristics. Also this study and that of Shires et al. (47) are limited by their short duration and in being carried out only during the period of rapid growth in rats.

In an earlier study of the life-prolonging action of food restriction, McCay et al. (19) examined the effects of lifelong food restriction on the skeleton and observed that the femurs of the restricted rats were very fragile, crumbled in the course of dissection, and floated in water as a result of their low density. However, the extent of McCay's food restriction was extreme. He used the "staircase" method in which the restricted animals were held at a constant weight by being starved for a period of weeks, then allowed to make a slight weight gain by being fed restricted amounts of food followed by another period of starvation until "members of the group seemed to be failing from the deficiency of calories" (19). It is clear that the fragility of the femurs must have been secondary to calcium deficiency, and general nutrient malnutrition due to the extreme nature of the food restriction. McCay et al. (19) started food restriction immediately postweaning, and it is unknown what the skeletal effects of life-prolonging food restriction would be in mature and old animals.

As a result of the uncertainties of previous studies, some years ago we started an evaluation of the effects of food restriction on the skeleton (33, 37). The study was part of a broad survey of the actions of life-prolonging food restriction, of which some of the results have been discussed earlier in this chapter. The studies on bone were designed (1) to evaluate the effects of aging and life-prolonging food restriction, without malnutrition, on rat skeleton; (2) to determine whether any changes in bone due to aging and food restriction are associated with alterations in the plasma levels of the hormones that regulate calcium and skeletal metabolism, parathyroid hormone, and calcitonin; (3) to assess whether the effects of food restriction on bone and the calcium-regulating hormones are due to the reduced protein intake or to restricting food intake only during the period of rapid growth; and (4) to determine whether food restriction started after the attainment of adulthood is as effective as lifelong food restriction.

To address these questions five groups of F344 male rats were studied from 6 weeks of age and on. Since the details of the experimental design have been presented earlier, only the salient features will be reiterated to enhance an understanding of the skeletal studies. Group 1 rats were fed *ad libitum* throughout life. Group 2 rats were fed 60 percent of the mean food intake of Group 1 rats for the rest of their lives. The food of Group 2 rats was similar to that of Group 1 animals but was fortified with vitamins, sodium, phosphorus, and calcium so that Groups 1 and 2 animals had similar daily intakes of these substances. Group 3 rats were food-restricted like Group 2 rats but only until 6 months of age, when they were permanently switched to *ad libitum* feeding like Group 1 animals. Group 4 rats were fed *ad libitum* until 6 months of age, and then restricted like the Group 2 animals to 60 percent of the *ad libitum* food intake until death. Group 5 rats were fed *ad libitum* a diet that contained only 60 percent of the protein content of the diet of the Group 1 animals, and the caloric content was increased by the addition of dextrin so that the caloric intake of rats in Groups 1 and 5 was similar and the protein intake of rats in Groups 2 and 5 was similar. Ten rats were killed at 6 weeks of age to serve as baseline controls.

Skeletal Changes

In all groups the rate of skeletal growth was highest from 1.5 to 6 months of age, and by 12 months the length, weight, density, and calcium content of the bones had achieved their peak levels in the Groups 1 and 5 rats fed *ad libitum* throughout life (Fig. 4-7). These levels remained stable until 24 months of age, but by 27 months Groups 1 and 5 animals had lost some bone, as indicated by a decrease in their femur weight, density, and femur calcium content when compared to the peak level achieved at 12 months of age. Food restriction had a marked effect on the skeleton. From 6 to 24 months of age, the femurs of the Group 2 rats maintained on lifelong food restrictions were significantly shorter, lighter, and less dense and contained less calcium than bones from the lifelong *ad libitum*-fed rats of corresponding ages. However, a plateau level in femur characteristics was not achieved in the Group 2 rats until much later than in the *ad libitum*-fed rats. Switching Group 4 rats at 6 months of age from *ad libitum* feeding to 60 percent food restriction arrested their bone growth, and subsequently their femur char-

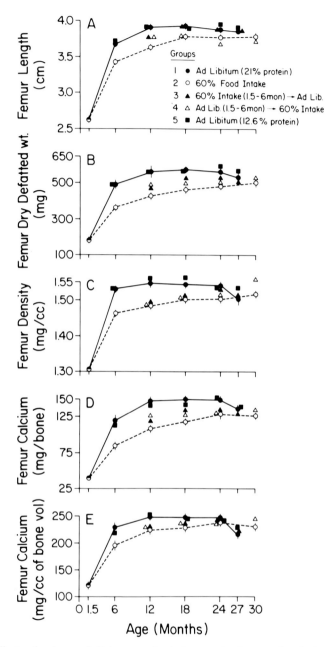

Fig. 4-7 Effects of aging and dietary manipulation on the femur of male F344 rats. Each point is mean of data from seven to 10 animals. The vertical bars are standard errors. Means for Group 2 rats are significantly lower than the corresponding means for Group 1 animals but are mostly similar to the means for Group 4 rats. Corresponding means for Groups 1 and 5 rats are similar, and the means for Group 3 rats mostly lagged behind those for Group 1 animals. [From Kalu et al. (37). With permission.]

acteristics were similar to those of the Group 2 animals. Conversely, switching Group 3 rats at 6 months of age from food restriction to *ad libitum* feeding enhanced their bone growth, and subsequently their femur characteristics approached but mostly lagged behind those of the lifelong *ad libitum*-fed rats.

In both the *ad libitum*-fed Group 1 and food-restricted Group 2 animals, the widths of the proximal epiphyseal growth plate were considerably reduced by 6 months of age and became irregular with advancing age. In the Group 1 animals aged 18 months and older, the growth plates of the tibiae had been sealed off by bone, most of the trabeculae had disappeared, and there were no longer obvious histologic signs of linear bone growth. In contrast, at 18 months of age the growth plates of the tibiae of the food-restricted Group 2 animals were still patent with cells in both the proliferative and hypertrophying zones and numerous trabeculae. In these animals the sealing off of the tibial growth plate by bone was delayed and became evident at 24 months of age.

It is striking and unexpected that the restricted animals did not suffer senile bone loss even at an older age than the *ad libitum*-fed animals. The smaller mass and lower density of the bones of the food-restricted animals cannot be due to dietary calcium deficiency, since their diet was fortified with calcium, phosphorus, and vitamins. Rather, food restriction might have decreased the rate of skeletal maturation of the rats, as is indicated by the longer time it took their bone length, weight, density, and calcium content to reach plateau levels and by the delayed sealing off of the tibial epiphyseal growth plate by bone. These findings are consistent with food restriction prolonging the life of the epiphyseal growth plates and at the same time modulating their activity such that the food-restricted rats had shorter bones than the *ad libitum*-fed controls.

The smaller mass and lower density of the bones of the animals on restricted food intake are most likely adaptive responses to the limited dietary energy and substrates made available to them, since it would be wasteful to divert a disproportionate amount of their limited resources to build a skeletal system as big and as dense as that of the *ad libitum*-fed animals, in order to support a body mass about 40 percent lighter. According to this view, the quality of the smaller bones of the restricted animals need not be compromised. Support for this view derives from the femur strength body weight ratios, which were significantly greater at all ages for the food-restricted animals than for the corresponding *ad libitum*-fed animals.

Parathyroid Hormone

The calcium-regulating hormones were measured to provide clues to the mechanism of the bone changes due to aging and food restriction. It was observed that serum immunoreactive parathyroid hormone increased with age (Fig. 4-8). In the lifelong *ad libitum*-fed Group 1 rats, the level increased gradually from 0.51 ± 0.12 ng/ml (mean $\pm$ SE) at 1.5 months of age to 3.23 ± 0.62 ng/ml in the 24-month-old animals, followed by a marked increase to 14.8 ± 4.65 ng/ml at 27 months of age. In the lifelong food-restricted animals (Group 2), the increase with age in serum parathyroid hormone was almost completely suppressed, the highest level being only 1.01 ± 0.08 ng/ml at 30 months of age.

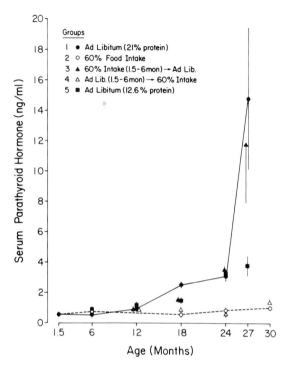

Fig. 4-8 Effects of aging and dietary manipulation on serum parathyroid hormone in male F344 rats. Each point is mean of data from seven to 10 animals, and the vertical bars are standard errors. [From Kalu et al. (37). With permission.]

Groups
1 ● Ad Libitum (21% protein)
2 ○ 60% Food Intake
3 ▲ 60% Intake (1.5-6mon) → Ad Lib.
4 △ Ad Lib. (1.5-6mon) → 60% Intake
5 ■ Ad Libitum (12.6% protein)

Serum Parathyroid Hormone (ng/ml)
Age (Months)

Starting food restriction at 6 months of age (Group 4) was as effective in suppressing the age-related increase in serum parathyroid hormone as lifelong food restriction. Switching Group 3 rats from food restriction to *ad libitum* feeding at 6 months of age caused an increase in their serum parathyroid hormone levels over those of Group 2 animals, and by 27 months their hormone levels were close to those of lifelong *ad libitum*-fed Groups 1 animals. The Group 5 animals, maintained *ad libitum* on food containing only 12.6 percent protein, showed a pattern of age-related increase in serum parathyroid hormone similar to that of Groups 1 and 3 animals up to 24 months of age, but unlike in Groups 1 and 3 rats, there was no further significant increase in their hormone levels at 27 months of age.

The reasons for the increase with age in serum parathyroid hormone are uncertain, but the increase may be secondary to age-related decrease in calcium absorption and/or progressive nephropathy, which are known to occur with aging in these rats, as discussed earlier. However, chronic nephropathy may only account for the second phase of the increase in serum parathyroid hormone, since in these rats severe renal lesions are not found at 12 and 18 months of age, when the parathyroid hormone levels had already increased two-fold and five-fold, respectively. Additional support for this view is the finding that the Group 5 rats, which had less severe renal pathology than the Groups 1 and 3 rats at advanced age, did not experience the terminal increase in parathyroid hormone levels. The plasma calcium and phosphorus levels (Figs. 4-9, 4-10) of these rats did not throw further light on the reasons for the age-related and dietary-modulated differences in circulating parathyroid hormone.

The bone loss suffered at advanced age by the Group 1 rats and to a lesser

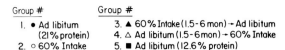

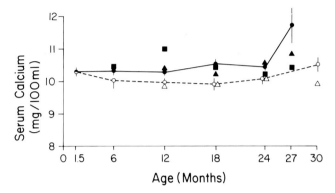

Fig. 4-9 Effects of aging and dietary manipulation on serum calcium in male F344 rats. Each point is mean of data from seven to 10 animals, and the vertical bars are standard errors. Mean values for Group 2 rats are not significantly lower than the corresponding means for Group 1 rats, except at 18 months ($p < .05$). Mean serum calcium for Group 1 rats is significantly higher at 27 than at 24 months of age ($p < .05$). [From Kalu et al. (33). With permission.]

extent by rats in Groups 3 and 5 is probably due to enhanced bone resorption secondary to augmented serum parathyroid hormone. In support of this view is the finding that in the Group 1 rats, where the bone loss was most severe and coincident with the terminal increase in parathyroid hormone, plasma calcium was significantly elevated as well. Whether the terminal bone loss in *ad libitum*-fed

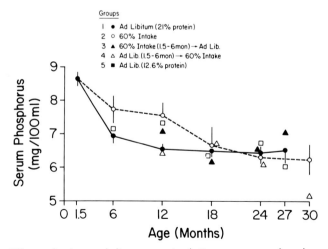

Fig. 4-10 Effects of aging and dietary manipulation on serum phosphorus in male F344 rats. Each point is mean of data from seven to 10 animals, and the vertical bars are standard errors. [From Kalu et al. (37). With permission.]

F344 male rats is analogous to the senile osteopenia that occurs late in life in humans remains to be determined. Our findings, however, indicate that moderate undernutrition without malnutrition may have beneficial effects on the skeleton by decreasing age-related hyperparathyroidism.

In a subsequent study we examined whether the salutary effects of food restriction and low protein diet on age-related chronic nephropathy and its sequalae can also be achieved by changing the protein source (49, 50). Soy protein was chosen as the alternative protein to casein, and serum parathyroid hormone (PTH) was measured with an intact N-terminal-specific radioimmunoassay (RIA) unlike in our earlier study in which we used a PTH RIA of uncertain regional specificity. From the observations made in this study we concluded that in male F344 rats, (1) an age-related increase in serum PTH precedes an age-related increase in serum creatinine concentration; (2) an age-related decline in renal function probably contributes to an age-related hyperparathyroidism which, in turn, contributes to senile bone loss; (3) food restriction inhibits age-related hyperparathyroidism and senile bone loss; (4) soy protein containing diet modulates an age-related decline in renal function and progressive hyperparathyroidism, and delays the onset but does not prevail senile bone loss. The latter findings indicate that to a great extent soy protein containing diet circumvents the confounding problem of renal disease when one uses the Fischer 344 rat as an aging model.

Calcitonin

Another calcium-regulating hormone that was evaluated in these studies is calcitonin, the hypocalcemic thyroid hormone that inhibits bone resorption. Serum calcitonin increased with age in all rats, but the increase started at a younger age and was much greater than the increase in parathyroid hormone (Fig. 4-11). In the lifelong *ad libitum*-fed Groups 1 and 5 and in the Group 3 animals switched from food restriction to *ad libitum* feeding at 6 months of age, the increase was progressive throughout life, but in Groups 2 and 4 animals the increase was markedly attenuated by food restriction. Thyroid calcitonin showed a similar pattern of age-dependent and dietary-modulated changes, and there was a high degree of positive correlation between serum calcitonin and thyroid calcitonin ($r = .917$, $p = .001$), presumptive evidence that the plasma calcitonin levels were determined, at least in part, by the size of thyroidal calcitonin pools. Since calcitonin levels are lower in young rats, our finding that food restriction-modulated age-related increase in calcitonin levels is in accord with other observations that restricting food intake maintains physiological processes toward more youthful levels in rodents (5–10, 31–34).

The mechanism by which food restriction mediates various effects is unclear, as discussed earlier. As a result of the dramatic nature of the effect of food restriction on plasma and thyroid calcitonin levels, the thyroid–plasma–calcitonin endocrine system may be a useful model for an in-depth exploration of the metabolic basis for the actions of food restriction. Such an exploration has been initiated in our laboratory with a detailed examination of the effects of life-prolonging food restriction on calcium metabolism, since plasma calcium is the physiological regulator of calcitonin secretion (51). These studies include the evaluation of total

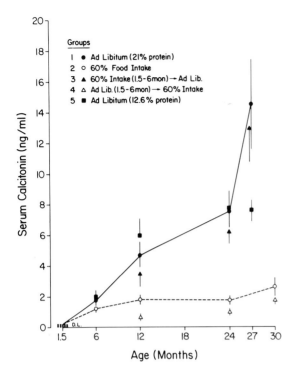

Fig. 4-11 Effects of age and dietary manipulation on serum calcitonin in male F344 rats. Each point is mean of data from seven to 10 animals, and the vertical bars are standard errors. [Adapted from Kalu et al. (33). With permission.]

and ionized blood calcium, gut transport of calcium, calcium balance, serum 1,25 $(OH)_2$ vitamin D_3, the hormonal regulation of intestinal absorption of calcium, and urinary calcium excretion.

We also evaluated the effects of food restriction on the clearance of calcitonin from plasma and on thyroidal calcitonin, calcitonin mRNA, and calcitonin-containing C cells (51). Animals were fed *ad libitum* or 60 percent of the *ad libitum* food intake from 6 weeks of age, and they were denied food for 15 h before each study. Food restriction decreased serum total calcium and calcitonin but caused no change in gut calcium transport or urinary calcium excretion. Although fecal calcium and the amount of calcium absorbed per day were less in the restricted than in the *ad libitum*-fed rats, the percentage of ingested calcium absorbed was unaltered by food restriction. Similarly, serum 1,25 $(OH)_2$ vitamin D_3 and blood ionized calcium, the physiologically active portion of plasma calcium, were not altered by food restriction, nor was the clearance of calcitonin from plasma.

In contrast, an age-related increase in thyroid calcitonin and the accumulation of calcitonin mRNA in the thyroid were suppressed by food restriction, as was the population of calcitonin-containing C cells (51). These findings suggest that the lowering of calcitonin levels by food restriction is likely to be due to a reduction in the population of calcitonin-secreting thyroidal C cells by a mechanism that appears not to be secondary to alterations in the regulation of extracellular calcium concentration. The finding of reduced thyroidal calcitonin mRNA in food-restricted rats indicates the need for additional studies to determine whether food restriction also modulates calcitonin levels by influencing the expression of the calcitonin gene.

SUMMARY

Food restriction markedly increases the life expectancy, median length of life, and life-span of rodents. In addition, it keeps the physiological systems youthful and retards or prevents the onset and progression of diseases associated with aging. The mechanisms by which food restriction mediates its effects have remained elusive. However, caloric restriction may be coupled to the aging process by its influence on endocrine control systems, the regulation of intermediary metabolism, or endocrine–metabolic interactions.

Undernutrition interacts with the calcium and skeletal systems in a complex manner that relates to the composition of the diet and the age of the animal. However, moderate undernutrition without malnutrition appears to slow down skeletal maturation without compromising the quality of bone and prevents senile bone loss, presumably by decreasing age-related hyperparathyroidism. The finding that food restriction markedly attenuates calcitonin levels makes the calcitonin endocrine system a useful model for an in-depth exploration of the metabolic basis of the action of food restriction.

Acknowledgments: Supported in part by grants AG01188 and AG07572.

REFERENCES

1. McCay, C. M., Crowell, M. F. (1934) Sci. Monthly 39:405–414.
2. Kirkwood, T. B. L., Holliday, R. (1979) Proc. Roy Soc. London B. 205:531–546.
3. Yu, B. P., Masoro, E. J., Murata, I., Lynd, F. T. Bertrand, H. A., (1982) J. Geront. 37:130–141.
4. Masoro, E. J. (1988) J. Gerontol. 43:859–864.
5. Masoro, E. J., Compton, C., Yu, B. P., Bertrand, H. (1983) J. Nutr. 113:880–892.
6. Reaven, E., Wright, D., Mondon, C. E., Solomon, R., Ho, H., Reaven, G. M. (1983) Diabetes 32:175–180.
7. Yu, B. P., Bertrand, H. A., Masoro, E. J. (1980) Metabolism 29:438–444.
8. Voss, K. H., Masoro, E. J., Anderson, W. (1982) Mech. Ageing Dev. 18:135–149.
9. Levin, P., Janda, J. K., Joseph, J. A., Ingram, D. K., Roth, G. S. (1982) Science 214:561–562.
10. Merry, B. J., Holehan, A. M. (1979) J. Reprod. Fertil. 57:253–259.
11. Berg, B. N., Simms, H. S. (1960) J. Nutr. 71:255–263.
12. Bras, G., Ross, M. H. (1964) Toxicol. Pharmacol. 6:246–262.
13. Nolen, G. A. (1972) J. Nutr. 102:1477–1493.
14. Saxton, J. A., Kimball, G. C. (1941) Arch. Path. 32:951–965.
15. Tucker, S. M., Mason, R. L., Beauchenne, R. F. (1976) J. Geront. 31:264–270.
16. Tannenbaum, A. (1945) Cancer Res. 5:616–625.
17. Ross, M. H., Bras, G. (1965) J. Nutr. 87:245–260.
18. Maeda, H., Gleiser, C. A., Masoro, E. J., Murata, I., McMahan, C. A., Yu, B. P. (1985) J. Geront. 40:671–688.
19. McCay, C., Crowell, M., Maynard, L. (1935) J. Nutr. 10:63–79.

20. Yu, B. P., Masoro, E. J., McMahan, C. A. (1985) J. Geront. 40:657–670.
21. Lew, E. A., Garfinkel, L. (1979) J. Chronic Dis. 32:563–576.
22. Stuchliková, E., Juricová-Horáková, J., Deyl, Z. (1975) Exp. Geront. 10:141–144.
23. Bertrand, H. A., Lynd, F. T., Masoro, E. J., Yu, B. P. (1980) J. Geront. 35:827–835.
24. Harrison, D. E., Archer, J. R., Astole, C. M. (1984) Proc. Natl. Acad. Sci. USA 81:1835–1838.
25. Sacher, G. A. (1977) In: Finch, C. E., Hayflick, L. (eds) *Handbook of the Biology of Aging.* New York: D. Van Nostrand pp. 582–638.
26. Harman, D. (1981) Proc. Natl. Acad. Sci. USA 78:7124–7128.
27. Masoro, E. J., Yu, B. P., Bertrand, H. A. (1982) Proc. Natl. Acad. Sci. USA 79:4239–4241.
28. McCarter, R., Masoro, E. J., Yu, B. P. (1985) Am. J. Physiol. 248:E488–E490.
29. Albright, F., Reifestein, E. C. (1948) *The Parathyroid Glands and Metabolic Bone Disease.* Baltimore: Williams and Wilkins.
30. Ross, M. H. (1969) J. Nutr. 97:565–601.
31. Cooper, B., Weinblatt, F., Gregerman, R. I. (1977) J. Clin. Invest. 59:467–474.
32. Gerbase-DeLima, M., Liu, R. K., Cheney, K. E., Mickey, R., Walford, R. L. (1975) Gerontologia 21:184–202.
33. Kalu, D. N., Cockerham, R., Yu, B. P., Roos, B. A. (1983) Endocrinology 113:2010–2016.
34. Simpson, M. E., Asling, C. W., Evans, H. M. (1950) Yale J. Biol. and Med. 23:1–27.
35. Berg, B. N., Harmison, C. R. (1957) J. Gerontol. 12:370–377.
36. Weiss, A. K., McBroom, M. J., Cornelison, Jr. R. L. (1969) J. Gerontol. 24:438–443.
37. Kalu, D. N., Hardin, R. H., Cockerham, R., Yu, B. P. (1984) Endocrinology 115:1239–1247.
38. Liu, C. C., Kalu, D. N. (1989) Bone Submitted for publication.
39. Bell, G. H., Cuthbertson, D. P., Orr, J. (1941) J. Physiol. 100:299–317.
40. Bachmann, G., Haldi, J., Wynn, W., Ensor, C. (1940) J. Nutr. 20:145–156.
41. Harrison, M., Fraser, R. (1960) J. Endocrinol. 21:197–205.
42. Harrison, M., Fraser, R (1960) J. Endrocrinol. 21:207–211.
43. Gershon-Cohen, J., Jowsey, J. (1964) Metabolism 13:221–226.
44. Rader, J. I., Baylink, D. J., Hughes, M. R., Safilian, E. F., Haussler, M. R. (1979) Am. J. Physiol. 236:E118–E122.
45. Frandsen, A. M., Nelson, M. M., Sulon, E., Becks, H., Evans, H. M. (1954) Anatomic Records 119:247–265.
46. El-Maraghi, N. R. H., Platt, B. S., Stewart, R. J. C. (1965) Br. J. Nutr. 19:491–509.
47. Shires, R., Avioli, L. V., Bergfeld, M. A., Fallon, F. D. Slatopolsky, E., Teitelbaum, S. L. (1980) Endocrinology 107:1530–1535.
48. Saville, P. D., Lieber, C. S. (1969) J. Nutr. 99:141–144.
49. Kalu, D. N., Masoro, E. J., Yu, B. P., Hardin, R. R., Hollis, B. W. (1988) Endocrinology 122:1847–1854.
50. Iwasaki, K., Gleiser, C. A., Masoro, E. J., McMahan, C. A., Seo, E.-J., Yu, B. P. (1988) J. Gerontol.: Biol. Sci. 43 (1): B5–B12.
51. Kalu, D. N., Herbert, D. C., Hardin, R. R., Yu, B. P., Kaplan, G., Jacobs, J. W. (1988) J. Gerontol.: Biol. Sci. 43(5): B125–B131.

5

Effects of Undernutrition on Skeletal Development, Maturation, and Growth

ALLEN W. ROOT

Malnutrition significantly impairs growth, skeletal development, and bone maturation. Nutritional deprivation may be generalized, such as protein–calorie malnutrition, or selective, involving a specific vitamin (e.g., vitamin A) or other dietary factors (e.g., essential amino acids) needed for growth and maturation of cartilage and bone, or suboptimal nutrition may deprive the subject of dietary components necessary for normal mineralization of cartilage (e.g., vitamin D, calcium, or phosphate). This chapter will discuss these two aspects of cartilage and bone growth and maturation and will attempt to define the mechanism(s) by which malnutrition inhibits normal bone development.

MALNUTRITION AND CARTILAGE AND BONE GROWTH AND MATURATION

Nutritional deprivation adversely affects linear growth and bone development in the growing subject (human or animal), often before the effects of undernutrition are noted upon other body systems (1). The skeletal "growth arrest line" is visual evidence of a prior period of undernutrition or of an acute or chronic illness. The cartilaginous growth plate consists of several zones which, listed from the epiphysis to the metaphysis of the long bone, are (1) zone of resting cells, (2) zone of proliferating chondrocytes, (3) zone of hypertrophic chondrocytes, (4) zone of provisional calcification, and (5) zone of capillary invasion (degenerative zone).

"Growth arrest lines" or arrest strata (1) are composed of dense, transversely or horizontally oriented, bony trabeculae (instead of the normally vertically oriented trabeculae) which appear radiographically denser than normal bone because of the superimposition of many calcified horizontal trabeculae upon each other. This area ressembles that of membrane calcification rather than of cartilaginous bone. Experimentally with (severe) nutritional deprivation the proliferative and hypertrophic zones of the epiphyseal cartilage atrophy, the degenerative zone disappears, and the ingrowth of capillaries and osteoblasts into the lowermost portions of the degenerative zone ceases, because the capillary–osteoblast complex is unable to penetrate the now quiescent proliferative zone. Consequently the osteoblasts on the undersurface of the impenetrable proliferative zone of the epiphyseal cartilage lay down bone in a horizontal manner along the undersurface of this zone, resulting in horizontal bony trabeculae. When the primary insult is removed, cartilage proliferation and normal bone formation recommence. The cartilagenous area "moves away" from the previous site of growth arrest, and the residual horizontal trabeculae are viewed radiographically as a "growth arrest line." In the human, histological examination of skeletal "growth arrest lines" reveals that calcified cartilage matrix (the terminal portions of the degenerative zone) is often incorporated into the arrest stratum. This occurs because the degree of insult causing cartilage growth arrest clinically is not usually so complete as to obliterate all of the degenerative zone prior to horizontal bony trabeculation.

The primary effect of generalized nutritional deprivation is to inhibit cartilage growth. Impairment of linear growth follows severe generalized protein–calorie malnutrition (i.e., marasmus) or primary protein deprivation (i.e., kwashiorkor). The mechanisms by which the effects of malnutrition on bone growth are mediated involve the growth hormone–somatomedin axis and possibly other skeletal and cartilage growth factors. Arrest striata develop in the hypophysectomized rat after treatment with growth hormone (GH) (1). In the human with hypopituitarism, "growth arrest lines" are visible radiographically after treatment with anabolic steroids or human GH.

The somatomedins (also termed insulinlike growth factors; IGF) are a group of peptides synthesized by the liver, kidney, cartilage, skin fibroblasts, and other cells (Table 5-1), which are under the primary control of pituitary GH. Their production is also regulated in part by insulin, thyroid hormone, prolactin, and diet (2). Somatomedins have insulinlike (anabolic) effects on protein, carbohydrate, and lipid metabolism and stimulate cartilage growth and metabolism. *In vitro* through specific receptors on chondrocytes, they enhance the incorporation of sulfate into cartilage proteoglycans, leucine, proline, and hydroxyproline into collagen and noncollagen proteins, thymidine into growth plate cartilage DNA, and uridine into RNA. *In vivo* somatomedins [particularly somatomedin C/insulinlike growth factor I (SmC/IGF-I)] promote growth in hypophysectomized rats and hypopituitary mice, stimulating increase in body weight and length and in sulfate uptake by cartilage in a manner comparable to that of GH itself (2, 3). Thus somatomedins stimulate both cell replication and differentiated cell functions (4). GH acts through systemic and locally synthesized somatomedins to stimulate anabolism, somatic cell growth and division, and bone, cartilage, and linear growth (3). The direct injection of GH into the epiphyseal cartilage of a rat's hind limb increases local somatomedin production and longitudinal growth of the GH-treated leg. It has been suggested that GH acts preferentially on prechondrocytes (stem cell or early proliferative chondrocytes) in the topmost area of the epiphyseal plate cartilage to stimulate cell division, while somatomedins enhance growth of already differentiated chondrocytes (69).

The GH–somatomedin axis is influenced by the nutritional state of the host. Although serum concentrations of GH are increased in nutritionally deprived sub-

Table 5-1   Somatomedins

Designation	Synonym	Molecular weight (daltons)
Insulinlike growth factor I	Somatomedin C	7,649
Insulinlike growth factor II	Multiplication stimulating activity Skeletal growth factor	7,471

jects (kwashiorkor, marasmus, anorexia nervosa, short-term starvation) (5–7), somatomedin levels, measured by bioassay or radioreceptor or radioimmunoassay, are decreased. Serum concentrations of somatomedin reflect the nutritional status of the host. They are low in malnourished humans and animals; in the nutritionally deprived subject, somatomedin levels cannot be increased by administration of exogenous GH (2, 8, 9). In fasted animals, bioactive somatomedin values decline to hypopituitary levels within 3 days, as does *in vitro* cartilage activity (measured by incorporation of radiolabeled sulfate), although the latter falls more slowly than do somatomedin levels (2). Upon refeeding, there is rapid increase in somatomedin levels followed shortly thereafter by increase in cartilage activity. *In vitro* perfusion of livers from rats starved for 2 days reveals significantly decreased somatomedin release, comparable to that observed from livers of hypophysectomized animals (10).

In infants with kwashiorkor (7) and marasmus (2), SmC/IGF-I concentrations are low. In human adults, acute starvation reduces plasma SmC/IGF-I within several days, and refeeding results in rapid increase in its synthesis and secretion (8). Specific dietary components, particularly protein, influence the rate of increase in plasma SmC/IGF-I concentrations after acute starvation. In experimental animals both total calories and the protein content of the diet are important in the restoration of somatomedin synthesis. Protein deficiency prevents a sustained rise in somatomedin values in starved rats even when total calorie intake is reasonable (2, 11). Clemmons et al. (12) fasted moderately obese adult volunteers for 10 days, during which period plasma SmC/IGF-I concentrations declined by 60–70 percent; the change in SmC/IGF-I values correlated with alterations in nitrogen balance. Refeeding of normal adult male volunteers starved for 5 days, in whom SmC/IGF-I levels had fallen, resulted in rebound increase in SmC/IGF-I concentrations to 68 percent of prefast values within 5 days when the diet contained 15 percent of the calories as protein. When a diet of similar isocaloric density (35.3 kcal/kg) but composed of only 5 percent protein was ingested, SmC/IGF-I values reached only 70 percent of the levels achieved by the diet of higher protein content (8).

In a similar experiment, refeeding of diets of identical caloric and nitrogen content but with supplementation of one diet with essential amino acids demonstrated that the amino acid-supplemented diet was associated with a significantly greater increase in SmC/IGF-I levels than was the nonsupplemented diet (13). These data indicate that both energy (calories) and proteins (essential amino acids) are necessary to enhance SmC/IGF-I generation (13, 14). It is likely that provision of a minimal amount of calories (11–18 kcal/kg) is necessary to spare tissue protein breakdown mandated by the basal energy needs of the body, increase SmC/IGF-I production, and enhance protein anabolism. The rise in plasma SmC/IGF-I concentrations during refeeding after starvation reflects efficient utilization of proteins. Plasma concentrations of IGF-II also decline during fasting and increase with refeeding (9), but the role of IGF-II in cartilage growth is unknown. It is probable that decreased synthesis of the somatomedins is of major pathogenetic importance in the arrest of growth and cartilage maturation observed in the nutritionally deprived state. In addition, an inhibitor of somatomedin bioactivity has been described in the serum of the starved animals, which is possibly also of hepatic origin (2, 15).

The mechanism by which acute starvation decreases somatomedin production is unknown, but a role for insulin, the secretion of which is also depressed by starvation, is suggested by the similarity between decreased somatomedin generation in starvation and in other insulin deficiency states, such as diabetes mellitus and hypopituitarism (2, 10). Insulin may provide intracellular nutrients necessary for somatomedin synthesis.

There are several other skeletal and cartilage-stimulating growth factors, some of which may be specifically or nonspecifically affected by nutritional deprivation. *In vitro* tri-iodothyronine (T_3), the most biologically active of the thyroid hormones, increases weight, protein content, cell number, cell size, and alkaline phosphatase activity of cultured (chick embryo) chondrocytes (16). Immunoneutralization of SmC/IGF-I attenuates the *in vitro* proliferative effects of T_3 on cartilage but has no effect on the differentiating and maturing effects of T_3 on chondrocyte size and alkaline phosphatase activity (4). These data suggest that T_3 has direct effects on epiphyseal cartilage maturation (increase in cartilage cell size and function) and indirect effects on chondrocyte proliferation mediated through somatomedin. T_3 induces DNA and messenger RNA coding for pituitary GH; in the absence of T_3, synthesis and secretion of GH are depressed, and somatomedin production is decreased (17, 18). There may also be a direct stimulatory effect of T_3 upon somatomedin generation by cartilage, since neutralization of SmC/IGF-I *in vitro* blocks the chondrocyte proliferative effects of T_3 as mentioned above (4).

The serum concentration of T_3 (the bulk of which is attributable to conversion of thyroxine to T_3 by the liver and kidney) is readily decreased by acute and chronic illness, trauma, surgery, and nutritional deprivation (19, 20). serum T_3 concentrations decline by 50 percent after 3 days of a complete fast in both normal and obese subjects (21). Dietary carbohydrate, but not protein, increases the synthesis of T_3 in the starved subject (22). In experimentally starved rats there is a decline in hepatic $5'$-monodeiodinase activity and consequent increase in the degradation of thyroxine to reverse T_3, a biologically inactive metabolite (19). In addition to decrease in hepatic $5'$-monodeiodinase activity, starvation also depletes intracellular cofactors necessary for enzyme activity and reduces hepatic cell uptake of thyroxine (19). In contrast to the effect of starvation on thyroxine metabolism in the liver, fasting does not affect renal uptake of thyroxine or its conversion to T_3 (23). Since insulin enhances hepatic conversion of thyroxine to T_3, it is possible that the effects of fasting on this system are in part attributable to the hypoinsulinemia of malnutrition (24). Thus, another major pathogenetic factor mediating the retarding effects of nutritional deprivation on growth, cartilage and skeletal maturation, is relative or absolute deficiency of T_3.

In addition to the recognized factors that regulate calcium homostasis such as parathyroid hormone, calcitonin, and 1,25-dihydroxy vitamin D_3, there are several other systemic, cartilaginous, and bone growth factors whose elaboration or activity might be influenced by the nutritional state of the host (25–27):

1. Systemic agents such as *epidermal, fibroblast,* and *platelet-derived growth factors*
2. Local skeletal products such as *transforming growth factor* β, derived from cultured bone explants which increases prostaglandin release and calcium mobilization (70); *bone-derived growth factor,* which stimulates bone DNA and collagen synthesis; cartilage *SmC/IGF-I; skeletal growth factor,* which is extractable from demineralized bone matrix and which links the processes of bone formation and resorption; *cartilage-derived growth factor,* which stimulates chondrocyte proliferation and may regulate linear skeletal growth; another *collagen-derived factor* with somatomedinlike activity and the ability to stimulate bone DNA, collagen, and noncollagen protein synthesis
3. Factors derived from bone matrix such as *bone morphogenetic protein,* which induces the proliferation and differentration of precursor mesenchymal cells into chondrocytes and osteoblast precursors; *cartilage-inducing factors,* possibly related to transforming growth factors; *osteonectin,* a 32,000-dalton peptide that binds collagen and inorganic bone mineral; and *osteocalcin,* a gamma carboxyglumatic acid (GLA)-containing 6,000-dalton peptide that inhibits matrix mineralization and regulates bone resorption

A *pituitary cartilage growth-promoting factor* has also been described, and there are several mononuclear cell products that also affect bone metabolism such as tumor necrosis factor (cachetin) which promotes bone resorption (71). Studies of the effects of suboptimal nutrition on these and other regulators of skeletal formation and modeling would be of interest.

The sex hormones, testosterone and estradiol, enhance cartilage growth and maturation and bone mineralization at adolescence (28). Nutritional deprivation delays the onset of sexual development by retarding maturation of pituitary gonadotropin secretion, primarily by altering the normal secretory dynamics of hypothalamic gonadotropin-releasing hormone (29, 30). However, even when malnutrition is relatively severe, pubertal development eventually ensues. Under such circumstances, sex hormones may advance epiphyseal maturation without increasing long-bone growth, resulting in epiphyseal fusion and shortening of adult stature (31).

MALNUTRITION AND MINERALIZATION OF CARTILAGE AND BONE

Normal mineralization of cartilage requires the integrated action of osteoblasts and osteocytes and a microenvironment of nutrients (primarily calcium and phosphate) that permits these cells to function optimally. Defective growth and mineralization may be due to primary abnormality of cartilage division or function (e.g., elaboration of an abnormal matrix) or to an abnormality in the concentrations of these micronutrients or the factors that ensure their availability (e.g., vitamin D and its metabolites). In the growing bone, abnormalities leading to defective mineralization result in the clinical, radiographic, and pathologic findings of rickets (28, 32) (Table 5-2).

Nutritional rickets leads to decreased linear growth and deformities of the rapidly growing cranial bones, long bones, and ribs (28). There are frontal bossing, craniotabes, a rachitic rosary at the costochondral junction, and flaring of the metaphyses of the radial, ulnar, femoral, tibial, and fibular long bones and ultimately valgus or varus deformities of the upper and lower extremities. There are often muscle weakness and hypotonia and occasionally hypocalcemic tetany and laryngeal stridor. Radiographically, there are delay in epiphyseal ossification, widening of the epiphyseal cartilage, irregular calcifications and cupping of the epiphyses, varus and valgus deformities of the legs, and thinning of the diaphyseal cortex. Other radiographic signs attributed to the bone resorption due to secondary hyperparathyroidism are also visible. Histologically, in rachitic bones there are increased numbers of mature but disorganized chondrocytes near the zone of cal-

Table 5-2   Nutritional Disorders of Bone Mineralization

  I. Deficiency of vitamin D
     A. Dietary
        1. Parenteral nutrition
        2. Prematurity
     B. Hepatobiliary disease
     C. Malabsorption syndrome
     D. Intestinal resection: bypass surgery
     E. Anticonvulsant drugs
 II. Deficiency of calcium
     A. Dietary
     B. Malabsorption
     C. Excessive loss
III. Deficiency of phosphate
     A. Dietary
        1. Very low birth weight
        2. Parenteral nutrition
        3. Excessive intake of aluminum hydroxide
     B. Decreased absorption
     C. Excessive loss
 IV. Inhibitors of mineralization
     A. Flouride
     B. Diphosphonate
  V. Miscellaneous
     A. Deficiencies
        1. Vitamin A
        2. Vitamin C
        3. Copper
     B. Excess
        1. Aluminum

cification, but the zones of resting and proliferating chondrocytes appear normal. With vitamin D deficiency there is an increase in unmineralized osteoid.

The serum concentrations of calcium and phosphate ions exceed their solubility product but are held in metastable equilibrium by inhibitors of calcification such as pyrophosphate (28). Bone formation is influenced by a variety of growth factors (26) that stimulate osteoblast differentiation, replication, and function. The osteoblasts elaborate an organic matrix upon which mineralization occurs. Mineralization may be initiated by alkaline phosphatase secreted by osteoblasts, which increases local phosphate concentrations by cleaving phosphate from organic phosphoproteins or by decreasing local levels of calcification inhibitors such as pyrophosphate. With local increase in the calcium $\times$ phosphate product and a proper matrix, deposition of hydroxyapatite (calcium phosphate) occurs. Calcium- and phosphate-containing organelles (matrix vesicles) may be present in the organic matrix and may serve as the nidus upon which mineralization takes place, perhaps influenced by the noncollagenous matrix proteins osteonectin or osteocalcin. However, the importance and even the presence of matrix vesicles have been questioned (33). The initial mineral phase in organic matrix may be simply heterodispersed particles of calcium phosphate. Once initiated, mineralization occurs rapidly at first and then more slowly. The primary mineralization phase, which accounts for 60–70 percent of the total mineral deposited in bone, is completed in 6–12 hours, whereas the secondary mineralization phase may require 1–2 months for completion (28).

DEFICIENCY OF VITAMIN D

The biological effects of vitamin D_3 are mediated through the active metabolite 1,25-dihydroxyvitamin D_3 [1,25 $(OH)_2D_3$] (32, 34). 1,25 $(OH)_2D_3$ increases intestinal absorption of calcium and phosphate and hence ambient levels of these ions. It has no direct effects on the mineralization process, although it may affect osteoblastic production of matrix osteoid. Specific nuclear receptors for 1,25 $(OH)_2D_3$ are present in osteoblasts and osteoprogenitor cells, suggesting that 1,25 $(OH)_2D_3$ may influence the composition of organic bone matrix and thus mineralization (34). 1,25 $(OH)_2D_3$ also affects bone levels of collagen, hyaluronic acid, phosphoproteins and alkaline phosphatase activity (72). This metabolite has direct effects on bone resorption, however. At high doses, 1,25 $(OH)_2D_3$ actually inhibits bone mineralization in the rachitic and intact rat (73, 74).

Brommage and DeLuca (34) have presented data that indicate that only 1,25 $(OH)_2D_3$ is necessary in the vitamin D-deficient animal to restore bone mineralization and histology to normal and that it does so indirectly by increasing intestinal absorption and serum concentrations of calcium and phosphate. Maintenance of rats on an absolute vitamin D-deficient diet and only 1,25 $(OH)_2D_3$ through two generations results in normal growth and skeletal mineralization in rapidly growing, mature, pregnant, and lactating female rats and in their suckling pups. Histologic examination of bones from these animals reveals normal longitudinal and transverse bone growth, mineralization of epiphyseal growth plate cartilage, endochondral bone formation, and endosteal and periosteal bone mineralization.

Although it has been suggested that another metabolite of vitamin D_3, 24,25 $(OH)_2D_3$, acts in the epiphysis and that 1,25 $(OH)_2D_3$ is active in the diaphysis of long bones (32), the data of Brommage and DeLuca (34) indicate that only the latter metabolite is necessary for histologically normal bone mineralization in the vitamin D-deficient rat. That the effect of 1,25 (OH_2D_3) on skeletal mineralizations is exerted indirectly by its maintenance of a normal serum calcium $\times$ phosphate product is supported by the observation that continuous infusion of calcium and phosphate into vitamin D-deficient rats to maintain normal circulating levels of calcium and phosphate results in normal bone mineralization, histologically indistinguishible from the bone morphology of vitamin D-replete animals. However, bone mineral content is increased in this animal model, evidence of a direct effect of 1,25 $(OH)_2D_3$ on bone resorption.

The majority of serum 25-OHD (the major circulating metabolite of vitamin D_3) is a product of cholecalciferol (vitamin D_3) which itself is derived from skin after conversion of 7-dehydrocholesterol by ultraviolet (sun) light and heat to this prohormone. Vitamin D_3 is then hydroxylated in the liver to form 25-OHD$_3$. It is estimated that as little as 10 min of exposure of an adequate skin surface area to sunlight each day is sufficient to generate the daily requirement of D_3 (10 µg/ day = 400 IU) of an adult or child. Dietary vitamin D_2 (ergocalciferol) is important when adequate exposure to sunlight is unavailable. This occurs in northern climes during the winter, in immobile children and adults housed indoors throughout the year, in populations where the body is shielded from sunlight by excessive clothing, and similar situations. When there is year-round exposure of the skin to adequate amounts of sunlight, dietary vitamin D_2 is of little importance in the integrity of the vitamin D–endocrine system and normal bone mineralization and growth.

However, even in year-round sunny climes such as the southern United States or the Middle East, it is possible to become vitamin D deficient. Root et al. (35) described a 13-month-old black male infant resident of Florida who presented with seizures and hypocalcemia (total calcium 5.1 mg/dl), undetectable serum concentrations of 25-OHD, and increased immunoreactive parathyroid hormone (PTH) values. Because of recurrent "allergic" upper respiratory symptoms, he had been maintained since 4 months of age indoors and on a diet of vegetables, cereals, tea, gelatin, and occasionally meat. Addition of vitamin D-fortified milk and 500 mg/day of calcium lactate to the diet and daily outdoor play resulted in rapid correction of the hypocalcemia, increase in 25-OHD concentrations, and decline in PTH levels. Interestingly this patient had no radiographic evidence of rickets, although serum alkaline phosphatase activity was elevated. It was postulated that lack of both calcium and vitamin D resulted in hypocalcemia without obvious rickets. In experimental rats rickets develops only when vitamin D deficiency is accompanied by increased intake of calcium and decreased intake of phosphate (36).

In northern climes, supplementation of the diet of children with vitamin D is essential, as the vitamin D content of unfortified foods is low. Milk and other foods are usually supplemented with sufficient vitamin D to provide adequate dietary intake. However, in premature infants, in breast-feeding infants whose mothers remain indoors and are not ingesting vitamin D-fortified foods, in children receiving parenteral nutrition, and in physically or mentally incapacitated subjects not exposed to sunlight, vitamin D deficiency may occur. Where vitamin D supplementation of milk is not practiced, as in Europe or England, rickets may occur in dark-skinned children with limited exposure to sunlight. In children ingesting anticonvulsants, which enhance the catabolism and excretion of vitamin D, additional dietary intake of vitamin D (2,000 units/day) is usually recommended (32).

Infants ingesting human breast milk without supplementary vitamin D are at risk for developing deficiency of this nutrient, because human breast milk contains only 20 IU/L of vitamin D_3 (37). It is possible to increase the vitamin D_3 content of human milk (to 130–140 IU/L) by administering orally 2,400 IU of vitamin D_3 daily to the lactating woman or by exposing her to ultraviolet light (38, 75). The dark-skinned person is less able to synthesize endogenous vitamin D_3 when exposed to ultraviolet light than the light-skinned individual (39). Therefore, the infant of the black lactating woman is at greater risk for developing hypovitaminosis D than is that of the white woman.

In 1979–80 there appeared four reports of 34 predominantly breast-fed children (30 of whom were black and four were white) with nutritional rickets and vitamin D deficiency, the majority of whom were members of religious communities who were vegeterians and who dressed in long garments through which ultraviolet sunlight was unable to penetrate (40–43). These infants had been breast-fed by mothers with marginal vitamin D intake and were weaned to diets with little vitamin D and no supplemental vitamin D. Krieger (1985) described 13 children with nutritional rickets seen at the Children's Hospital of Michigan (Detroit) over a 3-year period; all were black, none had received supplemental vitamin D, 11 had been breast-fed for prolonged periods, 11 were from lower socioeconomic strata, and in 11 the diagnosis of rickets was made between February and May, indicating lack of sunlight exposure. Thus nutritional vitamin deficiency remains a significant threat to certain populations of children (76).

Abnormal absorption of vitamin D_2 from the gastrointestinal tract because of primary enteropathies (celiac gluten-sensitive enteropathy) or hepatobiliary dysfunction may result in vitamin D deficiency. The primary factors in the pathogenesis of hepatobiliary osteodystrophy are reduced exposure to sunlight and decreased intake and malabsorption of dietary vitamin D; parental but not oral administration of vitamin D results in healing of rickets in these children (45). Hepatic hydroxylation of 25-OHD$_3$ is normal in patients with a variety of primary hepatic disorders (46). However, an element of end-organ resistance to or increased catabolism of 1,25 (OHD)$_2$D$_3$ may be present in such patients, as fourfold larger doses of 1,25 (OH)$_2$D$_3$ are required for healing of the rickets associated with biliary obstruction than that due to nutritional deficiency of vitamin D (47).

Resection of large segments of the intestine in infants with volvulus or other anomalies or in older subjects with chronic inflammatory bowel disease may impair absorption of vitamin D and calcium leading to metabolic bone disease. Bypass surgery for obesity may lead to similar complications. The biochemical hallmark of vitamin D deficiency is a decreased serum concentration of 25-OHD ($<$ 6 ng/ml) (32). Plasma concentrations of 1,25 (OH)$_2$D$_3$ are almost always inappropriately low for the borderline or low values of serum calcium and phosphate.

Serum osteoblastic alkaline phosphatase activity is usually high. Vitamin D deficiency rickets may be treated by exposure to ultraviolet (sun) light or more frequently by oral administration of vitamin D_2 or D_3 (5,000 units/day) and calcium. The latter nutrient is essential because after ingestion of vitamin D and synthesis of 1,25 $(OH)_2D$, there are intense intestinal absorption of calcium and phosphate and initiation of the process of bone mineralization, resulting in loss of serum calcium, which is replenished by its intestinal absorption. With adequate treatment serum concentrations of 25-OHD_3 and 1,25 $(OH)D_3$ increase, the latter often to supraphysiologic values transiently (150 pg/ml), alkaline phosphatase activity increases further and then decreases, and serum concentrations of calcium and phosphate increase. Calcification of unmineralized osteoid occurs rapidly.

DEFICIENCY OF CALCIUM

Adequate dietary calcium is particularly important for normal bone mineralization throughout infancy, childhood, and adolescence. It is the very low birth weight (<1,250 g), premature (<32 weeks' gestation) infant in whom the skeletal demand for calcium is greatest. The rate of calcium accretion by the fetus increases from 130 mg/kg/day at 28 weeks to 150 mg/kg/day by 36 weeks' gestation (37). If this amount of calcium is not provided in the enteral or parenteral diet, severe osteopenia, rib and long-bones fracture, and rickets may develop. Skeletal accretion of calcium continues at a relatively steady rate throughout childhood and then increases rapidly during the adolescent growth spurt. Krabbe and Christiansen (48,49) demonstrated that bone mineral content in the forearm of adolescent males increases 35 percent between 10.6 and 14.6 years and most rapidly at the time of peak height velocity. The increase in bone mineral content is preceded by rapid increase in the serum concentration of testosterone and alkaline phosphatase activity, suggesting that testosterone first stimulates osteoblast activity and then bone mineralization. Krabbe et al. (50) hypothesize that skeletal growth and maturation at puberty are related to increased secretion of GH induced by gonadal sex hormones, which in turn generates somatomedin, thereby enhancing cartilage cell division and growth, and which also increases 1,25 $(OH)_2D_3$ production, resulting in enhanced intestinal absorption of calcium and phosphate. The sex hormones complement the action of GH by directly stimulating osteoblast activity.

Lack of dietary calcium may adversely affect skeletal mineralization at any age. The rickets of prematurity is primarily due to decreased intake of calcium and/or phosphate, sometimes in association with vitamin D_3 deficiency (37). However, in the majority of premature infants with rickets, serum concentrations of 25-OHD_3 and 1,25 $(OH)_2D_3$ are normal or even elevated. Mineral deficiency in this group of very low birth weight infants is the consequence of several factors, including (1) decreased stores of calcium and phosphate at birth, because the majority of mineral accretion occurs in the last trimister; (2) restricted oral or parenteral intake of calcium and phosphate; (3) increased urinary loss of calcium due to diuretics such as furosemide or the urinary excretion of large acid loads due to parenteral hyperalimentation; (4) cholestasis and impaired intestinal absorption of vitamin D and hence of calcium and phosphate; (5) decreased absorption of dietary calcium and phosphate due to the feeding of soybean formulas that impair this process; and (6) the feeding of human milk, which is relatively phosphate deficient, hence resulting in hypercalciuria because of inability to utilize calcium for mineralization (37).

Rickets due to an isolated deficiency of dietary calcium in the presence of normal endogenous stores of vitamin D_3 has been recorded. Kooh et al. (51) reported a 1-year-old infant with rickets who had for 10 months ingested a lamb-base formula (initially introduced on a temporary basis because of gastroenteritis) that contained 1.0 mg/dl of calcium and 17.0 mg/dl of phosphate. He also received 800 IU of vitamin D_2 daily. It was estimated that the infant's diet provided 600 mg of phosphate but only 180 mg of calcium each day. Further investigation revealed hypocalcemia (7.6–8.4 mg/dl) and hypophosphatemia (2.5–3.2 mg/dl), increased alkaline phosphatase activity, high PTH levels, and normal serum concentrations of 25-OHD. Treatment of this child with a vitamin D-free skim milk formula (calcium content 700 mg/day; phosphate 600 mg/day) without supplementary vitamin D resulted in rapid increase in serum calcium and phosphate levels, decline in alkaline phosphatase activity and PTH values, and radiographic healing of the rickets within 3 weeks, whereas serum 25-OHD values changed little. A similar patient was described by Maltz et al. (52). A 16-month-old black infant female had ingested a diet adequate in phosphate (600 mg/day) and vitamin D (400 IU/day) that contained only 21–36 mg calcium per day. Clinical and radiographic signs of rickets were present by 16 months of age. Serum calcium levels were normal (9.1 mg/dl). With supplemental calcium (45 mg/kg/day), clinical, biochemical, and roentgenographic healing of the rickets occurred. These observations indicate that addition of dietary calcium without increase in phosphate intake or added vitamin D healed the rickets of these infants and support the suggestion that their metabolic bone disease was due to isolated calcium deficiency. The hypophosphatemia may be attributed to hyperphosphaturia induced by secondary hyperparathyroidism.

Calcium deficiency and metabolic bone disease have been observed in black South African school-aged children. Pettifor et al. (53) reported nine rural (black) children (4.6–13 years of age) with chemical, roentgenographic, and biochemical signs of rickets who were ingesting a low-calcium diet (<500 mg/day) and had normal serum concentrations of 25-OHD and no demonstrable cause of rickets. Their skeletal lesions healed with a normal daily dietary intake of calcium (1000 mg/day) without supplemental vitamin D. Histologic examination of bone biopsies from these patients revealed osteopenia and increased osteoid volume, surface, and thickness and decreased calcification rate, findings consistent with abnormal bone mineralization (54). Further investigation (55) demonstrated that perhaps as many as 40 percent of rural black South African children had biochemical evidence of metabolic bone disease (increased alkaline phosphatase activity) and that 13.2 percent had hypocalcemia. Those children with biochemical abnormalities ingested a diet containing only 15 percent of the recommended daily allowance of calcium, because they drank little milk. When such children received supplemental calcium (500 mg daily), the biochemical abnormalities reverted to normal.

Rickets due to combined dietary deficiencies of calcium and vitamin D has been observed in a 2-year-old Canadian white male in whom cow's milk was not tolerated and who received human breast milk for 1 year and no milk thereafter and who had never received supplementary vitamin D (56). The estimated daily intake of calcium was 80 mg, phosphate 400 mg. Serum concentrations of calcium were normal, of phosphate low, and of 25-OHD undetectable. Repletion of either calcium or vitamin D alone (although the latter was associated witih normalization of 25-OHD values) did not heal either the biochemical (elevated alkaline phosphatase activity, low calcium × phosphate product) or the radiographic signs of rickets. With addition of both calcium (900 mg/day) and vitamin D_2 (400 IU/day), there were rapid correction of serum chemistries and healing of the metaphyseal lesions.

DEFICIENCY OF PHOSPHATE

Dietary deficiency of phosphate and the ensuing disturbances of mineral homeostasis and skeletal mineralization are observed most frequently in very low birth weight infants, in subjects receiving phosphate-deficient parental hyperalimentation, and in patients ingesting antacids that complex phosphate in the intestinal tract, preventing its absorption. Since phosphate is found in many foods, it is different to select a phosphate-deficient diet (28).

The phosphate content of human breast milk is low (11–20 mg/dl) and insufficient for the needs (75 mg/kg/day) of the very low birth weight infant. Phosphate depletion in such infants is characterized by hypophosphatemia, hypophosphaturia, hypercalcemia, hypercalciuria, and rickets (57–60). Serum concentrations of 25-OHD are normal or elevated in these patients. With decrease in serum concentrations of phosphate, the calcium × phosphate product falls below levels required to initiate the process of mineralization, resulting in osteopenia and rickets. Hypophosphatemia may induce hypercalcemia and hypercalciuria by increasing bone mineral resorption and intestinal absorption of calcium, perhaps by enhancing the activity of renal 25-OHD-1-α-hydroxylase, thereby increasing production of 1,25 $(OH)_2D_3$, an osteolytic agent that may contribute to the metabolic bone disorder of hypophosphatemia (61, 62).

Serum levels of PTH are usually normal in phosphate-depleted subjects. Supplementation of the diet with phosphate orally on an intermittent schedule (59) or by continuous nasogastric infusion (63) results in normalization of serum concentratons of phosphate and calcium and healing of the rickets. Intermittent oral phosphate therapy may be associated with the risk of hypocalcemia, as the episodically very high levels of phosphate initiate bone mineralization and skeletal deposition of calcium. In some infants treated in this manner, it is necessary to provide calcium supplements also (57). Continuous nasogastric infusion of phosphate may avoid this problem (63).

Parenteral hyperalimentation may result in defective mineralization by providing too little calcium, phosphate, vitamin D, or other essential nutrient, through associated cholestasis, which may interfere with absorption of enteral vitamin D_3, or by increased urinary loss of calcium (64).

MISCELLANEOUS NUTRITIONAL DEFICIENCIES

Deficiency of Vitamin A

Arrest strata ("growth arrest lines") develop in the rat with vitamin A deficiency (1). In the vitamin A-deficient subject there are abnormal bone development and altered cartilagenous incorporation of radiolabeled sulfate, perhaps due to abnormal generation or biologic activity of somatomedin (65). Vitamin A in excessive amounts also induces bone lesions; this biologic rachitic-like effect may be due to antagonism of the metabolism or action of vitamin D (66). Its role in human bone maturation is uncertain.

Deficiency of Vitamin K

Osteocalcin is a bone protein secreted by osteoblasts that is under the control, in part, of 1,25 $(OH)_2D_3$. This peptide (MW 6,000–12,000 daltons) contains the vitamin K-dependent amino acid gamma-carboxyglutamic acid (GLA) (67). It binds ionized calcium and hydroxyapatite and may inhibit mineralization of bone matrix. Its plasma concentrations reflect the metabolic activity of bone and are increased in disorders with increased bone turnover (Paget's disease, rickets, hyperparathyroidism). In the vitamin K-deficient state an abnormal osteocalcin is formed, because glutamate cannot be converted to gamma-carboxyglutamic acid and thus cannot bind hydroxyapatite. However, in experimental animals with low blood and bone osteocalcin levels, no abnormality of bone histology or mineralization has been observed (67).

Deficiency of Vitamin C

The osteopathy of vitamin C deficiency (scurvy) is characterized by subperiosteal and bone marrow hemorrhages, which stimulate formation of irregular new bone, and by disruption of endochondral calcification due to defective synthesis of organic matrix collagen (64). Ascorbic acid is important as a cofactor for the enzyme (collagen-prolyl hydroxylase) that converts proline to hydroxyproline.

Aluminum

Osteodystrophy due to aluminum accumulation in bone has been observed in two groups of patients—those undergoing renal dialysis with high aluminum content of dialysis fluid, and those receiving total parenteral nutrition (77). Osteodystrophy may also occur after excessive ingestion of aluminum-containing antacids by mouth (78). Aluminum impairs mineral deposition in bone.

Copper

In infants who become copper deficient owing to low birth weight, unsupplemented parental nutrition, or malnutrition, an osteopoathy similar to that observed in vitamin C deficiency is observed. Copper is a cofactor for lysyl hydroxylase, an enzyme necessary for normal collagen synthesis (64).

Zinc

This trace metal is important for the sensations of taste and smell. Deficiency of zinc results in anorexia and decreased caloric intake, poor weight gain, decreased linear growth, delayed adolescence, and retarded skeletal maturation (68). Zinc deficiency may occur because of decreased dietary intake, abnormal intestinal absorption [as in patients with chronic inflammatory bowel disease or in (Middle and Far Eastern) regions where dietary zinc is rendered nonabsorbable by complexing to dietary phytate] or increased loss (as in patients with sickle cell anemia or in diuretic-treated subjects in whom there is hyperzincuria). It is likely that many trace metals (e.g., magnesium, manganese) play important roles in growth and skeletal development and that deficiency of one or more of these micronutrients may impair these processes.

Acknowledgments: The author expresses his appreciation to Ms. Sue Fine and Ms. Cheryl Cooper for competent and supportive secretarial assistance.

REFERENCES

1. Park, E. A. (1964) Pediatrics 33:815–862.
2. Phillips, L. S., Vassilopoulou-Sellin, R. (1980) N. Engl. J. Med. 302:371–380, 438–446.
3. Zapf, J., Schoenle, E., Froesch, E. R. (1985) In: Hintz, R. L., Underwood, L. E. (eds) *Somatomedins and Other Growth Factors: Relevance to Pediatrics,* Ross Laboratories 89th Conference on Pediatric Research, Columbus, pp. 47–54.
4. VanWyk, J. (1985) In: Hintz, R. L., Underwood, L. E. (eds) *Somatomedins and Other Growth Factors: Relevance to Pediatrics,* Ross Laboratories 89th Conference on Pediatric Research, Columbus, pp. 38–44.
5. Parra, A., Garza, C., Garza, Y., Saravia, J. L., Hazlewood, C. F., Nichols, B. L. (1973) J. Pediatr. 82:133–142.
6. Smith, S. R., Edgar, P. J., Pozehsky, T., Chhetri, N. K., Prout, T. E. (1974) J. Clin. Endocrinol. Metab. 39:53–62.
7. Hintz, R. L., Suskind, R., Amatayakul, K., Thanangkul, O., Olson, R. (1978) J. Pediatr. 92:153–156.
8. Clemmons, D. R., Underwood, L. E. (1985) In: Hintz, R. L., Underwood, L. E. (eds) *Somatomedins and Other Growth Factors: Relevance to Pediatrics,* Ross Laboratories 89th Conference on Pediatric Research, Columbus, pp. 56–62.
9. Merimee, T. J., Zapf, J., Froesch, E. R. (1982) J. Clin. Endocrinol. Metab. 55:999–1002.
10. Miller, L. L., Schalch, D. S., Draznin, B. (1981) Endocrinology 108:1265–1271.
11. Prewitt, T. E., D'Ercole, A. J., Switzer, B. R., VanWyk, J. J. (1982) J. Nutr. 112:144–150.
12. Clemmons, D. R., Klibansky, A., Underwood, L. E., McArthur, J. W., Ridg-

way, E. C., Beitins, I. Z., VanWyk, J. J. (1981) J. Clin. Endocrinol. Metab. 53:1247–1250.

13. Clemmons, D. R., Seek, M. M., Underwood, L. E. (1985) Metabolism 34:391–395.

14. Isley, W. L., Underwood, L. E., Clemmons, D. R. (1983) J. Clin. Invest. 71:175–182.

15. Bomboy, J. D. Jr., Burkhalter, V. J., Nicholson, W. E., Salmon, W. D. Jr. (1983) Endocrinology 112:371–377.

16. Burch, W. M., Lebovitz, H. E. (1982) J. Clin. Invest. 70:496–504.

17. Burstein, P. J., Draznin, B., Johnson, C. J., Schalch, D. S. (1979) Endocrinology 104:1107–1111.

18. Chernausek, S. D., Underwood, L. E., Utiger, R. D., VanWyk, J. J. (1983) Clin. Endocrinol. 19:337–344.

19. Cavalieri, R. R. (1980) Thyroid Today 3(7):1–6.

20. Chopra, I. J., Hershman, J. M., Pardridge, W. M., Nicoloff, J. T. (1983) Ann. Intern. Med. 98:946–957.

21. Vagenakis, A. G., Burger, A., Portnay, G. I., Rudolph, M., O'Brian, J. T., Azizi, F., Arky, R. A., Nicod, P., Ingbar, S. H., Braverman, L. E. (1975) J. Clin. Endocrinol. Metab. 41:191–194.

22. Burman, K. D., Dimond, R. C., Harvey, G. S., O'Brian, J. T., Georges, L. P., Bruton, S., Wright, F. D., Wartofsky, L. (1979) Metabolism 28:291–299.

23. Ferguson, D. C., Hoenig, M., Jennings, A. S. (1985) Endocrinology 117:64–70.

24. Sato, K., Robbins, J. (1981) J. Clin. Invest. 68:475–483.

25. Canalis, E. (1983) Endocrinol. Rev. 4:62–77.

26. Raisz, L. G., Kream, B. E. (1983) N. Engl. J. Med. 309:29–35, 83–89.

27. Centrella, M., Canalis, E. (1985) Endocrinol. Rev. 6:544–551.

28. Aurbach, G. D., Marx, S. J., Spiegel, A. M. (1985) In: Wilson, J. D., Foster, D. W. (eds) Textbook of Endocrinology. 7th Edition. Philadelphia: W. B. Saunders, pp. 1218–1255.

29. Vigersky, R. A., Andersen, A. E., Thompson, R. H., Loriaux, D. L. (1977) N. Engl. J. Med. 297:1141–1145.

30. Marshall, J. C., Kelch, R. P. (1979) J. Clin. Endocrinol. Metabl. 49:712–718.

31. Root, A. W., Powers, P. S. (1983) J. Adol. Hlth. Care 4:25–30.

32. Root, A. W. (1985) In: Colon, A. R., Ziai, M. (eds) Pediatric Pathophysiology. Boston: Little Brown, pp. 97–125.

33. Landis, W. J., Glimcher, M. J. (1982) J. Ultrastruct. Res. 78:227–268.

34. Brommage, R., Deluca, H. F. (1985), Endocrinol. Rev. 6:491–511.

35. Root, A. W., Vargas, A., Duckett, G. E., Hough, G. (1980) J. FL. Med. Assoc. 67:933–934.

36. Harrison, H. E., Harrison, H. C. (1979) Disorders of Calcium and Phosphate Metabolism in Childhood and Adolescence. Philadelphia: W. B. Saunders, p. 48.

37. Greer, F. R., Tsang, R. C. (1986) Perinatol-Neonatal 10:14–21.

38. Tsang, R. C. (1983) Lancet 1:1370–1372.

39. Clemens, T. L., Adams, J. A., Henderson, S., Holick, N. F. (1982) Lancet 1:74–76.

40. Bachrach, S., Fisher, J., Parks, J. S. (1979) Pediatrics 64:871–877.

41. Dwyer, J. T., Dietz, W. H., Jr., Hass, G., Suskind, R. (1979) Am. J. Dis. Child 133:134–140.

42. Rudolf, M., Aulananthan, K., Greenstein, R. M. (1980) Pediatrics 66:72–76.

43. Zmora, E., Gorodischer, R., Bar-Ziv, J. (1979) Am. J. Dis. Child 133:141–144.

44. Krieger, I. (1985) Pediatr. Consultant 8:113–114.

45. Kooh, S. W., Jones, G., Reilly, B. J., Fraser, D. (1979) J. Pediatr. 94:870–874.

46. Editorial (1982) Lancet 1:943–944.

47. Heubi, J. E., Tsang, R. C., Steichen, J. J., Chan, G. M., Chen, I. W., DeLuca, H. F. (1979) J. Pediatr. 94:977–982.

48. Krabbe, S., Christiansen, C. (1984) Acta Paediatr. Scand. 73:745–749.

49. Krabbe, S., Hummer, L., Christiansen, C. (1984) Acta Paediatr. Scand. 73:750–755.

50. Krabbe, S., Transbol, I., Christiansen, C. (1982) Arch. Dis. Child 57:359.

51. Kooh, S. W., Fraser, D., Reilly, B. J., Hamilton, J. R., Gall, D. G., Bell, L. (1977) N. Engl. J. Med. 297:1264–1266.

52. Maltz, H. E., Fish, M. D., Holliday, M. A. (1970) Pediatrics 46:865–870.

53. Pettifor, J. M., Ross, P., Wang, J., Moodley, G., Couper-Smith, J. (1978) J. Pediatr. 92:320–324.

54. Marie, P. J., Pettitor, J. M., Ross, F. P., Glorieux, F. H. (1982) N. Engl. J. Med. 307:584–588.

55. Pettifor, J. M., Ross, P., Moodley, G., Shueyane, E. (1979) Am. J. Clin. Nutr. 32:2477–2483.

56. Fraser, D., Kooh, S. W., Reilly, B. J., Bell, L., Duthie, D. (1980) In: DeLuca, H. F., Anast, C. S. (eds), *Pediatric Diseases Related to Calcium*. New York: Elsevier, pp. 257–267.

57. Miller, R. R., Menke, J. A., Mentser, M. I. (1984), J. Pediatr. 105:814–817.

58. Rowe, J. G., Wood, D. H., Rowe, D. W., Raisz, L. G. (1979) N. Engl. J. Med. 300:293–296.

59. Rowe, J., Rowe, D., Horak, E., Spackman, T., Saltzman, R., Robinson, S., Philipps, A., Raye, J. (1984) J. Pediatr. 104:112–117.

60. Sagy, M., Birenbaum, E., Balin, A., Orda, S., Barzilay, Z., Brish, M. (1980) J. Pediatr. 96:683–685.

61. Chesney, R. W., Hamstra, A. J., DeLuca, H. F. (1981) Am. J. Dis. Child 135:34–37.

62. Steichen, J. J., Tsang, R. C., Greer, F. R., Ho, M., Hug, G. (1981) J. Pediatr. 99:293–298.

63. Koo, W. W. K., Antony, G., Stevens, L. H. S. (1984) Am. J. Dis. Child 138:172–175.

64. Paige, D. M. (1983) *Manual of Clinical Nutrition*. Pleasantville: Nutrition Publications, pp. 19.1–17.

65. Mohan, P. J., Rao, K. S. J. (1980) J. Nutr. 110:868–875.

66. Metz, A. L., Walser, M. M., Olson, W. G. (1985) J. Nutr. 115:929–935.

67. Price, P. (1983) In: Peck, W. A. (ed) *Bone and Mineral Research I*. Amsterdam: Excerpta Medica, pp. 157–190.

68. Lifshitz, F., Nishi, Y. (1980) In: DeLuca, H. F., Anast, C. S. (eds) *Pediatric Diseases Related to Calcium*. New York: Elsevier, pp. 305–321.

69. Isaksson, O. G. P., Isgaard, J., Nilsson, A., Lindohl, A. (1988) In: Bercu, B. B. (ed) *Basic and Clinical Aspects of Growth Hormone*. New York: Plenum, pp. 199–211.

70. Sporn, M. B., Roberts, A. B., Wakefield, L. M., Assoian, R. K. (1986) Science 233:532–534.

71. Strober, W., James S. P. (1988) Pediatr. Res. 24:549–557.

72. Beresford, J. N., Gallagher, J. A., Russell, R. G. G. (1986) Endocrinology 119:1776–1785.

73. Gallagher, J. A., Beneton, M., Harvey, L., Lawson, D. E. M. (1986) Endocrinology 119:1603–1609.

74. Wronski, T. J., Halloran, B. P., Bikle, D. D., Globus, R. K., Morey-Holton, E. R. (1986) Endocrinology 119:2580–2585.

75. Sprecker, B. C., Tsang, R. C. (1987) J. Pediatr. 110:744–747.

76. Hayward, I., Stein, M. T., Gibson, M. I. (1987) Am. J. Dis. Child 141:1060–1062.

77. Sedman, A. B., Klein, G. L., Merritt, R. J., Miller, N. L., Weber, K. O., Gill, W. L., Anand, H., Alfrey, A. C. (1985) N. Engl. J. Med. 312:1337–1343.

78. Clinical Nutrition (1987) Nutrition Rev. 45:72–74.

6

Osteoporotic Fractures

CHARLES W. SLEMENDA AND C. CONRAD JOHNSTON JR.

DEFINITION

Osteoporosis may be defined as the skeletal fragility and susceptibility to fracture that result from age-related bone loss. No absolute threshold exists to separate those with and without disease; rather, the risk of fracture increases, perhaps exponentially, with increasing bone loss (1, 2). This chapter attempts to address the discrepancies between the intuitively simple understanding of osteoporosis as an extreme manifestation of the normal, age-related thinning of bone and the more complex problem of deciding where on the continuum of bone loss treatment should be initiated. Both prevention of and treatment for osteoporosis are considered. Questions are raised regarding common attitudes toward this serious and costly condition.

What is known regarding osteoporosis is derived primarily from cross-sectional observations of bone mass and fracture patterns. Relatively few studies have been made of the process that yields osteoporotic fractures because of the slowly progressive nature of osteoporosis and the development only recently of adequate equipment to measure small change in bone mass. Also lacking is any ability to assess the quality of bone. Thus, osteoporosis resembles other serious, chronic diseases such as atherosclerosis, where availability of methodology is lacking, thereby limiting the ability to study certain important aspects of the condition—for example, the slow growth of arterial plaques.

FRACTURES

Those with osteoporosis have an increased risk for fractures of the vertebrae, femoral neck, radius, pelvis, and proximal humerus. Curiously, although Colles's fractures of the distal radius are considered to be osteoporotic, the incidence of such fractures does not increase with age past 65 years (3), despite the continuing decline in bone mass at this site. Conversely, the rate of hip fractures in females roughly doubles with every 5 years of increasing age. This contrast in fracture rates occurs despite well-documented and similar age-related declines in bone mass at both sites, based on cross-sectional associations (4). Thus, although osteoporosis is a phenomenon affecting almost the entire skeleton, other factors must also influence the clinical manifestation of this disease.

Fractures of the vertebrae are difficult to study, requiring spine X-rays for diagnosis, because many of these fractures are asymptomatic. Often classified into two groups, wedge and compression fractures (anterior vs. anterior and posterior crushing), vertebral fractures may produce relatively little disability and are responsible for the "dowager's hump," the hallmark of osteoporosis in older women.

Riggs and colleagues have offered the terms "Type 1 osteoporosis" to define the early, estrogen deficiency-related loss of trabecular bone (5), and the separation has been confirmed by others (6). Although vertebral fractures are a clear, early sign of osteoporosis, their utility in the study of this condition is currently limited. Few international data are available, these being limited to some Western European countries and Japan (7). More than 20 years ago, Nordin studied a small number of X-ray films from middle-aged women of various countries and found spinal osteoporosis to be most common among those from India and Japan (7). Films for women over age 65 were unavailable. Further, while the prevalence of such fractures may exceed those at all other sites, the incidence of vertebral fractures often goes unnoticed, and few data thus are available regarding fracture patterns or risk factors.

In contrast, the severity of hip fractures assures greater availability of data. The age-adjusted frequency of hip fractures among females ranges from 5 per 100,000 population per year among South African blacks to 98 per 100,000 per year in the United States (8). Even with the likelihood of some underreporting in South Africa, this 20-fold excess probably reflects real underlying differences. Generally, less developed countries have lower age-adjusted rates of hip fracture than developed nations. Rates in Singapore and regions of Yugoslavia are less than 20 percent of those in the United States and New Zealand (8) and exhibit female:male ratios of less than 1. This contrasts with ratios of about 2 for the United States and Western Europe.

These differences are thought to reflect genetic differences, contrasting lifestyles, environmental influences, and differing underlying causes. The greater levels of physical activity, exposure to sunlight, genetic factors, and osteomalacia are the most often cited issues. Dietary factors also provide an interesting contrast. The intake of calcium in the populations of underdeveloped countries is generally considerably lower than that in most developed nations, and dairy products are a minor part of most adult diets. However, with regard to nutrition, it should also be noted that diets in developed nations are also generally much higher in protein and that high-protein diets may have detrimental effects on calcium balance (9).

Within the United States, osteoporosis, as manifested by fractures or low bone mass, is most common among white females. This probably reflects differences in skeletal size at maturity. Rates of bone loss may or may not differ by race (10), and in all racial groups, females lose bone faster than males. It is likely that both peak bone mass and rates of bone loss contribute to the public health burden of osteoporosis, although either factor may dominate in an individual.

SKELETAL DEVELOPMENT

Skeletal development includes two periods of rapid growth, during early child-hood and adolescence, followed by a period of stabilization from about ages 20 to 35, followed by a decline in bone mass that continues into the ninth decade of life (11). At about this time bone mass may actually begin to increase again as periosteal apposition of bone exceeds endosteal loss.

Emphasis has only recently been focused on the earlier phases of this process which determines peak skeletal mass. If, as all data suggest, the risk of fracture is proportional to bone mass, and if rates of bone loss are similar, then those with greater peak mass reach each successive level of risk some period of time after those with lower peak mass (as shown in Fig. 6-1). Whether or not those with greater peak bone lose bone at the same rate as those with less bone at maturity is unknown. No prospective data have been published with a long enough follow-up to ascertain whether there is any relationship between peak mass and long-term rates of loss.

In this hypothetical example, those with 5 percent greater peak mass would have approximately a 5-year lag (rate of loss 1% per year) in reaching successively lower levels of bone mass. Given that the incidence of hip fractures in the United States doubles every 5 years among the elderly, the implications of increased peak bone mass are clear. Many factors may contribute to the development of peak skeletal mass, including genetic makeup, diet, exercise, obesity, stature, and perhaps pregnancy and lactation (12). A frequently cited cross-sectional study of bone mass and dietary calcium from Yugoslavia found a higher peak bone mass and a lower hip fracture incidence in the region with the greater consumption of calcium (13). The region studied, however, demonstrated similar apparent rates of bone loss based on cross-sectional measurements of individuals across the spec-trum of ages, but the data were less definitive. This finding might correspond to the pattern shown in Fig. 6-1.

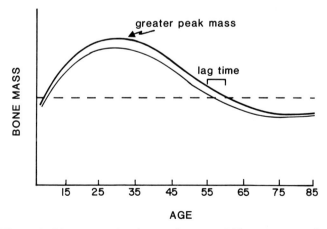

Fig. 6-1 Theoretical bone mass levels over the normal lifespan, comparing a higher with a lower peak bone mass.

A relationship between self-reported calcium consumption during childhood, adolescence, and young adulthood and adult bone mass has also been reported by several authors (14, 15). All of the studies examined adults, retrospectively assessed calcium intake, and measured radial and vertebral bone mass. Thus, three studies using different methodologies for measuring dietary calcium intake and for estimating skeletal size have reached similar conclusions about this relationship.

It has been shown that diseases of starvation, not surprisingly, result in loss of approximately 10 percent of tibial cortical bone (16). Data regarding skeletal recovery from malnutrition suggest at least retarded bone growth (17), although controversy exists regarding ultimate catchup growth and the effects of later childhood environments. The quality of diet in infancy has not been carefully studied, but in the rat the quantity and type of protein (animal or vegetable) have been shown to affect skeletal development only little (18). As will be discussed, animal models have serious weaknesses which adversely affect how the results of such studies are to be interpreted. Other studies have examined determinants of bone mass among young adults in caloric deficit. Those with anorexia nervosa have been shown to have reduced bone mass compared with controls (19–21), although high levels of activity may afford these subjects some protection against reduced bone mass (20).

Unfortunately, the findings from studies of extreme undernutrition offer little insight into the importance of dietary factors in ordinary osteopenia; the subjects in these studies were deficient in all nutrients save, perhaps, phosphorus (19). The female subjects also often became amenorrheic. Although serum estrogen concentrations were not correlated with bone mass (20), this has little relevance in cross-sectional studies because of the strong influences of stature and age, which might obscure weaker effects in studies with small sample sizes.

This possible protection offered by activity (20) introduces another important factor, physical activity, which probably affects bone directly, as well as indirectly through hormonal and dietary effects. It has been shown that whereas amenorrheic runners had less vertebral bone than the eumenorrheic runners, their average bone mass may not have been different from that of sedentary controls (22, 23). In this study, the amenorrheic, "osteopenic" group had significantly reduced estrogens and consumed 330 less kcal/day (not significant) than the eumenorrheic group.

Marcus et al. (24) have reported similar findings, with amenorrheic athletes having more bone than inactive women with amenorrhea. Again, among the athletes, the osteopenic, amenorrheic group was consuming 450 less kcal/day with 400 mg less calcium. This pattern of reduced bone mass among amenorrheic athletes has been reported many times, and lower caloric intakes are commonly reported in the amenorrheic groups (22). Recovery from activity-related amenorrhea has been reported to result in an increase in bone mass, although perhaps not to the level of eumenorrheic athletes (23). In groups not threatened by the possibility of cessation of menses, physical activity may offer some benefits. These factors are discussed later in this chapter. Thus, while activity among young females is thought to be protective against bone loss, "excessive" activity may have deleterious effects on the skeleton through alterations in hormones.

Controversy exists regarding the influence of pregnancy and lactation and nutrition during these periods on bone mass (25–27). Calcium absorption, however,
is improved during these periods, and it appears unlikely that, with adequate nutrition, mothers are at any increased risk of osteoporosis.

The public health implications of the changes in diet and exercise are unclear.
The increasing prevalence of eating disorders, the decline in consumption of dairy
products among teenagers, and the cultural obsession with thinness seem likely
to tip the balance toward lower peak skeletal mass, but the increased interest in
exercise may tend to counteract these influences. Other potential influences on
peak bone mass, poorly studied thus far, include increased use of alcohol and
tobacco, oral contraception, and earlier and later pregnancy. It must be stressed
that most of the studies cited here have examined the extremes of behavior and,
as such, may not relate to more moderate forms of exercise, dieting, and other
behaviors.

MECHANISMS OF BONE LOSS

Sex Hormones

At some point, probably around age 40, a slow loss of bone begins. In females,
bone loss is more rapid and may have an earlier onset if menopause is premature.
The possibility that nutritional factors, such as alterations in calcium absorption,
are involved in this process is considered below. Regardless of the mechanism,
certain characteristics of bone loss during this period of life are clear. Those who
undergo oophorectomies suffer rapid bone loss, which begins immediately after
surgery and which can be slowed or stopped by the administration of estrogen
(28). The association of rapid bone loss with menopause, and the well-established
slowing of bone loss with estrogen therapy has led to many studies of the roles
of hormones in osteoporosis (29, 30), although most studies have focused on
therapeutic rather than endogenous estrogens.

Cross-sectional studies have shown that postmenopausal females with greater
serum concentrations of estrone have greater bone mass (31). Such women, however, are usually more obese, and the obese have greater bone mass and perhaps
slower rates of bone loss, and, although it has long been postulated that the protection from osteoporosis due to obesity was the result of enhanced peripheral
aromatization of androgens to estrogens, there are data to suggest that weight
bearing itself is important in maintaining skeletal integrity. Specifically, both prolonged bed rest and the weightlessness of space travel have been associated with
rapid loss of bone (32, 33). Thus, although estrogen replacement is a useful treatment of age-related bone loss, the protection of obesity may be due, at least in
part, to another mechanism. In the spectrum of factors that affect postmenopausal
bone loss, circulating estrogen concentrations or therapeutic estrogen use must
rank first in importance, dwarfing by contrast any known nutritional or exercise
effects.

Other hormones have also been studied. Progesterone may be associated with slower rates of bone loss (34), and production of testosterone has been shown to be lower in those with vertebral crush fractures (35). The role of androgens in bone metabolism is an area worthy of further study. However, a recent longitudinal study measured estrone, estradiol, testosterone, and androstenedione at 4-month intervals for more than 3 years. Although mean testosterone concentrations were associated with slower rates of bone loss, estrogen concentrations were better predictors, and in multivariable models only the estrogens were consistent predictors of bone loss at both midshaft and distal radius (36). Despite these results, it is possible that androgens are important. Conceivably, in older woman, those with greater androgen concentrations might produce more estrogens via peripheral aromatization in adipose tissue.

The mechanism for the effect of estrogen on bone loss is not understood. It has been postulated that bone remodeling (resorption) is accelerated in females when estrogen concentrations decline (37), and estrogen replacement therapy has been shown to reduce remodeling (38). In the previously cited longitudinal study of estrogens and bone loss, estrone and estradiol were negatively correlated with serum Gla-protein (osteocalcin), a marker of bone remodeling (36). Thus, although it appears that estrogens have an effect on rates of bone remodeling, it is not known how this occurs.

Other possible mechanisms by which estrogen may affect bone include alterations in intestinal calcium absorption (39), changes in serum levels of parathyroid hormone (40), calcitonin (41), and vitamin D metabolites (42). The possible alterations in intestinal absorption and vitamin D metabolism appear to be less important effects than those that alter apparent rates of remodeling. However, the dominating action of estrogen remains too poorly understood to eliminate any reasonable explanation.

Calciotropic Hormones

Calcium homeostasis is maintained through the actions of parathyroid hormone, calcitonin, and vitamin D, with the skeleton as the ultimate reservoir for calcium. The precise mechanism by which bone provides calcium for critical functions such as blood clotting and transmission of electrical impulses is not completely understood, although it almost assuredly requires a process more rapid than resorption by osteoclasts. Whatever the immediate process, transient alterations in serum calcium trigger the calcium homeostatic mechanism. In healthy adults, PTH and vitamin D work in concert to increase serum calcium concentration when it declines, but it is unclear how this affects net skeletal calcium balance. While stimulating resorption of bone, thus decreasing its mineral content, simultaneous effects yield increased calcium absorption from the gut and decreased urinary excretion of calcium. Calcitonin, conversely, inhibits resorption of bone. Under ideal conditions this system should function to maintain skeletal integrity, increasing calcium absorption and retention as needed. It is possible, however, to envision minor derangements of this system, which might adversely affect the skeleton. These might include (1) renal dysfunction, which could reduce the availability of the active form of vitamin D, thereby reducing intestinal calcium absorption; (2) failure of the kidneys to conserve calcium during periods of increased bone resorption; and (3) resorption of bone at rates beyond the capabilities of compensatory mechanisms.

Insufficient data exist to choose from among these possibilities. Osteomalacia, which might result if vitamin D deficiencies are common, does not appear to be as prevalent as would be required to support the first mechanism as the major cause of hip fracture in the United States, but data are lacking. In particular, it is theoretically possible that slight deficiencies in vitamin D concentrations might cause secondary hyperparathyroidism and increased bone resorption. Increased resorption of bone and increased serum concentrations of PTH (impaired renal PTH metabolism?) have been reported to occur with aging (43), but the contribution of this process to osteoporosis is not known. Other factors must also be important.

Nutritional Calcium

Potential environmental influences on bone in addition to diet include activity, exposure to sunlight (vitamin D), medications and others. The intuitive appeal of dietary calcium as a key player in the development or prevention of osteoporosis is evident. The skeleton contains 99 percent of the body's calcium and provides the storage pool for ionized calcium in the blood. Because of the essential functions of calcium ions, bone is resorbed in preference to allowing unchecked declines in serum calcium, thereby allowing a steady efflux of calcium from bone.

Balance studies in young adults have demonstrated positive or zero calcium balance to be possible at intakes much less than 800 mg/day (U.S. RDA) (44). However, these studies do not address this issue for older females—those most prone to osteoporosis. The studies discussed previously focused on early nutrition without surprising results. Greater calcium intake during periods of growth appears beneficial to skeletal development (14, 15), and severe dietary restriction (anorexia) is associated with lower bone mass. Amenorrhea secondary to intense athletic training is also associated with low bone mass and with reduced caloric intake. Among older females a different picture emerges.

Calcium balance, the net difference between absorbed calcium and obligatory losses, must be zero or positive to preserve skeletal calcium. Calcium absorption is in part determined by vitamin D, which controls active transport across intestinal membranes and probably improves passive diffusion as well. Studies have shown that calcium absorption is lower in older people—perhaps as much as 30–50 percent lower (45), and thus, more dietary calcium is probably required to avoid negative calcium balance (46).

However, despite the intuitive simplicity of increasing calcium intake to reduce bone loss, the evidence in favor of increased dietary or calcium supplementation is meager. Two recent large studies of calcium and bone loss showed similar rates of bone loss in the high- and low-intake groups (47, 48). Although other less-comprehensive studies have also failed to find an association between calcium, bone mass, and osteoporosis, positive effects of calcium on the prevention or reduction of bone loss are reported along with, significantly, "mixed findings" (49). A supplement might be of value for those individuals whose dietary calcium intake is normally very low.

Unlike in the United States, osteoporotic fractures are uncommon in many cultures with very low calcium intakes. Furthermore, dietary calcium has not always been shown to be related to rates of bone loss. The question remains: What is the role of calcium in age-related bone loss? The answer must be that as a general influence in older women, it can be only a weak factor, and that the efficacy of supplementation remains to be demonstrated. As an influence in youth, the potential benefits seem greater.

Similarly, therapies with forms of vitamin D are intuitively logical. We know that the serum concentrations of the active $1,25(OH)_2D_3$ metabolite of vitamin D declines with age (50) and that an increase in this factor should both improve calcium absorption and prevent the bone loss due to secondary hyperparathyroidism. Again, however, the results of clinical trials have been disappointing. Although increased calcium absorption results (51), changes in bone mass only occasionally favor the vitamin D-supplemented groups (52). The potential for vitamin D supplementation is not, however, limited to alterations in calcium absorption alone, but extends to the prevention or correction of osteomalacia.

In Britain, osteomalacia may be an important determinant of hip fracture incidence (53). A case control study from Finland found significantly lower concentrations of $1,25(OH)_2D_3$ in patients with hip fractures (54), and the authors summarized several other similar studies with both positive and negative results. Among the studies with appropriate controls, those that indicated an important role for vitamin D deficiency were from more northern areas, such as Finland and Britain, thereby suggesting the possibility that inadequate exposure to sunlight may be involved. Thus, although vitamin D supplementation may not be effective in the prevention of osteoporosis, it offers some promise in those limited circumstances where osteomalacia may be involved in the genesis of fractures. Before further advances can be made in this area, careful histological studies (required for unequivocal diagnosis of osteomalacia) will be necessary. Indiscriminate large-scale supplementation with vitamin D is probably inappropriate because there may be some irreversible loss of bone in osteomalacia (55).

Other Dietary Factors

Other possible dietary influences include protein, caffeine, phosphorus, and other minerals. Balance studies have shown high-protein diets to have a detrimental effect on calcium balance, and ecological comparisons show groups with high protein intake generally to be those with greater prevalence of osteoporosis (56). However, such ecological evidence is not convincing, and the balance studies offer more direct evidence. Caffeine had a slight negative effect on calcium balance in the same study (9), and high coffee and tea consumption has been shown in one study to be associated with greater rates of bone loss over 1 year (although caffeine itself was not studied) (36). Phosphorus has been the subject of numerous studies with conflicting results. Although large amounts of dietary phosphorus may slightly reduce calcium absorption, its net effect on calcium balance is probably positive. Parfitt has reviewed the effects of these and other dietary components on bone (57).

Sodium fluoride and vitamin D have been shown to affect calcium metabolism or bone under certain circumstances, and trace elements may also play some role. The methodologic difficulties in studying these dietary components are considerable. Two related problems beset studies that attempt to relate any nutrient to a disease: first, there is a large within-person variability, and second, we lack knowledge regarding the distribution of micronutrients in our foods. Methods exist to deal with the first problem, but the study of trace elements will be seriously limited until means are developed to deal with the latter problem.

Hyper–Hypokinesia

Another almost universally accepted "environmental" influence is physical activity. But the data base constitutes the results of studies of extreme behavior. Prolonged bed rest produces osteopenia (58), as does the gravity-free environment of space travel (59), and there is some evidence that these effects are more pronounced in trabecular bone (60). At the opposite extreme, tennis players have been shown to have greater bone mass in their playing arms (61), and strenuous exercise, such as distance running (62), has been shown to have a beneficial effect in postmenopausal women.

As mentioned previously, exercise may also blunt the bone-damaging effects of amenorrhea, so exercise is widely recommended as a safe preventive measure for osteoporosis. However, there are aspects of these studies that make such recommendations questionable. Thus far, no truly randomized trials have shown positive results of exercise, allowing for the possibility that these findings reflect selection biases. In a randomized trial of a walking program, rates of radial bone density loss did not differ between the groups over the first 3 years of the trial (63), but walking is the exercise most frequently suggested for postmenopausal women. The lack of an effect in this study could reflect the fact that a non-weight-bearing site was measured or that the intensity of the exercise was not great enough to yield systemic effects. Still, it was a negative outcome. Moreover, there are scant data to support any simple, linear relationship between bone and activity (across the usual spectrum of activity).

The reasons for such findings include the possibility that no such relationships exist, or the difficulties in (1) distinguishing levels of activity (especially in populations where the level of activity is very low), (2) measuring rates of loss of bone over a relatively short time-span, and (3) achieving large differences between the exercise and control groups. Thus, although extremes of activity or inactivity in nonrandom groups can have dramatic effects on the skeleton, it remains unclear whether moderate increases in activity are beneficial.

Inconsistent results have been reported for factorial designs of the effects of exercise and calcium on bone in older women (64). Whereas those receiving only exercise or only calcium (plus vitamin D) gained bone, those receiving both lost bone. Furthermore, this was not a randomized trial, but rather a matched design. This same problem of a nonrandom design similarly reduces the interpretability of other exercise studies. Physical fitness, as estimated by maximum oxygen uptake and presumably reflective of habitual physical activity, has been shown to be associated with femoral–neck and lumbar–spine bone mass (65) and with forearm bone mass (66) in postmenopausal women.

These results suggest the possibility that more intense, long-term physical activity prevents or slows bone loss in older women. However, it may be that the associations seen here reflect lifetime activity patterns or selection biases that may have increased peak bone mass. It is plausible that women who are now more physically fit may be an exceptionally athletic group. Some evidence for this was presented in a study by Chow et al. (66), who showed that the more fit group with greater bone mass also had greater upper-body strength and leg strength.

Effects of Pharmacologic Intervention

Various medications are also known to influence bone. *Corticosteroids* have been shown to cause loss of trabecular and possibly cortical bone (67). This findings is somewhat complicated by the possibility that the disease processes for which corticosteroids are given may also cause skeletal degeneration. For example, individuals with rheumatoid arthritis may have less bone mass than comparison groups before treatment with steroids, and such groups may have greatly reduced levels of physical activity as a result of chronic pain (68). Despite these potentially confounding influences, corticosteroid therapy is generally detrimental to skeletal integrity.

The mechanism for this loss of bone probably involves alterations in calcium metabolism, although these effects may not be seen in all corticosteroid-treated patients. A comparison of patients treated with corticosteroids with similar doses for similar durations showed those with osteoporotic fractures (one or more vertebral crush fractures) to have only about half the fractional calcium absorption of those without fractures (69). The fracture group also had significantly higher calcium:creatinine and hydroxyproline:creatinine ratios, indicative of increased urinary calcium excretion and bone turnover. Thus, corticosteroid-induced osteoporosis probably results from at least two possibly related alterations in calcium metabolism. The reports of a bone-sparing corticosteroid are preliminary and require further study.

Anticonvulsant therapy is also associated with an increased fracture incidence (70), but the cause of these fractures is not clearly osteoporosis or osteomalacia. Among fracture patients receiving anticonvulsant therapy, serum alkaline phosphatase is elevated, and resorptive activity in trabecular bone is increased; additionally, there is increased osteoid (70). The bone disease that develops in those individuals who receive anticonvulsants therefore appears to have characteristics that defy simple classification.

Nonsteroidal antiinflammatory drugs (NSAIDs) have also been associated with an unusual form of bone damage. Acetabular damage was noted in osteoarthritic patients after treatment with many different NSAIDs (71). This effect did not appear to reflect merely a more severe underlying disease; those with and without damage had similar pain and walking ability scores, and many of those not using NSAIDs took other analgesics. While this association could have been due to excessive activity following pain relief, this explanation is less plausible than one based on some direct drug-related effect. The relevance of this association to osteoporosis is marginal, but it suggests the possibility that some "osteoporosis" may be damage due to other causes.

Not all medication effects on bone are negative. *Thiazides* are known to reduce urinary calcium concentrations (72) and thus should theoretically improve calcium balance. The data, however, are inconsistent and may relate to design differences and a relatively weak effect of thiazides (73). In retrospective studies, it is impossible to control for the conditions that lead to treatment with thiazides, primarily mild diastolic hypertension, although no association between bone mass and hypertension has been reported. Randomized trials of a thiazide effect on bone loss have been equivocal, perhaps suggesting a transitory effect (74).

Smokers generally have less bone than nonsmokers, but this relationship also is not straightforward (75, 76). Smokers are thinner than nonsmokers, and obesity protects against osteoporosis. Smokers may also have less adequate diets than nonsmokers. Furthermore, smokers have an earlier onset of menopause and thereby lose the protection of ovarian estrogens on the average of 1–2 years before non-smokers. Thus, although there is no question that smokers have reduced skeletal mass, this reduction may be mediated through several previously recognized mechanisms, including thinness and lack of ovarian function. It is also possible that smoking has other antiestrogenic effects (77). A recent publication has shown that smokers have a significant increase in 2-hydroxylation of estradiol, thereby decreasing the availability of free estrogens (78). Beyond these observations it is not clear what effects, if any, smoking has on bone. However, it is clear that, whatever the mechanism, the skeleton may be added to the list of organs adversely affected by smoking.

TREATMENT

If osteoporosis is defined as the clinical manifestation of fractures, a cure for osteoporosis does not exist. Nor is it likely that a "cure" will be developed in the foreseeable future. Once a vertebral body collapses or the neck of the femur is fractured, the best that can be hoped for is the stabilization of the existing fracture and the prevention of future deterioration. Thus, therapy for osteoporosis is focused primarily on the prevention of further deterioration and may include, alone or in various combinations, calcium, vitamin D, estrogen, fluoride, and calcitonin. No therapy, with the exception of fluoride has been shown to replace lost bone.

Fluoride therapy, alone or with other agents, remains investigational (see Mariano-Menez et al., Chapter 14).

Although fluoride does appear to reduce vertebral fracture rates and may actually increase trabecular bone mass, the effects on cortical bone may be negative (79), and femoral fractures may actually increase (80). Moreover, although stabilization of bone seems to result, the quality of bone may be changed, and the effects of this process on fracture risk are unclear. Fluoride can also be toxic (81), and it is associated with gastric or rheumatologic side effects in many patients (82). In summary, fluoride may have a limited but important potential in the treatment of osteoporosis for selected patients, but general use is almost certainly inappropriate.

Therapy with various forms of vitamin D has been reported to be effective

(51, 52) although not consistently so. Such benefits may result from increased calcium absorption and decreased net bone resorption (as evidenced by reduced excretion of hydroxyproline) (51). These improvements may be limited to those with deficiencies of vitamin D (due to changes in kidney function, lack of exposure to sunlight, etc.), although the prevalence of such deficiencies has not been assessed in U.S. populations. Some fractures attributed to osteoporosis may be due instead to unrecognized osteomalacia. In Britain, such cases may be relatively common (53), although this is thought not to be the case in the United States.

ADFR

A more complex theoretical approach to therapy has been termed ADFR (activate–depress–free–repeated) (83). It is based on the theory that current therapies can only stabilize remaining bone by reducing resorption and that a net increase in bone mass is possible by (1) *a*ctivation of the bone remodeling cycle, (2) *d*epression of the resorption phase, (3) a *f*ree period to allow formation of bone, and (4) *r*epetition of this process. Adequate tests of this approach in humans are lacking, although one small study has been completed (84).

Using inorganic phosphates to activate remodeling and etidronate to depress resorption, large increases in trabecular volume were observed in four or five patients after six 90-day cycles of treatment. Other approaches thought to have the potential to increase bone mass include therapy with parathyroid hormone (85) or phosphates, but neither of these modalities has been adequately tested.

Calcitonin has been tested with fairly consistent positive results (86). However, some studies reporting positive results have lacked placebo-treated controls and thus cannot be taken as supportive of beneficial effects—especially when the outcome is based on a subjective measure (87).

Anabolic steroids have been suggested as a therapy to reduce bone loss during immobilization or space flight (88). Although there is some potential for this approach, long-term studies have not been performed to assess the safety of this category of hormones. It is believed, however, that the long-term use of anabolic steroids is inappropriate because of possible hepatic and cardiovascular side effects.

Recent studies have begun to examine areas not previously considered. Greater serum concentrations of manganese, for example, have been shown to be associated with decreased bone resorption (89).

Lone bone mass, however, is not the only factor involved in fractures among the geriatric population. Little work has been done to investigate the quality of bone, to determine whether important qualitative changes occur, and to determine whether such changes affect the fracture risk. For example, microfracture healing probably slows with aging, and an accumulation of microdamage may be involved in vertebral and other fractures, but the importance of this and other qualitative factors is unknown. Trauma, however, is a well-recognized risk factor for fracture, and it occurs with increasing frequency among the aged. Minor trauma, such as occurs with falls from standing height or less, is associated with fracture and death among the very old (90). It is unclear whether the fall precipitates the events that follow or the fall is a reflection of some general deterioration.

FUTURE RESEARCH

The most obvious study of osteoporosis is the study of fractures. Unfortunately, despite their high cumulative frequency, most fractures have low incidence rates, thereby making prospective studies long and costly. Retrospective fracture studies are less valuable because of the possible impact of the fracture on mental status, activity patterns, and other factors associated with bone mass and other musculoskeletal characteristics.

Because of these difficulties, most studies have focused on correlates of bone mass and density measurements. Measurements can be made at almost any site, and in fact, some total body calcium data exist. For various reasons, the radius and the spine have been the most commonly measured sites, but technological advancement has recently permitted evaluation of the femoral neck. Early studies of bone "mass" employed radiographs of the hand, from which estimates of total bone width, cortical bone width, and other parameters were made. These estimates were crude but sufficiently accurate to establish many of the basic patterns in bone growth and development (91).

Photon absorptiometry permits the quantitative estimation of the mineral content. Although not a true density measurement, this method estimates density. Photon absorptiometry with photons at a single energy level (SPA) is best suited for measurement of the radius or the os calcis, sites where relatively little fat is present, and dual photon absorptiometry (DPA; photons at two energy levels) is appropriate for sites such as the spine and the hip, where more nonbone tissues are present. Computed tomography (CT) offers another precise method for estimating bone mineral. This approach differs from photon absorptiometry in that it provides a direct estimate of density by assessing the absorption of energy in a cross section with a defined thickness. Other approaches, such as Compton scattering, have been used but are not at present well established or practical.

The reproducibility of the methods referred to above is on the order of 2 percent in repeated measures of phantoms or excised bone specimens. Given the range of bone mineral content in healthy populations, this level of precision assures adequate cross-sectional assessments. However, most studies are designed to estimate rates of change, perhaps as a natural process or perhaps in response to a therapeutic agent. This becomes a more difficult task. Even during periods of "rapid" bone loss, rates exceeding 2 percent per year are the exception. Thus, changes in bone mineral content over 2 years would be within the error of the method. This possibility would not adversely influence estimates of bone loss in a population but would indicate a need for caution in the interpretation of sequential studies for individuals. In a group where zero change was the true value for everyone, methodological errors would yield rates of loss or gain for portions of the population simply because of the distribution of values about the mean. This logic implies that those technologies are well suited to population studies but are ill advised when the individual is the unit of interest. The exception would be in the case of a single assessment made as the basis for a therapeutic decision, such as whether to provide estrogen to a postmenopausal patient. Single measurements are highly reproducible since these do not involve assessments of small changes. Given the limitations of current technology, this decision would necessarily be based solely on absolute bone mass rather than on rates of loss.

SUMMARY

Osteoporosis is a common, chronic condition with serious consequences for at least one-third of older females and perhaps 15–20 percent of older males. Prevention of the most dangerous sequelae, fractures, is probably best achieved by preservation of bone mass and by the development of greater skeletal mass at maturity. For females beyond menopause, therapeutic estrogens at the time of menopause appear to be the safest, most effective means of preserving skeletal mass, and physical activity and an adequate diet are less certain but potential factors. Achievement of greater peak skeletal mass through diet, activity, or supplements is untested but appears to hold potential, based on observational studies. Therapies for those with manifest disease thus far offer less promise beyond the stabilization of remaining bone tissue.

REFERENCES

1. Melton, L. J. III, Wahner H. W., Richelson L. S., O'Fallon, W. M., Riggs, B. L. (1986) Am. J. Epidemiol. 124:254.

2. Melton, III L. J. and Riggs, B. L. (1986) In: *Current Concepts of Bone Fragility*. Proc. Conference on Bone Fragility in Orthopaedics and Medicine, Ottawa, May 16–18, 1985. Berlin: Springer-Verlag.

3. Melton, L. J., Cummings, S. R. (1986) Bone and Mineral (In press).

4. Mazess, R. B., Barden, H. S., Ettinger, M., Johnston, C., Dawson-Hughes, B., Baron, D., Powell, M., Notelovitz, M. *Bone and Mineral* (In press).

5. Riggs, B. L. and Melton III, L. J. (1983) Am. J. Med. 75:899.

6. Johnston, C. C., Norton, J., Khairi, M. R. A., Kernek, C., Edouard, C., Arlot, M., Meunier, P. J. (1985) J. Clin. Endocrinol. Metab. 61:551.

7. Nordin, B. E. C. (1966): International Patterns of Osteoporosis. Clin. Orthop. 45:17.

8. Cummings, S. R., Kelsey, J. L., Nevitt, M. C., O'Dowd, K. J. (1985) Epidemiol. Reviews 7:178.

9. Heaney, R. and Recker, R. (1982) J. Lab. Clin. Med. 99:46.

10. Cohn, S. H., Abesamis, C., Yasumura, S., Aloia, J. F., Zanzi, I., Ellis, K. J. (1977) Metab. 26:171.

11. Hui, S. L., Wiske, P. S., Norton, J. A., Johnston, C. C. (1982) J. Chron. Dis. 35:715.

12. Cummings, S. R., Kelsey, J. L., Nevitt, M. C., O'Dowd, K. J. (1985) Epidemiol. Rev. 7:178.

13. Matkovic, V., Kostial, K., Simonovic, I., Buzine, R., Brodarec, A., Nordin, B. E. C. (1979) Am. J. Clin. Nutr. 32:540.

14. Sandler, R. B., Slemenda, C. W., LaPorte, R. E., Cauley, J. A., Schramm, M. M., Barresi, M. L., Kriska, A. M. (1985) Am. J. Clin. Nutr. 42:270.
15. Anderson, J. J. B., Tylavsky, F. A. (1984) In: Christiansen, C., Arnaud, C. D., Nordin, B. E. C., Parfitt, A. M., Peck, W. A., Riggs, B. L. (eds) *Osteoporosis*. Department of Clinical Chemistry, Glostrup Hospital, Glostrup, pp. 299.
16. Akamaguna, A. I., Odita, J. C., Ugbodaga, C. I., Okolo, A. A. (1986) Pediatr. Radiol. 16:40.
17. Alvear, J., Artaza, C., Vial, M., Guerrero, S., Muzzo, S. (1986) Arch. Dis. Child. 61:257.
18. Bohannon, F., Ranhotra, G. (1985) Nutri. Reports Intl. 31:1291.
19. Crosby, L. O., Kaplan, F. S., Pertschuk, M. J., Mullen, J. L. (1985) Clin. Orthopaed. 201:271.
20. Rigotti, N. A., Nussbaum, S. R., Herzop, D. B., Neer, R. M. (1984) New Engl. J. Med. 311:1601.
21. Matthews, B. J., Lacey, J. H., Cleeve, H. (1985) Lancet 1:1431.
22. Nelson, M. E., Fisher, E. C., Catsos, P. D., Meredith, C. N., Turksoy, R. N., Evans, W. J. (1986) Am. J. Clin. Nutri. 43:910.
23. Fisher, E. C., Nelson, M. E., Frontera, W. R., Turksoy, R. N., Evans, W. J. (1986) J. Clin. Endocrinol. Metab. 62:1232.
24. Marcus, R., Cann, C., Madvig, P., Minkoff, J., Goddard, M., Bayer, M., Martin, M., Gaudiani, L., Haskell, W., Genant, H. (1985) Ann. Intern. Med. 102:158.
25. Wardlaw, G. M., Pike, A. M. (1986) Am. Jr. Clin. Nutr. 44:283.
26. Aloia, J. F., Vaswani, A. N., Yeh, J. K. (1983) Arch. Intern. Med. 143:1700.
27. Smith, R. W. (1967) Fed. Proc. 26:1736.
28. Lindsay, R., Hart, D. M., Forrest, C., Baird, C. (1980) Lancet 2:1151.
29. Riis, B. J., Rodbro, P., Christiansen, C. (1986) Calcif. Tissue Int. 38:318.
30. Gotfredsen, A., Nilas, L., Riis, B. J., Thomsen, K., Christiansen, C. (1986) Br. Med. J. 292:1098.
31. Cauley, J. A., Gutai, J., Sandler, R. B., LaPorte, R. E., Kuller, L. H., Sashin, D. (1986) Am. J. Epidemiol. 124:752.
32. Minaire, P., Meunier, P., Edouard, B., Bernard, J., Coupron, P., Bourret, J. (1974) Calcif. Tissue Res. 17:57.
33. Rambant, P. C., Smith, M. C., Mack, P. B., Vogel, J. M. (1978) In: *Biomedical results of Apollo*. NASA SP-368:303.
34. Johnston, C. C. Jr., Norton, J. A. Jr., Khairi, R. A., Longcope, C. (1979) In: Barzel, U. S. (ed) *Osteoporosis* II. New York: Grune & Stratton, pp. 91.
35. Longcope, C., Baker, R. S., Hui, S. L., Johnston, C. C. Jr. (1984) Maturitas 6:309.
36. Slemenda, C. W., Hui, S. L., Johnston, C. C., Longcope, C. (1986) Am. J. Epidemiol. 124:526.
37. Heaney, R. P., Recker, R. R., Saville, P. D. (1978) J. Lab. Clin. Med. 92:964.
38. Aitken, J. M., Hart, D. M., Smith, D. A. (1971) Clin. Sci. 41:233.
39. Gallagher, J. C., Riggs, B. L., DeLuca, H. F. (1980) J. Clin. Endocrinol. Metab. 51:1359.
40. Heaney, R. P. (1965) Am. J. Med. 39:877.
41. Stevenson, J. C., Hillyard, C. J., Abeyasekera, G., Phang, K. G., MacIntyre, I. (1981) Lancet 1:693.
42. Gallagher, J. C., Riggs, B. L., DeLuca, H. F. (1980) J. Clin. Endocrinol. Metab. 51:1359.
43. Francis, R. M., Peacock, M., Barkworth, S. A. (1984) Age and Ageing 13:14.

44. Nordin, B. E. C., Horsman, A., Marshall, D. H., Simpson, M., Waterhouse (1979) Clin. Orthop. Rel. Res. 140:216.
45. Gallagher, J. C., Riggs, B. L., Eisman, J., Hamstra, A., Arnaud, S. B., DeLuca, H. F. (1979) J. Clin. Invest. 64:729.
46. Heaney, R. P., Recker, R., Saville, P. D. (1978) J. Lab. Clin. Med. 92:953.
47. Riggs, B. L., Wahner, H. W., Melton, L. J., O'Fallon, W. M., Judd, H. L., Richelson, L. S. (1986) Am. Soc. Bone Min. Res. meeting, June 1986. J Bone Min. Res. 1(S-1):Abs #167.
48. Riis, B., Thomsen, K., Christiansen, C. (1987) N. Engl. J. Med. 316:173.
49. Recker, R. R., Saville, P., Heaney, R. (1977) Ann. Intern. Med. 87:649.
50. Tsai, K. S., Heath, H., Kumar, R., Riggs, B. L. (1984) J. Clin. Invest. 73:1668.
51. Riggs, B. L., Nelson, K. I. (1985) J. Clin. Endocrinol. Metab. 61:457.
52. Nordin, B. E. C., Baker, M. R., Horsman, A., Peacock, M. (1985) Am. J. Clin. Nutr. 42:470.
53. Peach, H. (1984) Community Med. 6:20.
54. Harju, E., Sotaniemi, E., Puranen, J., Lahti, R. (1985) Arch. Orthop. Trauma Surg. 103:408.
55. Parfitt, A. M., Rao, D. S., Stanciu, J., Villanueva, A. R., Kleerekoper, M., Frame, B. (1985) J. Cln. Invest. 76:2403.
56. Mazess, R. B., Mather, W. (1974) Am. J. Clin. Nutr. 27:916.
57. Parfitt, A. M. (1983) Lancet 1:1181.
58. Donaldson, C. L., Hulley, S. B., Vogel, J. M., Hattner, R. S., Bayers, J. H., McMillan, D. E. (1970) Metab. 19:1071.
59. Whedon, G. D. (1984) Calcif. Tissue Int. (Supp.) 36:146.
60. Young, D. R., Niklowitz, W. J., Brown, R. J., Jee, W. S. S. (1986) Bone 7:109.
61. Jones, H. H., Priest, J. D., Hayes, W. C. (1977) J. Bone Joint Surg. 59A:204.
62. Aloia, J. F., Cohn, S. H., Bab, T. (1978) Metab. 27:1793.
63. Cauley, J. A., Sandler, R. B., LaPorte, R. E., Kriska, A., Horn, D., Sashin, D. (1986) Am. J. Epidemiol. 124:525.
64. Smith, E. L., Reddan, W., Smith, R. E. (1981) Med. Sci. Spts. Exer. 13:60.
65. Pocock, N. A., Eisman, J. A., Yeates, M. G., Sambrook, P. N., Eberl, S. (1986) J. Clin. Invest. 78:618.
66. Chow, R. K., Harrison, J. E., Brown, C. F., Hajek, V. (1986) Arch. Phys. Med. Rehabil. 67:231.
67. Adinoff, A. D., Hollister, J. R. (1983) N. Engl. J. Med. 309:265.
68. Hancock, D. A., Asiedu-Offei, S., Atkinson, P. J., Reed, G. W., and Wright, V. (1978) Rheumatol. and Rehab. XVII:65.
69. Need, A. G., Philcox, J. C., Hartley, T. F., Nordin, B. E. C. (1986) Aust. NZ J. Med. 16:341.
70. Nissan, O. S., Lindholm, T. S., Elmstedt, E., Lindback, A., Lindholm, T. C. (1986) Arch. Orthop. Trauma Surg. 105:146.
71. Newman, N. M., Ling, R. S. M. (1985) Lancet 1:11.
72. Lamberg, B. A., Kuhlback, B. (1959) Scand. J. Clin. Lab. Invest. 11:351.
73. Lemann, J. Jr., Gray, R. W., Maierhofer, W. J., Cheung, H. S. (1985) Kidney Int. 28:951.
74. Transbol, I., Christensen, M. S., Jensen, G. F., Christiansen, C., McNair, P. (1982) Metab. 31:383.
75. Daniell, H. W. (1976) Arch. Intern. Med. 136:298.
76. Jensen, G. F. (1986) Eur. J. Clin. Invest. 16:239.
77. Baron, J. A. (1984) Am. J. Epidemiol. 119:9.

78. Michnovicz, J. J., Hershcopf, R. J., Naganuma, H., Bradlow, H. L., Fishman, J. (1986) N. Engl. J. Med. 315:1305.

79. Riggs, B. L., Seeman, E., Hodgson, S. F., Taves, D. R., O'Fallon, W. M. (1982) N. Engl. J. Med. 306:446.

80. Gerster, J. C., Charhon, S. A., Jaeger, P., Boivin, G., Briancon, D., Rostan, A., Baud, C. A., Meunier, P. J. (1983) Br. Med. J. 287:723.

81. Ad Hoc Committee Strategy Workshop for Osteoporosis Research, NIH, Bethesda; Editorial (1978) J. Am. Med. Assoc. 240.

82. Riggs, B. L. (1984) NIH Abstracts of Presentations of Health Consensus Development Conference on Osteoporosis: #167, p. 55 (abs).

83. Frost, H. M. (1979) Clin. Orthop. 143:227.

84. Anderson, C., Cape, R. D. T., Crilly, R. G., Hodsman, A. B., Wolfe, B. M. J. (1984) Calcif. Tissue Int. 36:341.

85. Reeve, J., Meunier, P. J., Parsons, J. A., Bernat, M., Bijvoet, O. L. M., Courpron, P., Edouard, C., Klenerman, L., Neer, R. M., Renier, J. C., Slovik, D., Vismans, F. J. F. E., Potts, J. T. Jr. (1980) Br. Med. J. 161:1340.

86. Aloia, J. F., Vaswani, A., Kapoor, A., Yeh, J. K., Cohn, S. H. (1985) Metab. 34:124.

87. Gennari, C., Chierichetti, S. M., Bigazzi, S., Fusi, L., Gonnelli, S., Ferrara, R., Zacchei, F. (1985) Current Therapeutic Res. 38:455.

88. Stepaniak, P. C., Furst, J. J., Woodward, D. (1986) Aviat. Space Environ. Med. 57:174.

89. Stern, P. H. (1985) Endocrinol. 117:2044.

90. Baker, S. P., Harvey, A. H. (1985) In: *Falls in the Elderly: Biological and Behavioral Aspects.* Philadelphia: W. B. Saunders, Clinics in Geriatric Medicine 1:501.

91. Garn, S. M. (1970) *The Earlier Gain and the Later Loss of Cortical Bone.* Springfield, IL.: Charles C. Thomas.

7

Magnesium Metabolism

RUTH SCHWARTZ

In 1932 Kruse et al. established the essentiality of magnesium by inducing magnesium deficiency in rats (1). One of the now classical series of articles that followed contained a description of the effects of magnesium depletion on bone (2). Despite marked retardation in overall growth, the magnesium-deficient rats had significantly heavier bones than controls, with greater ash and calcium content. Since the appearance of these reports, alterations in calcium metabolism and skeletal abnormalities have been among the most frequently cited aspects of magnesium deficiency. The varied and often contradictory changes reported include elevated or lowered plasma calcium levels (3–9); soft-tissue and, in particular, renal calcinosis (9–11); increased bone density (2, 4, 6, 12, 13); apparent defects in skeletal mineralization (12, 14–16); brittle or weak bones and teeth (15, 17, 18); abnormal bone morphology (4, 6, 13, 19, 20); and disturbances in parathyroid gland (PTG) function (3, 9, 21–24).

The published discrepancies in effects of magnesium deficiency on the skeleton and the processes that maintain its integrity can partly be ascribed to species differences and variations in experimental protocols. A major source of confusion in the past was the predominant use of rats in magnesium deficiency studies (6, 9, 11, 12, 14, 15, 18, 19). These provided the basis for the hypothesis—held long after observations made in other species proved it untenable—that magnesium and calcium shared homeostatic control mechanisms (9, 24). No evidence for hormonal regulation of magnesium homeostasis has emerged yet. It is becoming increasingly apparent, however, that magnesium participates in numerous reactions that regulate the homeostasis of calcium (23–28) and is a critical factor in bone formation, structure, and function (13–15, 19). What is not clear is whether the severe effects observed in experimental magnesium depletion can be extrapolated, as has been suggested, to implicate marginal magnesium status in the etiology of chronic bone diseases in human beings (29, 30).

MAGNESIUM HOMEOSTASIS

Body Distribution

The adult human body contains about 22–40 mg magnesium (31). Two-thirds of this amount is in the skeleton. About 19 percent is contained in skeletal muscle, and all but 1 percent of the remainder is distributed among the soft tissues (Table 7-1). The extracellular fluids and blood plasma account for the remaining 1 percent (31, 32). Fluid and tissue concentrations, also given in Table 7-1, range from 0.85–1.0 mM in plasma to 40–50 mM in bone (32, 33). Soft-tissue concentrations vary between 4 and 9 mM, depending partly on their content of connective tissue, which is relatively low in magnesium (31), and the metabolic level of a tissue. Organelles such as the nucleus, endoplasmic reticulum, or mitochondria are significantly higher in magnesium than the cytoplasm (34–37).

The first compartment to reflect magnesium depletion is plasma (8, 38). Red blood cell magnesium changes more slowly (32), possibly by dilution with newly formed magnesium-depleted erythrocytes. Skeletal and heart muscle magnesium can be diminished by 10 percent or more. Other soft tissues, including liver and kidney, retain normal or near normal magnesium concentrations, even during severe and prolonged magnesium depletion (24, 39). Whether any soft-tissue compartment can be regarded as a magnesium reserve is debatable (38). The relationship between skeletal and extracellular magnesium concentrations and its possible role in magnesium homeostasis will be discussed below.

Magnesium Absorption

Intestinal absorption appears of relatively minor importance in the regulation of magnesium homeostasis. Rates of magnesium absorption remain constant over a fairly wide range of dietary magnesium in man (40) or luminal magnesium concentration in rats (41, 42) and do not change measurably during magnesium depletion (40). At very low or high magnesium intakes or luminal concentrations, fractional absorption varies inversely with magnesium concentration, suggesting the presence of facilitated and saturable transport mechanisms (43, 45, 46).

Magnesium can be absorbed in man and rats from all segments of the gastrointestinal (GI) tract below the pyloric sphincter, as long as it is presented to the mucosa in soluble and available form (43, 47). When magnesium is consumed in the normal way, little or none seems to be absorbed from the colon, presumably

Table 7-1 Magnesium Content of Selected Tissue

Tissue	Species	Mg (mmole/kg)		Source
		Normal	Mg-deficient	
Plasma	Man	0.8	0.4	Walser, 1967 (32)
Erythrocytes	Man	2.1	1.6	Walser, 1967 (32)
Skeletal muscle	Man	8.3	—	Widdowson and Dickerson, 1964 (31)
Liver[a]	Rat[a]	9.1	8.4	—
Kidney	Rat[b]	8.2	8.8	—
Pancreas	Rat[c]	9.1	9.2	—
Bone	Rat	84	22	Jones et al., 1981 (53)

[a]Schwartz et al., 1969 (39).
[b]Kraeuter, 1975 (107).
[c]Greger and Schwartz, 1974 (106).

because it reaches the lower GI tract in nonabsorbable form (48). About 40–60 percent of dietary magnesium is absorbed from diets supplying 200–350 mg daily (40, 48). Endogenous fecal losses do not usually exceed 1–2 mmol/day (40, 49, 50).

Although magnesium absorption has been investigated in several species (42, 51–53), most of the data pertinent to absorption mechanisms in nonruminants were determined in rats by use of *in situ* ligated gut loops (43, 44, 53) or *in vitro* gut preparations (41, 42). Some data are available from kinetic studies in human beings using the short-lived radiotracer ^{28}Mg ($T^{1}/_{2}$ = 21.3 h) (45, 46, 48, 50) or by measuring luminal magnesium disappearance rates with intubation techniques (54, 55).

Mechanisms of magnesium absorption are incompletely understood. Areas of uncertainty include the relative rates and importance of magnesium absorption from segments of the small intestine (41, 42), whether magnesium transport is saturable or energy-dependent (40–45), is regulated by vitamin D status or its metabolites (54, 55), or whether magnesium competes with calcium for specific absorption sites (44). The rare, evidently genetically determined incidence of early-childhood hypomagnesemia with impaired magnesium absorption (17, 56) suggests the existence of magnesium-specific absorption site(s) or mechanism(s), at least during early development (53), but the location or nature of such a mechanism remains obscure. Currently, the most widely accepted concept of the characteristics of magnesium absorption is based on two studies by Behar (43, 44) in which ^{28}Mg transfer was measured *in situ* by perfusing ligated segments of rat ileum and colon. The data suggest a pattern of facilitated diffusion, augmented by solvent drag, with no evidence of a requirement for metabolic energy or for direct competition with calcium. Given the disagreement on the relative importance of the ileum in overall magnesium absorption (41, 42), it is important to enlarge these observations by comparative studies of magnesium absorption along different segments of the intestine.

Renal Excretion

The kidney is well established as a major locus of homeostatic control for magnesium. Plasma magnesium levels remain remarkably constant over a wide range of magnesium intake in individuals with unimpaired renal function. Normally, urinary magnesium closely matches the amount absorbed, changing rapidly as dietary magnesium levels are raised or lowered (8, 24, 57, 58). Particularly striking are the rapid excretion of injected magnesium and the reversal of elevated plasma magnesium levels in individuals with normal renal function (59). As far as is known, no hormone specifically regulates plasma magnesium or rates of renal excretion.

Mechanisms of renal tubular handling have been extensively investigated by micropuncture techniques (60, 61) and are fairly well established. Approximately three-fourths of the 70–80 percent of magnesium filtered through the glomerulus is free Mg^{2+} (60, 62). The remainder is complexed with phosphate and organic ligands (62). The data established so far on renal magnesium transport seem to relate only to total filtered magnesium without distinction between Mg^{2+} and other forms, although transfer rates may vary for different forms of magnesium.

About 20–30 percent of filtered magnesium is reabsorbed in passage through the straight proximal tubule, which is relatively impermeable to magnesium (60 percent of filtered water, sodium, and calcium is reabsorbed in this segment). Because of the relatively greater loss of water in the proximal tubule, the magnesium concentration of fluid entering the loop of Henle is 50–100 percent in excess of that of the glomerular filtrate (60, 61). No magnesium reabsorption has been observed in the descending limb of the loop of Henle, which may, in fact, add magnesium by secretion into the lumen when plasma magnesium is elevated (58), but this has not been confirmed. The major site of magnesium reabsorption is the thick ascending limb of the loop of Henle, where 50–60 percent of filtered magnesium is returned to the circulation. Additionally, 1–5 percent of the filtered load is transferred out of the distal tubule, the fraction varying inversely with luminal magnesium concentration (60).

An excellent review of renal tubular magnesium handling was published in 1986 by Quamme and Dirks (61). Whereas most of the studies on tubular magnesium transport were done in rats, the overall pattern appears to be similar in dogs and rabbits. It has not been possible so far to define cellular processes specifically linked to renal magnesium transport or to identify mechanisms of hormonal control. Parathyroid hormone and other peptide hormones whose action is mediated by cAMP have been found to increase reabsorption of magnesium in the loop of Henle of the hamster but apparently not in other species. Hypermagnesemia reduces magnesium reabsorption at this site by what has been termed a unique action at the contraluminal membrane. No tubular transport maximum for magnesium has been identified (60).

Skeletal Magnesium and Magnesium Homeostasis

Skeletal magnesium concentration can be 80 percent below normal in growing, severely magnesium-deficient animals (4, 6, 13, 32) (Table 7-2). Conversely, bone magnesium levels become elevated when plasma magnesium is raised, for instance, in rats fed excess magnesium (63) or in individuals with renal dysfunction (64, 65). The fraction of bone magnesium that can be released to the extracellular fluids varies with the age and stage of growth and with magnesium status (66, 67). The difference between exchangeable and nonexchangeable skeletal magnesium is not clear. However, the exchangeable fraction appears to be released or taken up by an entirely passive physicochemical process not dependent on biological regulation, suggesting that the labile fraction of bone magnesium is contained solely in the bone mineral phase.

Martindale and Heaton (68) found the amount of magnesium released *in vitro* to be of the same order from both boiled and live bone. Moreover, magnesium release from live bone was not significantly altered by parathyroid extract (PTE). When femurs from magnesium-depleted and control rats were incubated in solutions varying in magnesium content, bone magnesium loss or gain changed linearly with the concentration of magnesium in the medium. The slope describing

Table 7-2   Plasma and Bone Magnesium during Magnesium Depletion in Growing Rats

Days of depletion	Plasma Mg (mmole/l)	Bone Mg μmole/cm^3 (femur)
2	0.52 ± 0.03	55.3 ± 1.1
5	0.27 ± 0.04	39.1 ± 1.2
7	0.26 ± 0.02	22.7 ± 0.5
9	0.29 ± 0.03	22.1 ± 0.7
11	0.20 ± 0.01	23.7 ± 0.5
14	0.27 ± 0.01	23.4 ± 1.6
21	0.23 ± 0.01	21.8 ± 0.7
Control, day 21	1.03 ± 0.05	83.9 ± 2.5

Source: Jones et al., (6) (modified).

this relationship was similar for normal and magnesium-depleted bone, but the latter equilibrated (did not gain or lose magnesium) at a lower ambient magnesium concentration than control bone.

Similarly, Alfrey and Miller (64) found the release or gain of magnesium from iliac crest bone samples from normal and uremic individuals to relate almost linearly to the magnesium concentration of the bathing solution. In this instance, bone from uremics, which had a higher magnesium content than normal bone, equilibrated with medium more than twice as high in magnesium as did normal bone. Subsequently, Alfrey et al. (66) showed that the fraction of magnesium in rat femur was exchangeable *in vivo* with injected [28]Mg was directly proportional to the fraction that could be eluted *in vitro*. The elutable fraction was approximately 30, 26, and 16 percent in weanling, 2-month-old and 5 to 7-month-old rats, respectively. Magnesium depletion, which significantly lowered bone magnesium concentration, also decreased the *in vitro* elutable fraction and the fraction exchangeable with [28]Mg *in vivo*.

Data on the behavior of magnesium in synthetic crystalline hydroxyapatite (HAP) *in vitro* reinforce observations on exchangeable bone magnesium made *in vivo* and with live bone *in vitro*. The magnesium in synthetic HAP is thought to be surface bound by a physical force such as the zeta potential (69) or held in adherent hydration water (70). As HAP crystals age and enlarge, they extrude magnesium (71). Amorphous calcium phosphate (ACP), the precursor of HAP in *in vitro* systems, has a higher content of hydration water than ACP. Thus partially formed bone mineral, which may contain a relatively high proportion of ACP or other HAP precursors, can be expected to have a higher magnesium content in a form passively exchangeable with plasma magnesium than more mature bone mineral.

THE INFLUENCE OF MAGNESIUM ON BONE MINERAL

Formation of HAP from precursor phases *in vitro* is retarded by addition of magnesium to metastable calcium phosphate solutions (72, 73). In contrast to other HAP-retarding agents, such as ATP, diphosphonates, or pyrophosphates, which appear to prevent HAP crystal formation by surface poisoning, magnesium acts by stabilizing ACP and other HAP precursors. There is growing evidence that magnesium status exerts an effect on the rate of bone mineral formation and dissolution *in vivo*. The now well-substantiated resistance of magnesium-deficient bone to parathyroid hormone (PTH) stimulation (9, 23, 24, 74, 75) suggests the possibility of a shift of the equilibrium between bone HAP and its precursor forms. Unfortunately, no data are available on the crystallinity of magnesium-deficient bone mineral. On the other hand, mineral extracted from bones of hypermagnesemic rats and uremic patients has been found altered in crystal structure and behavior on heating (63, 64).

The influence of magnesium on HAP formation and crystal growth appears to be quite unique. Bone mineral, EDTA-extracted from bull femur diaphysis, increasingly lost calcium to solution as the medium magnesium concentration was raised (70). Uptake of calcium into the bone mineral was also increased by magnesium, suggesting surface exchange of magnesium for calcium on apatite crystals exposed to excess magnesium. In contrast, citrate, another ion that reduces bone mineral solubility, increases loss of calcium into ambient solution to a greater extent than equimolar magnesium but does not change calcium concentration in the crystalline phase. Unlike magnesium, citrate is incorporated into the HAP lattice, presumably by exchange with phosphate, and can be expected to alter crystallity by a change in apatite structure. Magnesium, on the other hand, primarily prevents or slows growth in crystal size and may further destabilize the crystal phase by surface exchange with calcium (70).

The effect of magnesium on apatite formation and stability is potentiated by interaction with ATP, which can retard apatite crystal growth by a process similar to that exerted by pyrophosphates or diphosphonates (72). These ions appear to absorb on surfaces of embryonic apatite crystals, hindering their growth and causing them to redissolve. In the process of interacting with the crystal surfaces, ATP is hydrolyzed and loses its influence on crystal growth. Magnesium stabilizes ATP by formation of $ATPMg^{2-}$, thereby enhancing the delay in crystal formation. The significance of this interaction in the regulation of bone mineralization is uncertain. It is thought to be an important mechanism for the prevention of intracellular calcification (72, 73). The presence of electron-dense, calcified mitochondria in myocardial tissue from magnesium-depleted rats (11) may be related to this mechanism.

A second group of substances of cellular origin that have been shown to interact with magnesium to retard HAP formation *in vitro* are calcium-acidic phospholipid phosphates (76, 77). The presence of these complexes in calcifying tissues and bone water suggests that they function in mineralization processes *in vivo*. Magnesium can compete with calcium for calcium-binding sites on phospholipids, although its affinity for them is much lower. To prevent formation of calcium-acidic phospholipid-phosphate complexes *in vitro* requries a magnesium:calcium ratio of 200:1, but HAP formation can be significantly retarded at lower magnesium concentrations by slowing the rate of formation of calcium phospholipid complexes. Once these are formed, magnesium ceases to affect phospholipid-induced HAP formation. *In vivo* magnesium probably prevents calcification at intracellular sites with exposed phospholipid residues where the magnesium:calcium ratio is high enough to hinder formation of calcium complexes. Whether magnesium similarly prevents the premature mineralization of matrix vesicles and modulates matrix vesicle-induced calcification in bone is not known.

MAGNESIUM AND CELLULAR METABOLISM

The rapid exchange of plasma magnesium with magnesium in bone (64–66) (see earlier), suggests that fluctuations in extraosseous magnesium concentration are transmitted to the bone fluid. That changes in bone fluid magnesium may influence bone cell development and function is still speculative, however, supported by observations on micro-organisms (78–81) and cultured fibroblasts (82, 83), an inconclusive study using bone cell culture (84), and information on the numerous and far-reaching roles of magnesium in cellular processes (85–94).

The most central role of magnesium in cells is its participation in reactions requiring $ATPMg^{2-}$ (85, 91, 93). In this role Mg participates in all biosynthetic reactions, glycolysis, energy-dependent transport processes, and the formation of cAMP (87, 90, 93). Free cytosolic magnesium, which varies inversely with pH and ATP concentration (87, 92), is thought to regulate important metabolic pathways by allosterically activating key enzymes such as brain glucokinase (90, 93). A high charge density and the resulting tendency to hydration distinguish magnesium from other divalent cations in the cell (95). Magnesium preferentially binds to phosphate groups, thereby stabilizing the double helix of DNA and other nucleoproteins and nucleic acids in both the nucleus (86, 89) and extranuclear organelles associated with protein synthesis (79, 88, 94). In fact, magnesium is essential for every step in the transmission of the genetic code. Although other divalent cations have been shown to substitute for magnesium in various enzymatic reactions *in vitro* (96), there is little doubt that magnesium is the element utilized *in vivo*. Not only are other divalent cations usually present in cells at concentrations too low for optimum activity, in many instances reactions carried out with substitute ions deviate from the normal course. An example is polymerization of DNA and RNA. When manganese or other divalent cations are substituted for magnesium, the rate of error nucleotide incorporation is greatly increased.

All cells in culture media have absolute requirements for magnesium to support growth and multiplication. This was first demonstrated with *E. coli* over 20 years ago (79) and, more recently, with a variety of micro-organisms (78, 80, 81). As reviewed by Walker (80), the cell division cycles of both prokaryotes and eukaryotic micro-organisms are intimately linked to the availability of magnesium and can be changed or arrested when magnesium is limiting. Of special interest are observations made on the fission yeast *Schizosaccharomyces pombe*, which undergoes characteristic morphological changes during the cell cycle, accompanied by alterations in cellular magnesium concentration that appear to be related to critical events before and during cell division (78).

Similar studies have not been feasible with cultured cells of higher organism that do not show such distinct morphological phases during the cell cycle. However, cultured chick embryo fibroblasts and BALB/c3T3 cells respond to extracellular magnesium deprivation by measurably decreasing the level of activities necessary for cell growth and division (82, 83). In this respect the effect of magnesium deprivation mimics the effects of changes in a number of growth effectors, for instance, elimination of serum, addition of cortisol, or increasing cell density. All such interventions induce a cascade of metabolic changes that include depression in hexose transport, glycolysis, and DNA and protein synthesis.

According to Rubin, the effect of magnesium deprivation is unique in that it alters the full cascade of reactions dependent on growth effectors (83). He proposed that magnesium was the central factor in cell growth and proliferation and that the action of other growth effectors was regulated by free intracellular magnesium via modulation of energy charge. He suggested further that the effects of calcium deprivation, which mimic those of magnesium restriction, could be the result of reductions in cytosolic magnesium due to magnesium binding to membrane binding sites freed by calcium (82). The inadequacy of current methods for measuring intracellular Mg^{2+} concentration has so far precluded tests of this interesting theory.

A magnesium-dependent cellular function with particular relevance to the sensitivity of bone cells to magnesium status is the regulation of hormone-sensitive adenylate cyclase (23, 25, 87). In addition to requiring $ATPMg^{2-}$ as a substrate, the receptor–cyclase complex, isolated from a number of different cells, including embryonic bone and osteosarcoma cells (23) has binding sites for Mg^{2+}. Grubbs and McGuire (87) have suggested that hormonal activation of the enzyme involves a form of the receptor cyclase complex that must include bound Mg^{2+}. However, dependence on $ATPMg^{2-}$ alone suggests a mechanism by which magnesium deprivation can blunt the sensitivity of osteocytes to parathyroid hormone, should intracellular Mg^{2+} become limiting.

SKELETAL ABNORMALITIES ASSOCIATED WITH MAGNESIUM DEPLETION

The most consistent finding in bones of magnesium-depleted animals is decreased magnesium content (4, 6, 13, 66). Other alterations frequently described are increased bone density and calcium content (2, 4, 13), defective or inadequate mineralization (12, 19), signs of severe growth retardation [both grossly and histologically (4, 14, 19)], deformed and exostotic bone (6, 7, 19), and the appearance of reduced bone resorption (4, 6, 7). Few attempts have been made to equalize growth rates in deficient and control animals. Moreover, with the exception of a few studies specifically designed to investigate the effects of marginal or subacute magnesium deprivation (6, 13, 15, 18), most observations were made in animals fed diets extremely low in magnesium. Such diets cause markedly reduced feed intakes and consequent undernutrition, which alone could account for some of the bone abnormalities ascribed to magnesium deprivation.

Although species other than the rat develop hypocalcemia as a result of magnesium depletion (7, 8, 9, 13, 24, 75), the rat has continued to be the preferred subject for magnesium deficiency studies. The tendency of this species to develop hypercalcemia when depleted of magnesium led to the hypothesis that hypomagnesemia stimulated hypersecretion of parathyroid hormone (PTH) (9, 97). Attempts were made to ascribe the changes in calcium homeostasis and bone morphology to secondary hyperparathyroidism until it became clear that PTH hypersecretion or parathyroid gland (PTG) hyperactivity was not a consistent feature of magnesium deficiency in rats (6, 16). So far no explanation has been advanced for the anomalous calcemic response of the magnesium-depleted rat. It has been suggested that the hypercalcemia frequently observed in hypomagnesemic rats may be due to the high calcium level of standard rat diets (9, 16), since hypocalcemia can be induced in rats only with diets deficient in calcium. Despite the species differences in calcium homeostasis, the bones of magnesium-deficient animals, including rats, show a number of common features suggesting that magnesium depletion rapidly alters the mineral as well as the cellular constituents of bone.

One of the earliest detailed accounts of histological manifestations of magnesium depletion in bone was published by Belanger in 1958 (14). He described severe growth retardation in rats with marked narrowing of the epiphyseal growth plate of the femur and significant reduction in radiolabeled sulfur and amino acid uptake at the plate. Later, he and his associates reported that the numbers of chondrocytes and newly formed trabeculae were reduced in the vicinity of the growth plate. The few osteocytes present appeared slim and inactive, surrounded by immature fibrillar matrix, suggesting reduced osteocytic osteolysis in addition to inadequate bone formation (19).

The rapid decrease in bone magnesium content of young growing magnesium-depleted animals (Table 7-2) (13, 32), suggests that bone cell development can occur in severely magnesium restricted environments. The possible consequence of lack of magnesium on newly forming bone is strikingly illustrated by the occurrence of massive subperiosteal hyperplasia which has so far been reported only in magnesium-depleted rats (6, 19). As first described by Hunt and Belanger (19) in weanling rats severely deprived of magnesium for 18–21 days, the lesion was confined to long bone-diaphyses at the point of muscle insertion. It appeared to consist of fibroblasts, collagen fibers, and sparse areas of ossification. Hunt and Belanger described the hyperplasia as an accumulation of inadequately differentiated osteoprogenitor cells. The lesion disappeared completely after only 7 days of magnesium repletion (19).

Subperiosteal hyperplasia, by all appearances similar to the lesion described by Hunt and Belanger, has been induced by Jones et al. (6) within a similar time frame in rats less severely deprived of magnesium. Although weight gains were only 20–25 percent less than those of rats fed an adequate diet *ad libitum,* plasma and bone magnesium levels decreased rapidly (Table 7-2). thickening of the periosteum was marked after only 7 days of magnesium depletion. By 21 days, the mass had progressed to a width that exceeded that of the femur and humerus shaft.

Whether subperiosteal hyperplasia is peculiar to the rat as a species or develops only when hypomagnesemia is accompanied by hypercalcemia is not known. It was not observed by Mirra et al. (16) in rats fed 10 ppm magnesium in a diet that contained only about 25–30 percent as much calcium as standard rat diets. Nor was subperiosteal hyperplasia seen in femurs of young magnesium-depleted chicks that otherwise showed morphological features similar to those found in comparably magnesium-depleted rats such as widened long-bone shafts and dense cortical bone with small, inactive-looking osteocytes (6, 13).

SKELETAL ABNORMALITIES ASSOCIATED WITH HYPERMAGNESEMIA

Few investigators have studied the skeletal effects of hypermagnesemia, possibly because it is difficult to induce elevations in plasma magnesium solely by dietary means. Excess magnesium in the diet or drinking water tends to produce diarrhea and depress food intake without consistently elevating plasma magnesium. One of the few investigations of magnesium excess was carried out by Alfrey and Miller (64) in uremic patients most of whom were also hypermagnesemic. Iliac crest bone from hypermagnesemic patients was found to contain a higher proportion of exchangeable magnesium than comparable bone from normomagnesemic people with or without uremia. There were, in addition, differences in crystal size and behavior of powdered bone upon heating.

Normal bone lost most of its capacity to take up magnesium from solution after being heated to 550°C. In contrast, bone from hypermagnesemic patients remained almost unchanged up to 550°C. At 550°C normal bone showed a sharp change in the X-ray diffraction pattern, suggesting an increase in crystallinity. Bone from hypermagnesemic uremics had to be heated to at least 25°C higher before similar changes in the X-ray diffraction pattern were seen. These findings are consistent with observations on the influence of magnesium on HAP formation *in vitro* (70, 72, 73) and were interpreted as showing that hypermagnesemic bone was relatively lower in HAP and higher in HAP precursors than normomagnesemic bone (64).

Two recent studies in which mice and rats were given large supplements of magnesium suggest that excess magnesium may, in addition, alter bone cell function (63, 99). The first, which was carried out in young mice (99), produced only minor, although significant, elevations in plasma and bone magnesium. At the same time, bone formation and resorption were significantly increased at the endosteal surfaces of caudal vertebrae. In the second study, Burnell et el. (63) fed diets containing about 10 times an adequate dietary level of magnesium supplemented with $AlPO_4$ to control the anticipated diarrhea. Plasma and bone magnesium increased by about 50 percent above normal levels. Periosteal bone formation was inhibited, and endosteal bone resorption increased. Mean crystal size of the bone mineral was significantly reduced by hypermagnesemia.

Additional research on the effects of hypermagnesemia with or without uremia would be desirable since hypermagnesemia is common in uremics (63, 64). Osteodystrophy, frequently associated with uremia, is usually ascribed to factors other than magnesium. However, the similarity of changes in the bones of uremic patients and hypermagnesemic rodents suggests at least a contributory role for hypermagnesemia in the etiology of skeletal abnormalities associated with renal dysfunction.

MAGNESIUM AND HORMONAL CONTROL OF CALCIUM HOMEOSTASIS

The hypothesis that magnesium homeostasis was regulated by parathyroid hormone (PTH) appeared to be supported by several observations. Magnesium-deficient parathyroidectomized rats did not develop hypercalcemia (9). Furthermore, plasma or medium magnesium concentrations were found inversely related to PTH output by perfused parathyroid glands (PTG) in vivo (9) or cultured PTG tissue in vitro (100–102). Frequently cited in support of the hypothesis is a study by Targovnic et al. (102) with cultured bovine PTG explants in media in which the total divalent cation concentration was kept constant while the ratio of calcium to magnesium was varied. The level of PTH in the medium did not vary significantly except at very low magnesium:calcium ratios when PTH output into the medium was reduced. Morrissey and Cohn (101) showed that magnesium could suppress PTH secretion but was only one-half to one-third as effective as equimolar calcium. Since the molar concentration of plasma magnesium is normally less than half that of calcium, PTH is unlikely to be effective in regulating plasma magnesium levels.

The theory that magnesium homeostasis depended on PTH remained viable for some time despite reports of hypocalcemia in magnesium-depleted animals (3, 5, 7) and man (8, 9, 21–24). As pointed out by Shils (9), its refutal was delayed by the inadequacy of early PTH assays and, when these became more reliable, by failure to relate precisely plasma PTH levels to plasma calcium. In patients with hypomagnesemia, for instance, plasma PTH levels have been reported normal (9, 22, 24), higher than normal (9, 22) and subnormal (21, 23). Decreased levels of PTH have been found in dogs (75) and hyperactivity of the PTG has been found in chicks (13). Since both of these species exhibit hypocalcemia when magnesium depleted, elevated PTH levels could indicate a normal PTG response. Low or normal PTH levels suggest PTG failure. It is now apparent that even elevated PTH levels may be inadequate relative to the severe hypocalcemia encountered in magnesium deficiency (9, 23, 75) and that, as indicated by the in vitro data reported by Targovnik et al. (102), normal PTG activity depends on a threshold level of ambient magnesium.

Shils (9, 24) suggested two discrete stages of parathyroid dysfunction during magnesium depletion. As plasma magnesium decreases, bone becomes resistant to the action of PTH by two mechanisms—the change in bone mineral as it becomes depleted of magnesium (see earlier) and the decreased ability of osteocytes to respond to PTH. The consequent decrease in plasma calcium initially triggers PTG hyperactivity and elevations in plasma PTH. With progressing magnesium depletion, the PTG may become exhausted, and plasma PTH levels may become low to undetectable. Thus contradictions in the literature regarding plasma PTH levels in magnesium deficiency may merely reflect different stages of magnesium depletion.

Intravenous injection of magnesium can increase plasma PTH within minutes in magnesium-deficient subjects (23). Such rapid response argues against PTG exhaustion and suggests, instead, that PTH secretion depends directly on extracellular magnesium concentration. Recent studies on the characteristics of PTG adenylate cyclase, which is thought to mediate PTH secretion support this suggestion (23, 25). The concentration of extracellular magnesium critically influences PTH secretion by parathyroid tissue *in vitro* (25). Like other adenylate cyclases (87), the PTG enzyme requires magnesium as $ATPMg^{2-}$ and free Mg^{2+} for activation of the membrane-bound enzyme GTP complex (23, 87).

Calcium suppresses the activity of adenylic cyclase, apparently by binding to one of two calcium-binding sites—a high-affinity site with a K_m of about 1.5– 2.0 μM, a concentration close to that in cell cytosol, and a low-affinity site with a K_m of about 250 μM. Maximum inhibition of PTH secretion and binding to the high-affinity calcium site occurs at medium magnesium concentrations of 0.5 mM or less. At successively higher magnesium levels, enzyme activity and PTH secretion are increased, and calcium binding is shifted toward proportionately greater predominance, of the low-affinity binding site (23). These data were obtained *in vitro* with isolated PTG membranes. The medium concentrations of calcium and magnesium were similar to plasma concentrations that could occur in magnesium depletion or excess, but they may not occur in the cell interior. The extent to which pathological intracellular deviations in plasma magnesium concentration influence activity is yet to be established.

The mechanism by which magnesium deficiency induces end organ resistance to PTH appears to be similar to that by which it exerts its effect on PTH secretion. Both renal and skeletal adenylate cyclase have been reported to be resistant to PTH stimulation in magnesium depletion (23). Like PTG adenylate cyclase, the membrane-bound enzyme of cells prepared from long-bone diaphyses of guinea pigs was found to be activated by GTP and magnesium and inhibited by calcium. It showed two calcium-binding sites with binding constants similar to those of the PTG enzyme complex, and similar quantitative responses to ambient calcium and magnesium concentrations.

RELATIONSHIP OF MAGNESIUM TO VITAMIN D

Magnesium absorption can be facilitated by vitamin D (54, 55). The effect is nonspecific, however, and does not appear to be linked to a mechanism for control of magnesium absorption. High doses of vitamin D have been reported to decrease plasma magnesium levels in rats by redistributing extracellular magnesium within the body (30), but the significance of these observations to the role of vitamin D in normal magnesium homeostasis is not clear. While vitamin D may not specifically regulate magnesium homeostasis, however, there is little doubt that magnesium status influences vitamin D metabolism. At the cellular level, magnesium is required for both steps in the hydroxylation of vitamin D (26, 103). Low serum concentrations of 1,25-dihydroxy vitamin D have been found in people with hypomagnesemia (27) and vitamin D-resistant rickets (104). Correction of hypomagnesemia corrected resistance to vitamin D.

A POSSIBLE ROLE FOR MAGNESIUM STATUS IN THE ETIOLOGY OF OSTEOPOROSIS

One of the characteristics of aging and osteoporotic bone is increased crystallinity (105). Cohen et al. (29) found mean bone mineral crystallinity, measured by infrared absorption spectrophotometry, higher in iliac crest biopsy samples from 19 postmenopausal osteoporotic women than in similar samples from 10 age-matched controls. Significantly lower mean crystallinity was found in iliac crest samples from five postmenopausal uremic patients who showed no signs of bone disease. Magnesium status, which was determined by bone magnesium and retention of an intravenous magnesium load, was found significantly lower than control in the osteoporotic group and significantly higher in the uremic patients.

These findings are provocative but need to be confirmed in larger numbers of patients. The link of low bone magnesium or increased crystallinity to osteoporosis is still tenuous. When undermineralized or apparently osteoporotic bone was seen in experimental magnesium deficiency, it occurred in growing animals after prolonged magnesium depletion with growth retardation (15, 16, 18). It is unlikely that magnesium depletion of comparable degree and duration could go undetected in the population at risk of developing osteoporosis.

SUMMARY

The numerous and far-reaching cellular roles of magnesium include all reactions involving ATP, the regulation of energy charge, energy-dependent transport, generation of cAMP, and transmission of the genetic code. Magnesium also influences critically the rate of formation and physical structure of hydroxyapatite (HAP). It is not surprising, therefore, that severe magnesium depletion or excess causes abnormalities in bone mineral as well as alterations in the cellular components of bone.

Two-thirds or more of body magnesium is in the skeleton, primarily in bone mineral, surface-bound on HAP crystals, or in adherent hydration water. The equilibrium between plasma and bone magnesium appears to be entirely physicochemical and not under biological control. Only a fraction of bone magnesium is accessible for exchange with magnesium in the plasma, however, the available portion decreasing with age and magnesium depletion.

Derangements in bone morphology and function, and disturbances in calcium homeostasis are among the earliest and most frequently reported consequences of magnesium depletion. Initially thought due to excess parathyroid hormone (PTH) secretion, it is now becoming apparent that lack of magnesium alone can account for many of the bone abnormalities. It is clear, moreover, that magnesium is required both for PTH secretion and for its interaction with renal and skeletal cells. Some of the features of experimentally induced hypomagnesemic or hypermagnesemic bone are seen in chronic diseases such as osteoporosis or the osteodystrophy associated with uremia. Further research is needed to evaluate the possible role of magnesium in the etiology of osteoporosis and osteodystrophy.

REFERENCES

1. Kruse, H. D., Orent, E. R., McCollum, E. V. (1932) J. Biol. Chem. 96:519–539.

2. Orent, E. R., Kruse, H. D., McCollum, E. V. (1934) J. Biol. Chem. 106:573–593.

3. Breitenbach, R. P., Gonnerman, W. A., Erfling, W. L., Anast, C. S. (1973) Am. J. Physiol. 225:12–17.

4. Chou, H. F., Schwartz, R., Krook, L., Wasserman, R. H. (1979) Cornell Vet. 69:88–103.

5. Dunn, M. J. (1971) Clin. Sci. 41:333–344.

6. Jones, J. E., Schwartz, R., Krook, L. (1980) Calcif. Tiss. Int. 31:231–238.

7. Reddy, C. R., Coburn, J. W., Hartenbower, D. L., Friedler, R. M., Brickman, A. S., Massry, S. G., Jowsey, J. (1973) J. Clin. Invest. 52:3000–3010.

8. Shils, M. E. (1969) Ann. NY Acad. Sci. 162:847–855.

9. Shils, M. E. (1980) Ann. NY Acad. Sci. 355:165–180.

10. Heaton, F. W., Anderson, C. K. (1965) Clin. Sci. 28:99–106.

11. Heggtveit, H. A., Herman, L., Mishra, R. K. (1964) Am. J. Pathol. 45:757–782.

12. Duckworth, J., Godden, W., Warnock, G. M. (1940) Biochem. J. 34:97–108.

13. Welsh, E. J., Schwartz, R., Krook, L. (1981) J. Nutr. 111:514–524.

14. Bélanger, L. F. (1958) J. Histochem. Cytochem. 6:146–153.

15. Heroux, O., Peter, D. W., Tanner, H. A. (1975) Can. J. Physiol. Pharmacol. 53:304–310.

16. Mirra, J. H., Alcock, N. A., Shils, M. E., Tannenbaum, P. (1982) Magnesium 1:16–33.

17. Milla, P. J., Aggett, P. J., Wolff, O. H., Harries, J. T. (1979) Gut. 20:1028–1033.

18. Watchorn, E., McCance, R. A. (1937) Biochem. J. 31:1379–1390.

19. Hunt, B. J., Bélanger, L. F. (1972) Calcif. Tiss. Res. 9:17–27.

20. Schwartz, R., Reddi, A. H. (1979) Calcif. Tiss. Int. 29:15–20.

21. Anast, C., Mons, J., Kaplan, S., Burns, J. (1972) Science 177:606–608.

22. Connor, T. B., Toskes, P., Mahaffey, J., Martin, L. G., Williams, J., Walser, M. (1972) Johns Hopkins Med. J. 131:100–117.

23. Rude, R. K., Oldham, S. B. (1987) In: Altura, B. M., Durlach, J., Seelig, M. S. (eds) *Magnesium in Cellular Processes and Medicine*. Basel: Karger, p 183.

24. Shils, M. E. (1988) Ann. Rev. Nutr. 8:429–460.

25. Mahaffee, D. D., Cooper, C. W., Ramp, W. K. (1982) Endocr. 110:487–495.

26. Carpenter, T. O., Carner, D. L. Jr., Anast, C. S. (1987) Am. J. Physiol. 253:E106–E113.

27. Rude, R. K., Adams, J. S., Ryzen, R., Enders, D. B., Hiroo, N., Horst, R. L., Haddad, J. G., Singer, F. R. (1985) J. Clin. Endocr. Metab. 61:933–940.

28. Tufts, E. V., Greenberg, D. M. (1938) J. Biol. Chem. 122:715–726.

29. Cohen, L., Laor, A., Kitzes, R. (1983) Magnesium 2:70–75.

30. Seelig, M. S. (1980) New York: Plenum, p 358.

31. Widdowson, E. M., Dickerson, J. W. T. (1964) In: Comar, C. L., Bronner, F. (eds) *Mineral Metabolism,* Vol 2, Pt A. New York: Academic Press, p 2.

32. Walser, M. (1967) Rev. Physiol. Biochem. Exp. Pharmacol. 59:185–296.

33. Lowenstein, F. W., Stanton, M. F. (1986) J. Am. Coll. Nutr. 5:399–414.

34. Greger, J. L., Schwartz, R. (1974) J. Nutr. 104:1618–1629.

35. Griswold, R. L., Pace, N. (1956) Exp. Cell Res. 11:362–367.

36. Rose, I. A. (1968) Proc. Nat. Acad. Sci. 67:1079–1086.

37. Thiers, R. E., Vallee, B. L. (1957) J. Biol. Chem. 226:911–920.

38. Elin, R. J. (1987) Clin. Chem. 33:1965–1970.

39. Schwartz, R., Wang, F. L., Woodcock, N. A. (1969) J. Nutr. 97:185–193.

40. Wilkinson, R. (1976) In: Nordin, B. E. C. (ed) *Calcium Phosphate and Magnesium Metabolism.* New York: Churchill Livingstone, p 36.

41. Aldor, T. A. M., Moore, E. W. (1970) Gastroent. 59:745–753.

42. Ross, D. B. (1962) J. Physiol. 160:417–428.

43. Behar, J. (1974) Am. J. Physiol. 227:334–340.

44. Behar, J. (1975) Am. J. Physiol. 229:1590–1595.

45. Danielson, B. G., Johansson, G., Jung, B., Ljunghall, S., Lundquist, H., Malmborg, P. (1979) Min. Electr. Metab. 2:116–123.

46. Graham, L. A., Caesar, J. J., Burgen, A. S. V. (1960) Metab. 9:646–659.

47. Chutkow, J. G. (1964) J. Lab. Clin. Med. 63:71–79.

48. Schwartz, R. (1984) In: Turnlund, J. R., Johnson, P. E. (eds) *Stable Isotopes in Nutrition.* ACS Symposium Series No. 258. Washington, DC: American Chemical Society, p 77.

49. Aikawa, J. K., Gordon, G. S., Rhoades, E. L. (1960) J. Appl. Physiol. 15:503–507.

50. Avioli, L. V., Berman, M. (1966) J. Physiol. 226:653–674.

51. Aikawa, J. K. (1959) Proc. Soc. Exptl. Biol. Med. 100:293–295.

52. Care, A. D., Van't Clooster, A. Th. (1965) J. Physiol. 177:174–191.

53. Meneely, R., Lepper, L., Gishan, F. K. (1982) Pediat. Res. 16:295–298.

54. Norman, D. A., Fordtran, J. S., Brinkley, L. J., Zerwekh, J. E., Nicar, M. J., Strowig, S. M., Pak, C. Y. C. (1981) J. Clin. Invest. 67:1599–1603.

55. Schmulen, A. C., Lerman, M., Pak, C. Y. C., Zerwekh, J., Morawski, S., Fordtran, J. S., Vergne-Marini, P. (1980) Am. J. Physiol. 238:G349–G352.

56. Paunier, L., Radde, I. C., Kooh, S. W., Fraser, D. (1965) Pediat. 41:385–402.

57. Fitzgerald, M. G., Fourman, P. (1956) Clin. Sci. 15:635–647.

58. Heaton, F. W. (1969) Ann. NY Acad. Sci. 162:775–785.

59. Nordin, B. E. C. (1976) In: Nordin, B. E. C. (ed) *Calcium, Phosphate, and Magnesium Metabolism.* New York: Churchill Livingstone, p 208.

60. Quamme, G. A. (1986) Magnesium 5:248–272.

61. Quamme, G. A., Dirks, J. H. (1986) Renal Physiol. 9:257–269.

62. Walser, M. (1973) In: Orloff, J., Berliner, R. W. (eds) *Handbook of Physiology. Renal Physiology.* Washington, DC: American Physiological Society, p 555.

63. Burnell, J. M., Liu, C., Miller, A. G., Teubner, E. J. (1986) Am. J. Physiol. 250:F302–F307.

64. Alfrey, A. C., Miller, N. L. (1973) J. Clin. Invest. 52:3019–3027.

65. Alfrey, A. C., Miller, N. L., Trow, R., Contiguglia, S. R. (1973) J. Clin. Res. 21:28.

66. Alfrey, A. C., Miller, N. L., Trow, R. (1974) J. Clin. Invest. 52:1074–1081.

67. Breibart, S., Lee, J. S., McCoord, A., Forbes, G. (1960) Proc. Soc. Exp. Biol. Med. 105:361–363.

68. Martindale, L., Heaton, F. W. (1965) Biochem. J. 97:440–443.

69. Brommage, R., Neuman, W. F. (1979) Calcif. Tiss. Int. 28:57–63.

70. Pak, C. Y. C., Diller, E. C. (1969) Calcif. Tiss. Res. 4:69–77.

71. Neuman, W. F., Mulryan, B. J. (1971) Calcif. Tiss. Res. 7:133–138.

72. Betts, F., Blumenthal, N. C., Posner, A. S. (1980) J. Crystal Growth 53:63–73.

73. Blumenthal, N. C., Betts, F., Posner, A. S. (1977) Calcif. Tiss. Res. 23:245–250.

74. Freitag, J. J., Martin, K. J., Conrades, M. B., Klahr, S., Slatopolsky, E. (1978) J. Clin. Invest. 64:1238–1244.
75. Levi, J., Massry, S., Coburn, J., Llach, F., Kleeman, C. (1974) Metabolism 23:323–335.
76. Boskey, A. L., Posner, A. S. (1980) Calcif. Tiss. Int. 32:139–144.
77. Wuthier, R. E., Eanes, E. D. (1975) Calcif. Tiss. Res. 19:197–210.
78. Duffus, J. H., Patterson, L. J. (1974) Z. Allg. Mikrobiol. 14:727–729.
79. McCarthy, B. J. (1962) Biochim. Biophys. Acta. 55:880–888.
80. Walker, G. M. (1986) Magnesium 5:9–23.
81. Walker, G. M., Duffus, J. H. (1980) J. Cell. Sci. 42:329–356.
82. Rubin, H. (1975) J. Cell. Physiol. 91:449–458.
83. Rubin, A. H., Terasaki, M., Sanui, H. (1979) Proc. Nat. Acad. Sci. 76:3917–3921.
84. Nielsen, S. P. (1973) Calcif. Tiss. Res. 11:78–94.
85. Eichhorn, G. L. (1973) In: Eichhorn, G. L. (ed) *Inorganic Biochemistry*. New York: Elsevier, p 1191.
86. Eichhorn, G. L. (1981) In: Eichhorn, G. L., Marzilli, L. G. (eds) Metal ions in genetic information transfer. New York: Elsevier/North-Holland, p 1.
87. Grubbs, R. D., McGuire, M. E. (1987) Magnesium 7:113–127.
88. Grunberg-Manago, M., Hui Bon Hoa, G., Douzow, P., Wishnia, A. (1981) In: Eichhorn, G. L., Marzilli, L. G. (eds) *Metal Ions in Genetic Information Transfer*. New York: Elsevier/North-Holland, p 193.
89. Kornberg, T., Gefter, M. L. (1971) Proc. Nat. Acad. Sci. 68:761–764.
90. Livingston, D. M., Wacker, W. E. C. (1976) In: Aurbach, G. D. (ed) *Handbook of Physiology*. Vol. 7. Washington, DC: American Physiological Society, p 215.
91. Mildvan, A. S. (1987) Magnesium 6:12–17.
92. Rasmussen, H., Goodman, D. P. B., Friedmann, N., Allen, J. E., Kurokawa, K. (1976) In: Aurbach (ed) *Handbook of Physiology*, vol. 7. Washington, DC: American Physiological Society, p 225.
93. Wacker, W. E. C. (1980) *Magnesium and Man*. Cambridge, MA: Harvard University Press, p 11.
94. Yi, Q. M., Wong, K. P. (1982) Biochem. Biophys. Res. Comm. 104:733–739.
95. Williams, D. R. (1971) *The Metals of Life: The Solution Chemistry of Metal Ions in Biological Systems*. New York: D. Van Nostrand, p 8.
96. Loeb, L. A., Mildvan, A. S. (1981) In: Eichhorn, G. L., Marzilli, L. G. (eds) *Metal Ions in Genetic Information Transfer*. New York: Elsevier/North-Holland, p 125.
97. Aikawa, J. K. (1981) *Magnesium: Its Biologic Significance*. Boca Raton, IL: CRC Press, p 51.
98. Burnell, J. M., Miller, A. G., Teubner, E. J. (1978) Clin. Res. 26:164.
99. Marie, P. J., Travers, R., Delvin, E. E. (1983) Calcif. Tiss. Int. 35:755–761.
100. Habener, J., Potts, J. (1976) Endocr. 98:197–202.
101. Morrissey, J. J., Cohn, D. V. (1978) Endocr. 103:2081–2090.
102. Targovnik, J. H., Rodman, J. S., Sherwood, L. M. (1971) Endocr. 88:1477–1482.
103. DeLuca, H. F. (1979) Nutr. Rev. 37:162–193.
104. Reddy, V., Sivakumar, B. (1974) Lancet I:963–965.
105. Baud, E., Pouezat, J., Tochon-Danguy, H. (1976) Calcif. Tiss. Res. 21:supp pp 452–456.
106. Greger, J. L., Schwartz, R. (1974) J. Nutr. 104:1610–1617.
107. Kraeuter, S. L. (1975) PhD Thesis. Cornell University, Ithaca NY.

8

The Vitamin D Endocrine System

HARRIET S. TENENHOUSE

The importance of the vitamin D endocrine system in the regulation of calcium homeostasis is well recognized. Studies over the past two decades have established that vitamin D must undergo two hydroxylation reactions, first in the liver and then in the kidney, before it can assume its physiological role as a major calciotropic hormone. The molecular events involved in the regulation of vitamin D hormone biosynthesis and the mechanisms whereby the vitamin D hormone elicits its biological response in target tissues require further definition. However, with recent technological advances in cellular and molecular biology, new insights into our understanding of the vitamin D endocrine system have been forthcoming. The following discussion reviews the current status of vitamin D chemistry, biology, and pathophysiology. To compensate for incompleteness, the reader is referred to a number of other surveys of vitamin D metabolism and function (1–13). These papers will be referred to when the primary citations are too numerous for the scope of the present review.

CHEMISTRY OF VITAMIN D

Vitamin D is a secosteroid in which the 9–10 carbon bond of the cyclopentano-perhydrophenanthrene B ring is broken, allowing the A ring to become inverted from the C and D rings with rotation occurring around the bond between C-7 and C-8 (see Fig. 8-1). The important aspects of vitamin D chemistry center about its *cis*-triene structure. This conjugated double-bond system (between C-19 and C-10, C-5 and C-6, C-7 and C-8) gives vitamin D a characteristic UV absorption maximum at 265 nm and absorption minimum at 228 nm. The ratio of absorbance at 265 nm to that at 228 nm serves as an index of vitamin D purity and is 1.8 for the purified crystalline compound. The molar extinction coefficient of vitamin D at 265 nm is 18,200. The *cis*-triene structure also confers on vitamin D its susceptibility to oxidation and other chemical transformations. Vitamin D is stable when stored in dry form in a moisture-free inert atmosphere and protected from light in a freezer. In solution, vitamin D undergoes a dynamic equilibrium between two chair conformations of the A ring. This interchange, which occurs

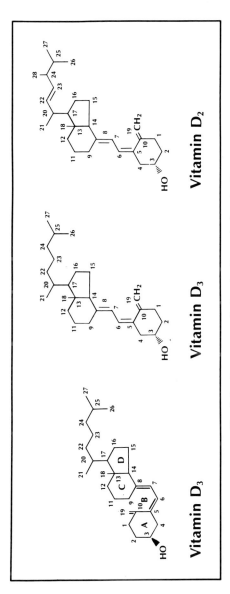

Fig. 8-1 Structures of vitamin D_3 and vitamin D_2.

several times per second, must be taken into account to understand the structure–function relationship of vitamin D.

Vitamin D occurs in two active forms, ergocalciferol (vitamin D_2) and cholecalciferol (vitamin D_3), which differ in the C-20 side chain structure (see Fig.8-1). Ergocalciferol, which has an extra methyl group on the 24th carbon and a double bond between the 22nd and 23rd carbons, is a synthetic metabolite made by UV irradiation of the plant sterol ergosterol. Cholecalciferol is formed in the skin by the action of UV irradiation on 7-dehydrocholesterol (see Biosynthesis of Vitamin D). Vitamins D_2 and D_3 are equally active in humans and other mammals, indicating that both metabolites are transported through the circulation and metabolized in a similar fashion. In birds, however, vitamin D_2 is virtually inactive.

BIOSYNTHESIS OF VITAMIN D

Vitamin D_3 is produced in the skin from 7-dehydrocholesterol, a final intermediate in cholesterol biosynthesis found in all of the epidermal strata (see Fig. 8-2). The conversion of 7-dehydrocholesterol to vitamin D_3 occurs by a nonenzymatic, photochemically mediated reaction with energy derived from environmental UV light between 290 and 315 nm (14). The 9–10 bond in the B ring of 7-dehydrocholesterol is thus cleaved to generate previtamin D_3 which undergoes thermal isomerization to vitamin D_3. Whereas the photolytic reaction producing previtamin D_3 is rapid, the isomerization to vitamin D_3 occurs by a slow, nonenzymatic rearrangement at a rate that is determined by skin temperature. In warm-blooded mammals, including man, it takes approximately 24 h for 50 percent of previtamin D_3 to isomerize to the thermally more stable vitamin D_3. At 37 °C the thermal

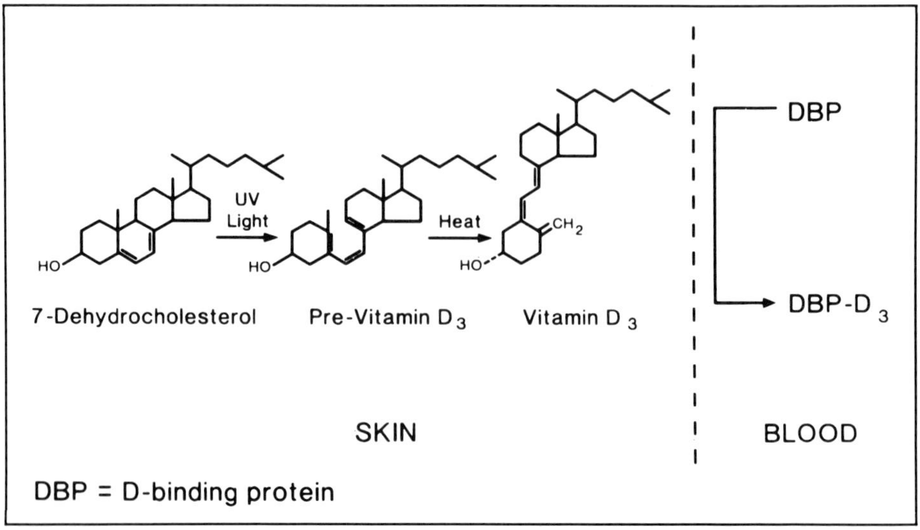

Fig. 8-2   Formation of vitamin D_3 in the skin. [From Audran and Kumar (12). With permission.]

isomerization of previtamin D_3 is more rapid *in vivo* than *in vitro*. This difference is presumed to be due to the translocation of vitamin D_3 from the skin into the circulation by a specific vitamin D-binding protein (DBP; see Transport of Vitamin D metabolites in Blood). Once 10–15 percent of 7-dehydrocholesterol in skin is photolytically converted to previtamin D_3, an equilibrium is established, and with further irradiation, previtamin D_3 readily isomerizes to lumisterol$_3$ and tachysterol$_3$, which are biologically inert products and have a very low affinity for DBP (15). It is therefore not likely that an intoxicating amount of vitamin D_3 is generated in the skin as a result of excessive exposure to sunlight.

The regulation of cutaneous synthesis of vitamin D_3 has been studied by Holick *et al.*, who reported that melanin is an effective UV radiation absorber and thereby competes with 7-dehydrocholesterol for UV photons, thus limiting previtamin D_3 production (15). Previtamin D_3 formation is also decreased in populations who infrequently go outdoors or who reside in northern latitudes (16). It has also been determined that aging significantly decreases the capacity of human skin to produce vitamin D_3 and that this may be related to an age-dependent decrease in 7-dehydrocholesterol stores in human epidermis, where greater than 85 percent of cutaneous previtamin D_3 is formed (16). These findings tend to implicate impaired UV-irradiated vitamin D_3 formation in the skin as one of the factors contributing to age-related diseases of calcium metabolism.

The skin also has the capacity to form 24-dehydrovitamin D_3 from the 24-dehydroderivative of 7-dehydrocholesterol, which accounts for 20–25 percent of total 7-dehydrocholesterol in the skin (17). The physiological role of 24-dehydrovitamin D_3, which, like vitamin D_3, is synthesized by photolytic and isomerization reactions in skin and is specifically translocated into the circulation by DBP, remains to be determined.

The demonstration of specific, high-affinity cytosolic receptors for $1,25(OH)_2D_3$, the active vitamin D hormone, in the skin of various species has led to the suggestion that skin is also a target organ for the vitamin D hormone. Indeed, Esvelt et al. reported that $1,25(OH)_2D_3$ caused a four-fold increase in rat skin 7-dehydrocholesterol, suggesting that the vitamin D hormone may exert positive feedback regulation on the production of vitamin D_3 in skin (18). In addition, it has been demonstrated that $1,25(OH)_2D_3$ has the potential of regulating the differentiation of receptor-positive keratinocytes in culture (19).

TRANSPORT OF VITAMIN D METABOLITES IN BLOOD

Because of their hydrophobic nature, the vitamin D metabolites (D_2 and D_3) are transported in the blood bound to a specific transport protein, vitamin D-binding protein (DBP). The identity of DBP with the polymorphic group-specific component (G_c) was recognized in 1975, and more than 120 variants of the GC/DBP system have since been described (20). DBP has been detected in the plasma of many species as well as in over 100,000 human sera so far examined, suggesting that DBP gene deletion would be a lethal mutation. DBP is an α-globulin which is synthesized in the liver and represents about 6 percent of the total α-globulin pool. It is a single polypeptide chain of 57 kD with approximately 1–2 percent carbohydrate and an isoelectric point of 4.6–4.9, determined in part by the sialic acid content. Each DBP binds one molecule of vitamin D sterol with the affinity for 25-OH-D$_3$ and 24,25(OH)$_2$D$_3$, somewhat higher than that for the vitamin D parent compound and 1,25(OH)$_2$D$_3$, the vitamin D hormone. Previtamin D has a low binding affinity for DBP and therefore remains in the skin. The plasma concentration of DBP is approximately 5 μM in man and does not appear to vary with vitamin D status, age, or sex. Various hormonal agents, however, have been shown to modulate circulating DBP in blood, and under normal conditions less than 5 percent of total DBP is saturated with ligand. The reason for such an abundance of DBP remains unknown (21).

DBP does not appear to facilitate the entry of vitamin D metabolites into specific target tissues, as is the case of other carrier proteins. In fact the unbound hormone is believed to permeate the lipophilic cell membrane freely before binding to cytoplasmic and/or nuclear receptors. As a result, it is the free and not the total hormone concentration that is thus available for cellular entry and induction of the cellular response. The free fraction of vitamin D metabolites represents 0.03–1 percent of the total pool (22).

In addition to binding and transport of vitamin D metabolites, DBP may facilitate the production of vitamin D in skin by displacing the equilibrium between previtamin D$_3$ and vitamin D$_3$ (see Biosynthesis of Vitamin D$_3$). The demonstration that DBP binds monomeric or G-actin with a high affinity has led to the suggestion that DBP may play an important role in the depolymerization of viscous F-actin, released after cell destruction (21). The demonstration of proteins immunologically related to DBP in tissues other than the liver has led to the speculation that DBP may have additional functions. The origin of immunologically reactive "DBP" in extrahepatic tissues is still open to question. It is reasonable to assume that the recent availability of a cloned full length cDNA probe for DBP will allow the systematic investigation of DBP gene expression and its regulation in both hepatic and extrahepatic tissues (23).

INTESTINAL ABSORPTION AND ENTEROHEPATIC CIRCULATION OF VITAMIN D METABOLITES

Ingested vitamin D is absorbed in the small intestine, and efficiency of absorption is determined by the composition of the luminal fluid. In the absence of bile salts or under conditions where chylomicron production is inhibited, intestinal absorption of vitamin D is markedly reduced. In an effort to understand the superior absorption of 25-OH-D$_3$ in patients with malabsorption, Sitrin et al. compared the *in vivo* absorption of physiological amounts of vitamin D$_3$ and 25-OH-D$_3$ from jejunal sacs in the rat (24). They found that absorption of 25-OH-D$_3$ was greater than absorption of vitamin D, that taurocholate enhanced absorption of vitamin D and 25-OH-D$_3$ in the presence of high luminal fat, whereas in the presence of low luminal fat, taurocholate was without affect, and finally that the majority of both metabolites was transported from the intestine into portal blood rather than lymph. In contrast, studies from another laboratory demonstrated that absorption of vitamin D and 25-OH-D$_3$ into the portal circulation plays only a minor role in their total absorption from the intestine (25). Furthermore, it was found that whereas 80 percent of vitamin D was recovered in the chylomicrons, 94 percent of 25-OH-D$_3$ was recovered in the protein fraction associated with α-globulin (25).

The intestinal absorption of 1,25 (OH)$_2$D$_3$ from *in vivo* jejunal sacs was also studied in the rat. Only 7 percent was recovered in lymph, indicating that 1,25(OH)$_2$D$_3$ is absorbed almost entirely *via* portal blood. In addition, the absorption of the vitamin D hormone was not dependent on bile salts and was not decreased by agents inhibiting chylomicron formation (26). These results may explain why oral 1,25(OH)$_2$D$_3$ is effective for correcting calcium malabsorption and treating metabolic bone disease in patients with gastrointestinal disorders associated with the malabsorption of lipid.

The role of the enterohepatic circulation on vitamin D economy has been the subject of considerable controversy. The demonstration by Arnaud et al. of considerable biliary excretion and enterohepatic cycling of intravenously injected [3]H-25-OH-D$_3$ suggested the existence of a large conservative enterohepatic circulation for 25-OH-D$_3$ in man (27). However, these investigators failed to determine how much of the biliary radioactivity appeared as 25-OH-D$_3$. In contrast, studies by Clements et al. in man (28) and by Gascon-Barré in rat (29) indicated that there was insufficient vitamin D or 25-OH-D$_3$ in bile for the reabsorption of these metabolites to make a significant contribution to normal vitamin D status. Therefore, interference with an enterohepatic circulation of vitamin D metabolites cannot be a cause of vitamin D deficiency, as was originally proposed, and cannot account for the vitamin D deficiency associated with malabsorptive disease and the consumption of high-fiber diets.

HEPATIC METABOLISM OF VITAMIN D AND EFFECT OF XENOBIOTICS

Vitamin D produced in the skin or ingested in the diet is hydroxylated at the C-25 position to form 25-hydroxyvitamin D$_3$ (25-OH-D$_3$), the major circulating vitamin D steroid (see Fig 8-3). It is generally agreed that the liver is the principal physiological site for the 25-hydroxylation of vitamin D, although evidence has accumulated for extrahepatic production of 25-OH-D$_3$ in several species (30). Whereas both hepatocytes and nonparenchymal cells prepared from rat liver can accumulate vitamin D, 25-hydroxlation *in vitro* was found to be carried out exclusively by hepatocytes (31). The nonparenchymal cells of liver may therefore serve as a storage site for vitamin D. The production of 25-OH-D$_3$ occurs in both the liver mitochondrial and microsomal fractions and appears to be catalyzed by a cytochrome P-450 mixed-function oxidase.

Cytochrome P-450, recently purified from rat liver microsomes, was shown to mediate specifically the 25-hydroxylation of vitamin D$_3$ and other C$_{27}$ steroids (32). The failure of this purified cytochrome P-450 to 25-hydroxylate vitamin D$_2$, a substrate that is 25-hydroxylated by rats *in vivo*, suggests that yet another mixed-function oxidase must be involved in the hepatic conversion of vitamin D to 25-OH-D$_3$. The recent findings that 25-hydroxylase activity is restricted to the mitochondrial fraction of human liver (33) and that the mitochondrial, but not microsomal, 25-hydroxylase activity correlates best with plasma levels of

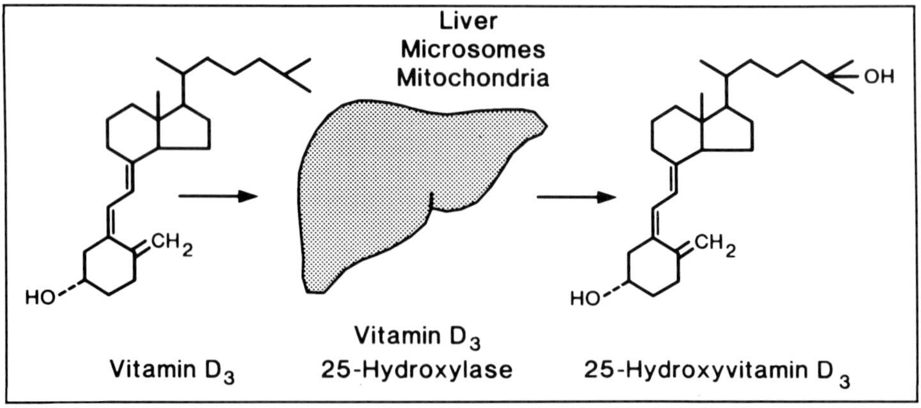

Fig. 8-3 Formation of 25-hydroxyvitamin D_3 in the liver. [From Audran and Kumar (12). With permission.]

25-OH-D_3 in the rat (34) are consistent with the notion that the principal site of hepatic 25-OH-D_3 synthesis may reside in the mitochondrial and not the microsomal fraction.

Little information is available regarding the regulation of liver 25-hydroxlase. The effect of vitamin D status on the kinetics of the enzyme was investigated in two laboratories. The demonstration of the twofold increase in K_m and a threefold increase in V_{max} associated with vitamin D repletion indicates that the 25-hydroxylase is not subject to substrate or product inhibition (35). Another study that showed no effect of vitamin D status on the kinetics of 25-hydroxylase in isolated rat hepatocytes also provided evidence for the absence of feedback regulation of 25-hydroxylation (31). In addition, *in vivo* studies in sheep and other species indicate that the plasma concentration of 25-OH-D_3 appears to be related to the administered dose of vitamin D precursor (36).

Recent studies in man and rat have implicated $1,25(OH)_2D_3$, the active vitamin D hormone, as a regulator of hepatic 25-OH-D_3 production. Bell et al. demonstrated that concomitant administration of $1,25(OH)_2D_3$ prevents the increase in serum 25-OH-D_3 after vitamin D challenge in normal adult human subjects (37). Although the authors conclude from their studies that $1,25(OH)_2D_3$ inhibits the hepatic synthesis of $25(OH)D_3$, support for this hypothesis can only be achieved by direct examination of the effect of $1,25(OH)_2D_3$ on hepatic 25-hydroxylase. Evidence for this hypothesis has been obtained in the rat by Baran and Milne, who showed that $1,25(OH)_2D_3$ directly inhibited production of $25(OH)D_3$ by isolated perfused liver and liver homogenates (38). In constrast, others have demonstrated that chronic $1,25(OH)_2D_3$ administration in the rat lowers the serum concentration of 25-OH-D by increasing the metabolic clearance of 25-OH-D_3— not by decreasing its production (39). Moreover, an increase in the renal production of $1,25(OH)_2D_3$ in calcium deprived rats also elicits an increase in the hepatic inactivation of 25-OH-D_3 (40). These findings suggest that calcium deficiency may promote vitamin D deficiency in individuals with an adequate exposure to sunlight and may be important in understanding the pathogensis or rickets and osteomalacia.

The effect of anticonvulsant drugs on the hepatic production of 25-OH-D$_3$ has received a lot of attention after several reports in the literature of osteomalacia and rickets in patients receiving chronic anticonvulsant therapy for seizure disorders. The demonstration of decreased plasma 25-OH-D$_3$ concentration in these patients has been attributed to drug-induced stimulation of hepatic mixed-function oxidases which alter the normal metabolism of vitamin D by favoring the production of more polar biologically inactive metabolites of vitamin D. In a rat model, Baran demonstrated that chronic administration of phenobarbital was associated with a significant decrease in hepatic production of 25-OH-D$_3$, in release of 25-OH-D$_3$ from the liver into the perfusate, and in plasma 25-OH-D$_3$ concentration (41). The discrepancies in the earlier literature regarding the effect of anticonvulsant drugs on hepatic vitamin D metabolism may be related to variations in duration of drug treatment. Indeed, short-term treatment with phenobarbital results in increased hepatic production of 25-OH-D$_3$ and a rise in plasma concentration of 25-OH-D$_3$ (41).

More recently, the effects of several other widely prescribed drugs known to interact with hepatic cytochrome P-450-dependent mixed-function oxidases have been investigated. Cimetidine, the histamine H$_2$ receptor antagonist given to patients to inhibit gastric secretion of acid, inhibited the *in vitro* production of 25-OH-D$_3$ when added to rat liver homogenates (42). In addition, cimetidine injected into rats 1 h prior to sacrifice resulted in decreased *in vitro* production of 25-OH-D$_3$ (42). In the same study, the effect of isoniazid, an antituberculous agent known to inhibit microsomal drug metabolism, was examined. Similar inhibition of 25-OH-D$_3$ synthesis *in vitro* was apparent after isoniazid administration (42). These results are compatible with the demonstration of reduced plasma levels of 25-OH-D$_3$ and inhibition of hepatic mixed-function oxidase in normal males treated with isoniazid (43). A similar fall in plasma levels of 25-OH-D$_3$ was associated with induction of hepatic mixed-function oxidase in normal males following administration of rifampicin, also used in the treatment of tuberculosis (44). These studies demonstrate how drug therapy can affect mineral metabolism in large segments of the population and should alert clinicians to the potential hazards of these powerful pharmacological agents, particularly in patients with poor nutritional status and limited exposure to sunlight.

RENAL METABOLISM OF 25-HYDROXYVITAMIN D$_3$

25-Hydroxyvitamin D$_3$ synthesized in the liver binds DBP and is transported through the blood to the kidney where it can undergo further hydroxylations to form either 1,25(OH)$_2$D$_3$, the active vitamin D hormone, or 24,25(OH)$_2$D$_3$, an abundant vitamin D metabolite, the physiological function of which is poorly understood (Fig. 8-4) (1). The kidney is believed to be the major site of 1,25(OH)$_2$D$_3$ and 24,25(OH)$_2$D$_3$ production, although several other tissues have been reported to support their synthesis (see Extrarenal Synthesis of 1,25-Dihydroxyvitamin D$_3$). The 1- and 24-hydroxylation reactions have been localized to the proximal tubule of chicken (45) and rat (46) kidney by microdissection studies and, by subcellular fractionation, to the inner mitochondrial membrane. The 25-OH-D$_3$-1-hydroxylase

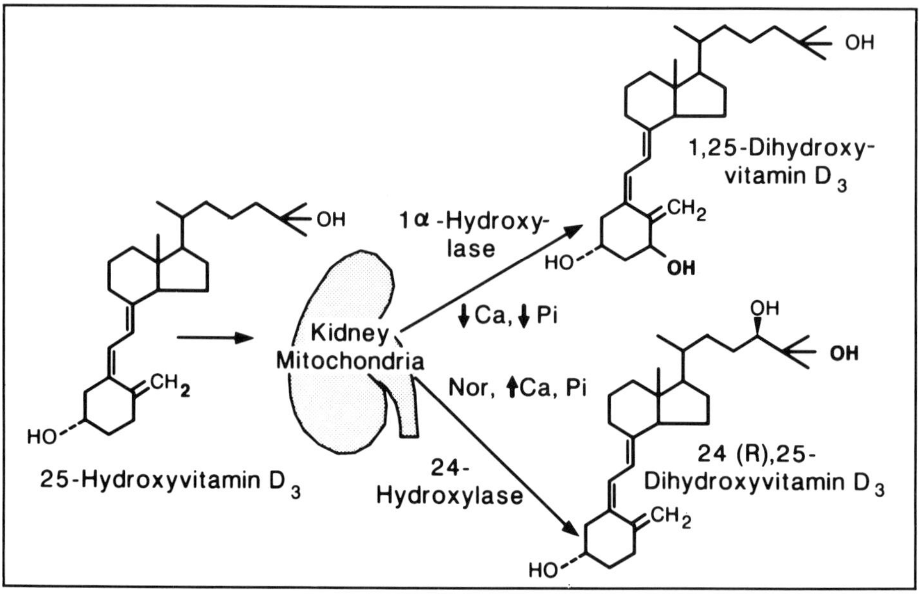

Fig. 8-4 Metabolism of 25-hydroxyvitamin D_3 in renal mitochondria. Ca, calcium; Nor, normal; Pi, inorganic phosphate. [From Audran and Kumar (12). With permission.]

(1-hydroxylase) and probably the 25-OH-D_3-24-hydroxylase (24-hydroxylase) are cytochrome P-450 mixed-function oxidases that require molecular O_2, NADPH, a flavoprotein reductase, and a non-heme iron protein (1). The renal 1-hydroxylase and 24-hydroxylase enzymes are subject to tight homeostatic regulation, unlike the hepatic 25-hydroxylase discussed above.

The most powerful determinants of $1,25(OH)_2D_3$ and $24,25(OH)_2D_3$ production are the vitamin D, calcium, and phosphate status of an animal (1). In vitamin D deficiency and in hypocalcemic and hypophosphatemic states, there is a marked increase in the rate of $1,25(OH)_2D_3$ production, and $24,25(OH)_2D_3$ synthesis is inhibited. In contrast, in vitamin D-replete animals with a normal calcium and phosphate dietary intake, $24,25(OH)_2D_3$ is the predominant metabolite produced by the kidney. This is reflected, in part, by the circulating levels of $1,25(OH)_2D_3$ and $24,25(OH)_2D_3$ in normal human plasma, where the concentration of $24,25(OH)_2D_3$ is 30- to 160-fold greater than that of $1,25(OH)_2D_3$ (Table 8-1). It should be noted that the disposition of these metabolites also contributes to their steady-state plasma level.

Table 8-1 Plasma Concentration of Vitamin D Metabolites

Metabolite	Concentration (nM)
25-Hydroxyvitamin D	25–125
24,25-Dyhydroxyvitamin D	2–20
1,25-Dihydroxyvitamin D	0.07–0.12

Source: D. Fraser (1).

The regulation of the renal hydroxylases has been investigated in a variety of experimental systems, both *in vivo* and *in vitro*, using isolated perfused kidney (47), nephron segments (48), cultured renal epithelial cells (49), cortical slices (50), renal homogenates (51), and isolated renal mitochondria (52). In order to elucidate the biochemical mechanisms involved in the regulation of these enzymes, attempts have been made to solubilize, purify, and reconstitute the catalytic activity associated with renal mitochondrial cytochrome P-450. However, this task has been difficult for the following reasons: (1) the concentration of cytochrome P-450 in the renal mitochondrial membrane is low; (2) the presence of other chromophores in mitochondria prevents the spectral quantitation of cytochrome P-450; and (3) the enzyme recovery is low and the catalytic rates of the enzyme are slow after solubilization of the membrane. Recently, cytochrome P-450 was purified from bovine renal mitochondria; the purified enzyme catalyzed the synthesis of $1,25(OH)_2D_3$ but not that of $24,25(OH)D_3$ and required NADPH, flavoprotein reductase, and non-heme iron protein (53). Cytochrome P-450 was also purified from renal mitchondria of vitamin D-replete and vitamin D-deficient rats. Both preparations catalyzed the production of $1,25(OH)_2D_3$ and $24,25(OH)_2D_3$, although the activity of the enzyme isolated from the deprived rats was 10-fold greater than that of the replete rats (54). In contrast to the bovine enzyme, the purified rat cytochrome P-450 catalyzed both 1- and 24-hydroxylations of 25-OH-D_3 in the absence of NADPH, flavoprotein reductase, and non-heme iron protein (55). On the basis of these and other findings, Warner concluded that purified rat renal mitochondrial cytochrome P-450 is acting like a dioxygenase rather than a mixed-function oxidase during the hydroxylation of 25-OH-D_3 (55). A subsequent study, however, questioned the authenticity of the $1,25(OH)_2D_3$ product which was produced by the partially purified cytochrome P-450 preparation described above (56). Using several chromatographic systems in combination with mass spectrometry, the product was identified as 19-oxo-19-nor-25-hydroxyvitamin D_3, a vitamin D metabolite which co-elutes with $1,25(OH)_2D_3$ on the traditional HPLC system used for separating vitamin D metabolites (56).

REGULATION OF RENAL 1,25-DIHYDROXYVITAMIN D₃ SYNTHESIS

Considerable effort has been devoted to the investigation of the factors involved in the regulation of vitamin D hormone biosynthesis and a brief summary of these studies is given below (see Table 8-2) (1–13).

PTH

PTH is an important regulator of renal 25-OH-D_3 metabolism and has been shown to mediate the increase in $1,25(OH)_2D_3$ synthesis in response to hypocalcemia (57). *In vivo* administration of PTH to intact or parathyroidectomized animals elicits a rapid rise in the plasma concentration of $1,25(OH)_2D_3$ and leads to an increase in renal 1-hydroxylase and a decrease in renal 24-hydroxylase activities measured *in vitro* (1). *In vitro* effects of PTH on renal 25-OH-D_3 metabolism have been demonstrated in primary cultures of chick kidney cells (49) and in

Table 8-2 Factors Affecting Renal 1-Hydroxylase or Plasma Concentration of 1,25(OH)$_2$D

Factor	Change	Reference
PTH	Increase	57–65
1,25(OH)$_2$D$_3$	Decrease	49,66,67
Calcium	Decrease	54,57,61,68–71
Phosphate	Decrease	57,72–80
Calcitonin	Increase, decrease, no effect	70,81–85
Sex steroids	Increase	86–89
Pregnancy	Increase	1,86
Insulin	Increase[a]	90–95
Growth hormone	Increase	96–103
Prolactin	Increase, no effect	103–105
Acidosis	Decrease	106,107
Alkalosis	Increase	108
Age	Decrease	109–114

[a]Effect of insulin was seen in diabetic rats (92).

cortical slices prepared from guinea pig (58) and rat kidney (59). Armbrecht et al. demonstrated that the effect of PTH on the renal 1-hydroxylase appears to be age-related; whereas PTH stimulated 1,25(OH)$_2$D$_3$ production only in young rats, it inhibited 24,25(OH)$_2$D$_3$ synthesis in both young and adult rats (59). In addition, the effect of PTH appears to be determined by the plasma calcium concentration (60). Hove et al. reported that whereas PTH infusion elicited a rise in plasma 1,25(OH)$_2$D$_3$ in hypocalcemic ruminants, it decreased circulating levels of 1,25(OH)$_2$D$_3$ when administered with calcium chloride, suggesting that hypercalcemia can effectively abolish the stimulatory effect of PTH on 1,25(OH)$_2$D$_3$ production (61).

The mechanism by which PTH acts on 25-OH-D$_3$ metabolism has not been completely elucidated. Horiuchi et al. demonstrated that cAMP could mimic the PTH-mediated increase in plasma 1,25(OH)$_2$D$_3$ following thyroparathyroidectomy in rats (62). Moreover, cAMP can mimic the PTH-mediated decrease in renal 24-hydroxylase activity in 1,25(OH)D$_3$-treated, parathyroidectomized rats (63). It has been shown that forskolin, which elevates intracellular cAMP levels by direct interaction with adenylate cyclase, mimics the effect of PTH on renal 1-hydroxylase and 24-hydroxylase in rat renal slices (64) and cultured chick kidney cells (65). These results suggest that cAMP plays an important intermediary role in the regulation of renal hydroxylases induced by exogenous and endogenous PTH. Although no evidence is yet available, it is conceivable that cAMP-dependent activation of specific protein kinases elicits the phosphorylation and activation of renal 1-hydroxylase and inhibition of the 24-hydroxylase.

1,25-Dihydroxyvitamin D$_3$

As described above, vitamin D status is a powerful determinant of renal 1-hydroxylase and 24-hydroxylase activities. Studies from numerous laboratories have documented that 1,25(OH)$_2$D$_3$ administered *in vivo* can profoundly affect the metabolism of 25-OH-D_3 measured *in vivo* and *in vitro* (1). The data in Table 8-3 demonstrate that treatment of vitamin D-deprived mice with 1,25(OH)$_2$D$_3$ markedly inhibits 1-hydroxylase and stimulates 24-hydroxylase in isolated renal mitochondria (66). In vitamin D-replete mice, stimulation of 24-hydroxylase is also achieved by 1,25(OH)$_2$D$_3$ treatment; however, no effect on 1-hydroxylase is detectable, primarily because the production of 1,25(OH)$_2$D$_3$ is extremely low in renal mitochondria from vitamin D-replete mice (Table 8-3) (66). It has also been demonstrated that 1,25(OH)$_2$D$_3$ can exert an effect *in vitro* when added to primary cultures of chick and mouse kidney cells. The addition of the hormone to the medium causes a decrease in 1-hydroxylase (49, 67) and an increase in 24-hydroxylase (49). Both effects are reversible and can be inhibited by cycloheximide and actinomycin D, which suggests a role for the expression of new genetic information and new protein synthesis in this process (49).

Calcium

It is well known from studies in many laboratories that a fall in plasma calcium is associated with increased renal 1-hydroxylase and a concomitant rise in the plasma concentration of 1,25(OH)$_2$D$_3$(1). These findings, however, do not distinguish whether control is exerted by the fall in calcium per se or by the consequent secretion of PTH in response to the fall in plasma calcium. The demonstration that thyroparathyroidectomized rats failed to exhibit the dramatic increase in plasma 1,25(OH)$_2$D$_3$ in response to calcium deprivation provided convincing evidence that PTH was essential in the mediation of this response (57). More recently, however, Trechsel et al. have shown that thyroparathyroidectomy of rats does not, in fact, abolish the increase in plasma 1,25(OH)$_2$D$_3$ in response to calcium restriction, providing evidence for a PTH-independent response of plasma 1,25(OH)$_2$D$_3$ to calcium restriction (68). In addition, studies in ruminants (61), dogs, and humans (69) indicated that calcium can modulate and often override the effect of PTH on renal 1-hydroxylase as assessed by measurement of the steady-state plasma level of 1,25(OH)$_2$D$_3$.

The effect of calcium on the metabolism on 25-OH-D_3 in primary cultures of renal cells has also been investigated. Lowering the medium calcium from 1.6 to .8 mM resulted in a 1.6-fold increase in 1,25(OH)$_2$D$_3$ production by primary cultures of mouse renal epithelial cells (70), whereas no effect of calcium was ob-

Table 8-3 Effect of 1,25(OH)$_2$D$_3$ Treatment on Renal Mitochondrial 25-OH-D_3 Metabolism in Vitamin D-Deprived (−D) and -Replete (+D) Mice

	Control	1,25(OH)$_2$D$_3$
−D: 1-Hydroxylase	.45 ± .03[a]	.03 ± .01[b]
24-Hydroxylase	.00 ± .00	.27 ± .13[b]
+D: 1-Hydroxylase	.01 ± .01	.02 ± .00
24-Hydroxylase	.20 ± .03	1.55 ± .12[b]

Source: Tenenhouse, H. S. and Jones, G. (66).

[a] pmol/mg prot min^{-1}.

[b] Significantly different from control, $p < .001$ by Student's t-test.

served in chick kidney cells (71). In the isolated perfused kidney, reducing the calcium concentration of the perfusate also failed to alter the pattern of $1,25(OH)_2D_3$ and $24,25(OH)_2D_3$ production (47). However, addition of .1 mM calcium to purified and reconstituted mitochondrial cytochrome P-450 elicited a two-fold stimulation of both 1-hydroxylase and 24-hydroxylase activities (54). Clearly, more work will be required to establish whether calcium plays a direct role in regulating $25(OH)D_3$ metabolism and to elucidate its mechanism of action on renal 1-hydroxylase and 24-hydroxylase activities.

Phosphate

The demonstration of an inverse relationship between the plasma concentration of phosphate with that of $1,25(OH)_2D_3$ led to the suggestion that plasma phosphate may be an important regulator of renal 1-hydroxylase activity (72). Recently, direct evidence has been obtained for increased production of $1,25(OH)_2D_3$ in renal homogenates prepared from phosphate-deprived mice (73), rats (74), and pigs (75). The persistence of this response after parathyroidectomy indicates that increased renal production of $1,25(OH)_2D_3$ is phosphate-deprived animals is independent of PTH action (57). The response to low-phosphate diets has been demonstrated in both vitamin D-deprived and vitamin D-replete rats and appears to be dependent on age and sex (76). Gray demonstrated that the plasma concentration of $1,25(OH)_2D_3$ achieved in response to phosphate deprivation of rats was highest in young males when compared with adult males and young and adult females (76). Studies in healthy men have shown that modulation of dietary phosphorus induced changes in serum levels of phosphorus which, in turn, mediated changes in the production rate and serum concentration of $1,25(OH)_2D_3$ (77).

The effect of phosphate on 25-OH-D_3 metabolism has also been examined *in vitro*. Reduction of phosphate in the culture medium from 3 to 1 mM was accompanied by a modest increase in $1,25(OH)_2D_3$ accumulation by mouse renal cells (70), whereas lowering the phosphate concentration of the perfusate failed to alter either $1,25(OH)_2D_3$ or $24,25(OH)_2D_3$ production by the isolated perfused kidney (47). The mechanism by which renal 1-hydroxylase is stimulated during phosphate deprivation is poorly understood and does not appear to be associated with changes in either content or distribution of renal cell phosphate pools as estimated by chemical methods and NMR spectroscopy (78). These studies suggest that some factor other than renal cell inorganic phosphate content must initiate the increase in renal $1,25(OH)_2D_3$ synthesis that occurs during phosphate deprivation. The role of insulin (79) and of the pituitary gland (80) in the renal 1-hydroxylase response to phosphate deprivation has been demonstrated and will be discussed below (see Insulin and Pituitary Hormones).

Calcitonin

Although several investigators had reported that calcitonin stimulates $1,25(OH)_2D_3$ accumulation *in vivo* (81), studies of the direct action of calcitonin on renal 1-

hydroxylase activity *in vitro* have yielded conflicting results. In chick renal tubules and primary cultures of chick renal cells, calcitonin failed to modulate 25-OH-D$_3$ metabolism (82). However, a more recent study reported that the addition of calcitonin to the culture medium modestly stimulated the production of 1,25(OH)$_2$D$_3$ in cultured mouse renal epithelial cells, suggesting a direct action of calcitonin on kidney vitamin D metabolism (70).

Using vitamin D-deficient rats, Kawashiwa et al. have demonstrated that calcitonin stimulates 1-hydroxylase activity by a cAMP-independent mechanism in the proximal straight tubule, a segment of the nephron where PTH has no observed effect on renal 1,25(OH)$_2$D$_3$ synthesis (83). It has been suggested that calcitonin-stimulated 1-hydroxylase in the proximal straight tubule may play a significant physiological role in the fetus where serum calcium concentrations are elevated and where 1,25(OH)$_2$D$_3$ is required for development of the skeleton. The recent demonstration of a positive correlation between calcitonin levels and postnatal increase in serum 1,25(OH)$_2$D in 5 day old infants provides further evidence that calcitonin plays an important role in the regulation of circulating levels of 1,25(OH)$_2$D$_3$ in the newborn (84).

The effect of chronic calcitonin infusion on plasma levels of 1,25(OH)$_2$D was recently examined in adult thyroparathyroidectomized rats (85). In rats fed either a calcium-free diet or a calcium-replete diet, calcitonin elicted a threefold increase in the circulating concentration of 1,25(OH)$_2$D without significantly affecting the plasma levels of 25-OH-D (85). Although these results suggest that calcitonin stimulates the renal production of 1,25(OH)$_2$D$_3$, the possibility that calcitonin exerts its effect by reducing the metabolic clearance of 1,25(OH)$_2$D$_3$ cannot be ruled out.

Sex Steroids

Reproduction-related activation of renal 1-hydroxylase in birds has been well recognized for over a decade. In chicks, the *in vivo* administration of estradiol, alone or in combination with testosterone or progesterone, greatly enhanced renal 1,25(OH)$_2$D$_3$ synthesis measured *in vitro* (86). In humans, the demonstration of a rise in the serum concentration of 1,25(OH)$_2$D$_3$ around day 15 of the menstrual cycle of adult women and the failure of women on oral contraceptives to manifest the midcycle peak in the 1,25(OH)$_2$D$_3$ levels suggest an influence of ovarian function and endogenous estrogens on the metabolism of 1,25(OH)$_2$D$_3$ (87). The precise mechanism for the effect of estrogens on renal vitamin D metabolism is poorly understood. The failure of estradiol to alter 25-OH-D$_3$ metabolism when added to primary cultures of chick kidney cells *in vitro* suggests that the effects of estrogens observed *in vivo* are not exerted directly on the renal cell (88). A recent report demonstrating that estradiol causes a marked increase in the number of renal PTH receptors and in catalytic subunit adenylate cyclase activity suggests that estrogens may modulate the response of the kidney to PTH, thereby leading to elevated 1-hydroxylase activity in the absence of changes in circulating PTH concentrations (89).

Insulin

The demonstration of decreased plasma concentration of $1,25(OH)_2D_3$ in children with insulin-dependent diabetes (90) as well as in experimental animal models of diabetes (91) suggested that insulin may play an important role in the renal production of vitamin D hormone. Subsequently, it was reported that streptozotocin-induced diabetes in the rat resulted in decreased 1-hydroxylase activity and increased 24-hydroxylase activity measured *in vitro* in renal cortical slices (92) and isolated renal mitochondria (93). The restoration of renal $25\text{-OH-}D_3$ metabolism to normal after treatment of diabetic rats with insulin suggested that insulin deficiency was in part responsible for reduced production of the vitamin D hormone in the streptozotocin-treated rats (92). Insulin also plays an important role in the renal 1-hydroxylase response to phosphate deprivation (79). Phosphate restriction of diabetic rats elicited an 8-fold increase in $1,25(OH)_2D_3$ production after insulin treatment, whereas only a 3.6-fold rise was apparent in untreated rats (79).

In vitro, the addition of insulin to primary cultures of chick kidney cells failed to show any direct effect on renal production of $1,25(OH)_2D_3$ (94). However, the presence of insulin in the culture medium was necessary for the stimulatory action of PTH on renal 1-hydroxylase activity (94). Furthermore, in insulin-treated diabetic rats, PTH stimulation of $1,25(OH)_2D_3$ production was markedly increased over that seen in untreated diabetic rats (95). In both the above studies, a normal cAMP response to PTH was observed in the absence of insulin, suggesting that insulin may exert its action on 1-hydroxylase activity distal to the generation of cAMP (94, 95).

Pituitary Hormones

There is evidence to suggest that the pituitary hormones play a role in the regulation of $25\text{-OH-}D_3$ metabolism. Hypophysectomy in the rat results in reduced renal production of $1,25(OH)_2D_3$ and elevated renal synthesis of $24,25(OH)_2D_3$ as measured in renal cortex slices *in vitro* (96). Administration of growth hormone to hypophysectomized rats can, to a large extent, overcome the effects of hypophysectomy; that is, the growth hormone increases renal 1-hydroxylase and decreases 24-hydroxylase by a mechanism that appears to be independent of PTH (96). These results suggest that growth hormone, either directly or indirectly, can modulate renal metabolism of $25\text{-OH-}D_3$.

In contrast, to these findings in the rat, growth hormone-deficient children show no increase in plasma $1,25(OH)_2D_3$ levels when given growth hormone replacement therapy (97). This apparent discrepancy may be due to the quantities of growth hormone involved. Whereas physiological doses of growth hormone were administered to the children (97), much larger quantities were used in the animal studies (96). Indeed, plasma levels of $1,25(OH)_2D_3$ are elevated in acromegaly, indicating an effect of supraphysiological doses of growth hormone on $1,25(OH)_2D_3$ production in man (98). Similarly, elevated plasma levels of $1,25(OH)_2D_3$ were reported in rats bearing growth hormone and prolactin-secreting transplantable pituitary tumors (99).

Hypophysectomized rats fail to show enhanced renal production of $1,25(OH)_2D_3$

in response to phosphate deprivation (100, 101). Administration of growth hormone to hypophysectomized rats fed a low-phosphate diet resulted in a 3.5-fold elevation in plasma $1,25(OH)_2D_3$ levels, but no such elevation was apparent after prolactin, ACTH, TSH, or triiodothyronine treatment (100). These results, as well as those showing normal plasma growth hormone levels in intact phosphate-deprived rats (102) and the failure of growth hormone to stimulate $1,25(OH)_2D_3$ production in intact rats (103), suggest that growth hormone plays a permissive role in the renal 1-hydroxylase response to phosphate deprivation.

The effect of prolactin on renal $25\text{-}OH\text{-}D_3$ metabolism has also been investigated. In primary chick kidney cell cultures, prolactin administration resulted in a modest increase in 1-hydroxylase activity and no change in 24-hydroxylase (104). However, no evidence is available regarding an effect of prolactin on $25\text{-}OH\text{-}D_3$ metabolism in rats (103) or humans (105).

Hydrogen Ion Concentration

The effect of metabolic acidosis on renal $25\text{-}OH\text{-}D_3$ metabolism has been investigated by several groups. Kawashima et al. demonstrated that metabolic acidosis, induced in the vitamin D-deficient rat by ammonium chloride, markedly suppresses renal 1-hydroxylase in the proximal convoluted tubule after 3 or 7 days of acidosis but not after 16 h of acidosis (106). Furthermore, PTH did not stimulate the suppressed renal 1-hydroxylase in acidotic rats, whereas cAMP was able to restore the enzyme activity to normal (106). These data suggest that metabolic acidosis suppresses renal 1-hydroxylase by inhibiting PTH-dependent adenylate cyclase activation. The data also indicate that metabolic acidosis does not affect the intracellular processes necessary for 1-hydroxylase stimulation following cAMP formation.

Reddy et al. demonstrated a similar reduction in $1,25(OH)_2D_3$ synthesis by perfused kidney from vitamin D-deficient acidotic rats, but no effect on $24,25(OH)_2D_3$ production in vitamin D-replete acidotic rats (107). These authors also reported that lowering the pH of perfusate from 7.4 to 6.8 did not directly affect 1-hydroxylase and 24-hydroxylase activity of perfused rat kidney from nonacidotic rats. In contrast, there was a highly significant correlation between 1-hydroxylase activity and the plasma pH in acidotic rats, suggesting that H^+ *in vivo* can modulate renal $25\text{-}OH\text{-}D_3$ metabolism.

Recently it was demonstrated that metabolic alkalosis, induced by feeding bicarbonate to rats, caused a substantial increase in the plasma concentration of $1,25(OH)_2D_3$ without a concomitant increase in calcium and phosphate absorption in the duodenum (108). More work will clearly be required to elucidate the mechanism for these effects.

Age

Because the metabolic requirement for calcium and phosphate varies with age, it is likely that age-related changes in the renal production of $1,25(OH)_2D_3$ are also apparent. To investigate this possibility, several groups have examined the effect of age on the steady-state plasma concentrations of vitamin D metabolites in man.

In one study, the circulating levels of $1,25(OH)_2D_3$ were found to be highest in infants of 4 days and lowest in adults (109). The demonstration of reciprocal data for the circulating concentration of $24,25(OH)_2D_3$ suggested that $1,25(OH)_2D_3$ synthesis has relative priority over $24,25(OH)_2D_3$ production during infancy compared with adulthood (109). In another study, the serum concentration of $1,25(OH)_2D_3$ was similar in children and young adults but was significantly decreased in older adults (110). An examination of the concentration of $1,25(OH)_2D_3$ in serum samples withdrawn at 30-min intervals for 28 h revealed that there are no large fluctuations in the circulating levels of the vitamin D hormone in man (111).

In experimental animals it has been possible to examine directly the effect of age on the renal production of $1,25(OH)_2D_3$. It was demonstrated in rodents, that, age is an important determinant of the magnitude of the adaptive renal 1-hydroxylase response to vitamin D and calcium deficiency (112, 113) and to PTH administration (59). The younger the animals at the initiation of vitamin D and calcium deprivation, the greater the fall in serum calcium and the greater the increase in renal 1-hydroxylase activity (113). Furthermore, whereas young animals could respond to vitamin D and calcium deprivation and to PTH stimulation with increased renal $1,25(OH)_2D_3$ synthesis as well as decreased renal $24,25(OH)_2D_3$ production, adult animals showed only the 24-hydroxylase response (59, 113).

The diminished gastrointestinal absorption of calcium associated with aging has been correlated with decreased renal 1-hydroxylase activity. Studies in vitamin D-replete rats demonstrated a specific decrement in $1,25(OH)_2D_3$ production (Fig. 8-5A) and increase in $24,25(OH)_2D_3$ synthesis (Fig. 8-5B) associated with aging. The decrease in 1-hydroxylase activity correlated with the age-dependent decline in serum $1,25(OH)_2D_3$ levels and in intestinal calcium transport (114). The precise contribution of age-related decrease in renal $1,25(OH)_2D_3$ synthesis to age-related bone disease requires further study (see Osteoporosis).

EXTRARENAL SYNTHESIS OF 1,25-DIHYDROXYVITAMIN D$_3$

Although it is generally accepted that the kidney is the major physiologic site of $1,25(OH)_2D_3$ production, 1-hydroxylase activity has been demonstrated in a number of other cell types. However, with the exception of the placenta, the biological significance of extrarenal $1,25(OH)_2D_3$ production remains to be established.

Tanaka et al. first provided evidence for the presence of 1-hydroxylase activity, measured *in vitro,* in placental tissue obtained from rat (115). More recently, $1,25(OH)_2D_3$ production was demonstrated in human decidual cells isolated from term placenta (116). The $1,25(OH)_2D_3$ produced had a mass spectrum identical to that of authentic $1,25(OH)_2D_3$, comigrated with authentic $1,25(OH)_2D_3$ in four chromatographic systems, and bound to the specific, high-affinity $1,25(OH)_2D_3$ cytosolic receptor (116). These and other studies documenting placental $1,25(OH)_2D_3$ synthesis could account for the increased circulating $1,25(OH)_2D_3$ levels throughout pregnancy. It remains to be established whether $1,25(OH)_2D_3$ produced by the placenta plays a role in the mineral homeostasis of the developing fetus or in the placental transfer of calcium and phosphorus from mother to fetus.

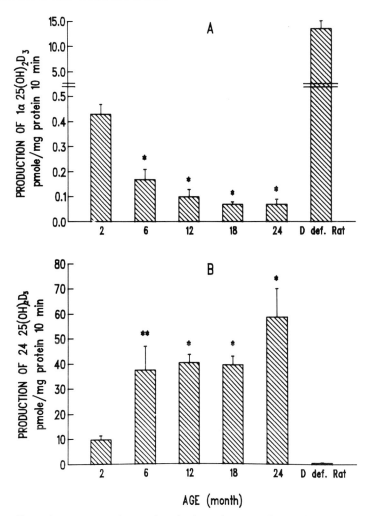

Fig. 8-5 Effect of age on renal mitochondrial production of 1,25-dihydroxyvitamin D_3 (A) and 24,25-dihydroxyvitamin D_3 (B) in rat kidney. (Unpublished results. With permission from B. Sacktor.)

The demonstration of detectable plasma levels of $1,25(OH)_2D_3$ in an anephric patient with sarcoidosis (117) led several investigators to examine the *in vitro* metabolism of 25-OH-D_3 by pulmonary alveolar macrophages. Adams et al. demonstrated that whereas pulmonary alveolar macrophages from patients with sarcoidosis could in fact convert 25-OH-D_3 to $1,25(OH)_2D_3$, pulmonary alveolar macrophages from patients with idiopathic pulmonary fibrosis could not synthesize $1,25(OH)_2D_3$ (118). These results indicated that in sarcoidosis the macrophage is a site of synthesis of the vitamin D hormone (118). In addition, it has been demonstrated that normal human bone marrow and pulmonary alveolar macrophages exhibit $1,25(OH)_2D_3$ production when cultured in the presence of recombinant γ-interferon (119). The biological significance of these findings is being investigated.

Cultured bone cells derived from chick calvaria and human iliac crest have been reported to synthesize $1,25(OH)_2D_3$ as well as $24,25(OH)_2D_3$ (120, 121). In both studies, the 1-hydroxylase and 24-hydroxylase activities could be regulated by pretreatment of cultures with $1,25(OH)_2D_3$. The demonstration of an inhibition of $1,25(OH)_2D_3$ production and an enhancement of $24,25(OH)_2D_3$ synthesis by $1,25(OH)_2D_3$ indicated that the bone hydroxylases were subject to the same regulatory control reported for the renal enzymes. It is postulated that vitamin D hormone synthesized in bone could act locally and therefore play a significant role in the regulation of mineral metabolism (120, 121).

Primary cultures of human foreskin keratocytes can convert 25-OH-D_3 to a number of metabolites including $1,25(OH)_2D_3$ (122). The identify of the vitamin D hormone product was established by several criteria including mass spectral analysis. The $1,25(OH)_2D_3$ produced remained mainly in the cell and would not be sufficient to contribute to or maintain circulating levels of the hormone *in vivo* (122). Accordingly, it is postulated that $1,25(OH)_2D_3$ formed by keratinocytes serves a function within the cell in which it is produced.

The demonstration of $1,25(OH)_2D_3$ and $24,25(OH)_2D_3$ synthesis in cells isolated from embryonic intestine has led those authors to speculate that all tissues involved in the net transmural transport of calcium ion contain an active or readily inducible 1-hydroxylase and 24-hydroxylase (123). Clearly, further investigation will be required to precisely elucidate the biological significance of extrarenal vitamin D hormone biosynthesis (124, 125).

CATABOLISM OF 1,25-DIHYDROXYVITAMIN D_3 AND 24,25-DIHYDROXYVITAMIN D_3

$1,25(OH)_2D_3$ and $24,25(OH)_2D_3$ appear to have similar pathways of catabolism (see Fig. 8-6). Studies in the rat by several groups indicate that the vitamin D hormone first undergoes 24-hydroxylation in the intestine, in the kidney, and perhaps in other target tissues (126, 127). The $1,24,25-(OH)_3D_3$ thus produced and $24,25(OH)_2D_3$ (128) can serve as precursors for the synthesis of 24-oxo-$1,25(OH)_2D_3$ and 24-oxo-25-OH-D_3. The 24-oxo derivatives are then hydroxylated at position C-23, yielding 24-oxo-$1,23,25(OH)_3D_3$ and 24-oxo-$23,25(OH)_2D_3$. It has been reported that the above-C-24 oxidation pathway is the predominant route of intestinal and renal $12,5(OH)_2D_3$ metabolism (126, 127) and of renal $24,25(OH)_2D_3$ metabolism (128). This pathway can be stimulated by prior treatment with $1,25(OH)_2D_3$, suggesting that target tissue catabolism of $1,25(OH)_2D_3$ may be an important mechanism for the inactivation of this biologically potent metabolite. The C-24 oxidation pathway has been demonstrated in LLC PK cells, a cultured pig kidney cell line that may prove to be a useful model system for the study of vitamin D metabolism (129). Recently, C-24 oxidation of $1,25(OH)_2D_3$ was examined in UMR-106 clonal osteoblast cells and evidence for the production of $1,24,25(OH)_3D_3$, 24-oxo-$1,25(OH)_2D_3$, 24-oxo-$1,23,25(OH)_3D_3$ and $1,23(OH)_2$-$24,25,26,27$-tetranor-D_3, the side chain cleavage product of $1,25(OH)_2D_3$, was obtained (130).

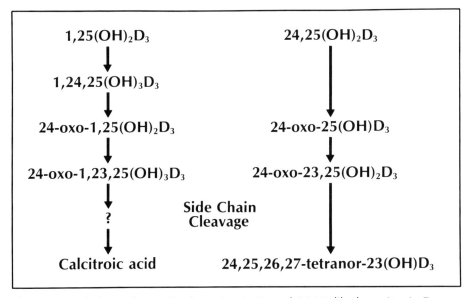

Fig. 8-6 Catabolism of 1,25-dihydroxyvitamin D_3 and 24,25-dihydroxyvitamin D_3.

In the chicken, the metabolic fate of 24,25$(OH)_2D_3$ appears to differ from that described above in the rat (131). In chick renal homogenates, 24-oxo-25-OH-D_3 is converted predominantly to 24-oxo-23,25$(OH)_2D_3$, 24,25$(OH)_2D_3$, and 23,24,25$(OH)_3D_3$, whereas in rat kidney, as described above, 24-oxo-25-OH-D_3 is converted to 24-oxo-23,25$(OH)_2D_3$, which then undergoes side-chain cleavage at C-23 to yield 23-OH-24,25,26,27-tetranorvitamin D_3 (128). No evidence for the production of C-23 derivatives of 24,25$(OH)_2D_3$ was obtained in chick kidney (131).

Evidence for side-chain cleavage of 1,25$(OH)_2D_3$ was obtained by administration of (^{14}C-26,27)1,25$(OH)_2D_3$ to rats and the subsequent demonstration that ~25 percent of the radiolabel was converted to $^{14}CO_2$ within 24 h. The rate of $^{14}CO_2$ production was significantly reduced by prior removal of the large and small bowel but was unaffected by nephrectomy (132). The side-chain cleaved sterol product of 1,25$(OH)_2D_3$ was identified as calcitroic acid and is most probably derived from 1,23$(OH)_2$-24,25,26,27-tetranor-D_3(133). Calcitroic acid is biologically inactive and rapidly excreted in the bile (134).

BIOLOGICAL ACTION OF 1,25-DIHYDROXYVITAMIN D₃

Intestine and bone are the major target organs for 1,25$(OH)_2D_3$. In the intestine, 1,25$(OH)_2D_3$ stimulates the absorption of both calcium and phosphate (2,4,7,10–13). Whereas the stimulation of calcium transport is greatest in the duodenum, with duodenum > jejunum > ileum > colon, phosphate absorption shows a different hierarchy of rates, with jejunum > duodenum > ileum in rat. There are three steps involved in the net transport of calcium and phosphate across the intestinal epithelial cell: uptake across the brush border membrane, transport across the cell, and efflux across the basolateral membrane. It is well known that $1,25(OH)_2D_3$ stimulates the production and/or activity of a wide variety of intestinal proteins and enzymes (2,4). However, their precise role in $1,25(OH)_2D_3$-stimulated transepithelial transport of calcium and phosphate remains to be established. The recent demonstration that $1,25(OH)_2D_3$ increases calmodulin binding to specific proteins in the chick duodenal brush border membrane suggests that calmodulin may play a role in $1,25(OH)_2D_3$-stimulated calcium movement across the intestinal brush border membrane (135).

Bone is a major target tissue for the action of vitamin D metabolites, and specific intracellular receptors for $1,25(OH)_2D_3$ have been described in bone homogenates as well as in bone cells in culture (136). However, it is still unclear whether the vitamin D hormone plays a direct role in the mineralization of osteoid or whether the effects of vitamin D on skeletal mineralization are mediated through the provision of suitable concentrations of calcium and phosphate in the extracellular fluid by the action of vitamin D on intestinal transport. The demonstration by De Luca et al. that skeletal parameters indicative of growth and mineralization were normalized in vitamin D-deficient rats infused with sufficient calcium and phosphate provided evidence against direct action of vitamin D metabolites on bone mineralization (13). Similar conclusions were reached in a study of vitamin D-deficient suckling and weaned rats fed high dietary contents of calcium and phosphorus (137).

It is well established that $1,25(OH)_2D_3$ is a potent stimulator of bone resorption both *in vivo* and *in vitro*. The bone-resorbing properties of $1,25(OH)_2D_3$ are independent of PTH and in many ways are similar to the direct action of PTH on bone. In *in vitro* studies utilizing calvaria, long bones, or bone cell lines in culture, it has been demonstrated that $1,25(OH)_2D_3$ is the most potent analog, and a striking correlation between the bone resorbing potency of vitamin D analogs and their ability to bind the intestinal cytosolic receptor has been reported (138). $1,25(OH)_2D_3$ increases the activity of acid phosphatase in monolayers of osteoclast-like but it decreases the synthesis of collagen and alkaline phosphatase activity in osteoblast-like cells (136).

The renal action of $1,25(OH)_2D_3$ has also been investigated in several laboratories. 1,25-Dihydroxyvitamin D_3 was shown to increase renal mitochondrial 24-hydroxylase activity (49, 66) and to stimulate phosphate uptake by isolated renal epithelial cells (139) and renal brush border membrane vesicles (140). However, it is not yet clear if $1,25(OH)_2D_3$ exerts a direct effect on the renal tubular transport of calcium. A recent *in vivo* study in thyroparathyroidectomized rats suggested the presence of dual effects of vitamin D_3 on renal handling of calcium: one to facilitate renal calcium reabsorption, and the other to enhance renal responsiveness to PTH (141).

1,25-Dihydroxyvitamin D_3 mediates its response in target tissues in a manner analogous to that of classical steroid hormones (Fig. 8-7) (142). Target tissues are defined by the presence of high-affinity intracellular receptor proteins that specifically bind the steroid hormone. The steroid hormone–receptor complex becomes tightly associated with chromatin in the nucleus and thereby selectively stimulates transcription of specific genes. The newly synthesized messenger RNAs

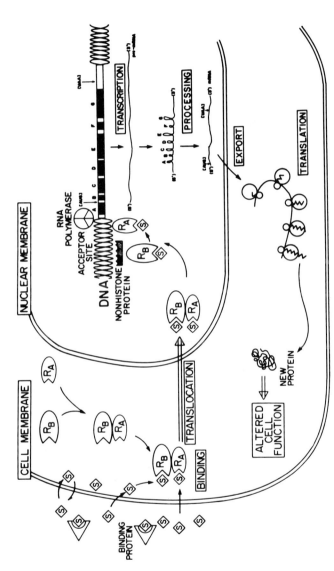

Fig. 8-7 Schematic representation of the pathway for steroid hormone action. The steroid hormone (S) binds to the receptor (R_A and R_B) and interacts with chromosomes. Gene activation occurs, and a large precursor mRNA is synthesized. The precursor is spliced and processed, and the mature mRNA is transported to the cytoplasm, where it is translated on ribosomes to produce proteins that alter cell function. [From O'Malley (142). With permission.]

are translated to produce proteins necessary to generate the biological response of the hormone in question. Although other mechanisms may serve to mediate the action of $1,25(OH)_2D_3$ (see Liponomic Action of 1,25-Dihydroxyvitamin D_3), the receptor-mediated genomic activation model is the most generally accepted mechanism for its action.

Target Tissues for 1,25-Dihydroxyvitamin D_3

In addition to the classical vitamin D target organs of intestine, bone, and kidney, a multitude of newer vitamin D target tissues have recently been described in both avian and mammalian species (2,4,10). Identification of these "nonclassical target organs" is based on the following criteria: (1) ability of tissue to concentrate specifically ^3H-$1,25(OH)_2D_3$ after intravenous administration; (2) presence of specific high-affinity intracellular receptors for $1,25(OH)_2D_3$; and (3) presence of vitamin D-dependent calcium-binding proteins (CaBP) as assessed by immunological procedures or Chelex binding assays. On the basis of one or more of these criteria, the following new target tissues for $1,25(OH)_2D_3$ have been reported (4,10): parathyroid gland, pancreas, pituitary, placenta, parotid, skin, mammary gland, testis, uterus, yolk sac, colon, thymus, brain, and, recently, muscle (143).

Biochemical Properties of 1,25-Dihydroxyvitamin D_3 Receptors

The chick intestinal receptor for $1,25(OH)_2D_3$ has been most thoroughly characterized (144). It is a 60-kDa protein with a sedimentation coefficient of 3.75 in 5–20 percent sucrose density gradients. It contains a cysteine residue in or near the ligand binding site that is essential for the maintenance of binding activity. It binds its ligand, $1,25(OH)_2D_3$, with very high affinity (e.g., $K_d = 10^{-11}M$). Structure–function studies indicate that the 1α-hydroxyl and 25-hydroxyl groups are critical for efficient receptor recognition. Unoccupied receptor for $1,25(OH)_2D_3$ partitions in nucleus and cytosol, with approximately 70 percent in the nuclear and 30 percent in the cytosolic fraction of intestinal cells. Binding of $1,25(OH)_2D_3$ to its receptor causes a physical chemical change in the receptor that increases its affinity for the chromatin of the target cell. Distinct molecular domains for $1,25(OH)_2D_3$ and DNA binding on the $1,25(OH)_2D_3$ receptor have been identified following trypsin cleavage of the receptor (145). Monoclonal antibodies raised against the chick $1,25(OH)_2D_3$ receptor were used to demonstrate $1,25(OH)_2D_3$-dependent phosphorylation of the receptor in mouse fibroblasts. These studies suggest that phosphorylation of the receptor may represent an important event in the functional activation of the $1,25(OH)_2D_3$ receptor (144).

Molecular cloning of complementary DNA encoding the $1,25(OH)_2D_3$ receptor from chick intestinal (146) and human jejunal (147) cDNA libraries was recently reported. Sequence comparisons demonstrated that the vitamin D receptor belongs to the steroid-receptor gene family and is closest in size and sequence to another member of this family, the thyroid hormone receptor. The cDNA for the

$1,25(OH)_2D_3$ receptor represents one of the rarest mRNA cloned to date in eukaryotes, as well as the first receptor sequence described for an authentic vitamin.

Vitamin D-Dependent Calcium-Binding Proteins

Since the initial demonstration of vitamin D-dependent CaBP in chick intestinal cytosol in 1966, vitamin D-dependent CaBPs have been identified and purified from a wide variety of mammalian and avian tissues (4). Based on molecular weight, two major subclasses of CaBPs have been defined. The 28-KDa CaBP from avian intestine and from various mammalian tissues has four high-affinity calcium-binding sites, and the 9-KDa CaBP from mammalian intestine and perhaps other tissues has two high-affinity calcium-binding sites. These two classes of CaBPs are immunochemically distinct, are localized in the cytosolic fraction of cells, and bind calcium in the physiologically important concentration range of intracellular calcium ($K_d = 1-10 \times 10^{-7}$ M).

The precise function of CaBP remains unknown, although a quantitative relationship exists between the degree of intestinal calcium absorption and intestinal CaBP concentration. It has been postulated that CaBP may facilitate the intracellular diffusion of calcium from the mucosal to the serosal surface of the intestinal epithelial cell, or it may serve as an intracellular calcium buffer during calcium absorption and thereby prevent the intracellular concentration of ionized calcium from reaching toxic levels. Recently, cDNAs for the 28-kDa and 9-kDa CaBPs have been cloned and used as probes to examine mechanisms for the regulation of CaBP gene expression in intestine and other tissues (148–151).

A vitamin D-dependent CaBP has also been identified in bone. This 6-kDa protein, known as osteocalcin or "bone gla protein," undergoes vitamin K-dependent post-translational carboxylation of glutamic residues that confer upon the protein its calcium-binding properties (K_d for calcium = $1-10 \times 10^{-7}$ M). The precise function of bone gla protein is not yet well understood. Whereas Hauscka et al. propose that it functions in bone mineralization, Price et al. maintain that bone gla protein inhibits the mineralization of bone by preventing excessive calcification of the growth plate (152). The plasma concentration of bone gla protein appears to be a sensitive indicator of changes in bone activity and may provide clinicians with a useful marker to assess chronic responses to different calciotropic hormones in selected patient groups.

Liponomic Action of 1,25-Dihydroxyvitamin D_3

The liponomic mechanism of $1,25(OH)_2D_3$ action in target tissues refers to rapid and direct effects of the vitamin D hormone on membrane lipid composition which in turn elicits alterations in ion transport at the membrane level (153). The liponomic effect of $1,25(OH)_2D_3$ occurs by mechanisms that are independent of genomic nuclear activation and *de novo* RNA and protein synthesis. Considerable evidence has accumulated to support a nongenomic mechanism of $1,25(OH)_2D_3$

action on calcium and phosphate transport across intestinal and renal brush border membranes (154, 155): (1) stimulation of ion transport by $1,25(OH)_2D_3$ occurs prior to detectable changes in mRNA and protein synthesis; (2) effects of $1,25(OH)_2D_3$ are not inhibited by actinomycin D or cycloheximide; (3) changes in membrane lipid composition can be induced by $1,25(OH)_2D_3$; and (4) agents known to modify cell membrane lipid composition and hence membrane fluidity also elicit changes in calcium and phosphate transport across the brush border membrane. These results suggest that $1,25(OH)_2D_3$ can exert a rapid action on the cell membrane. A recent study demonstrated that the rapid increase in intracellular in cGMP in $1,25(OH)_2D_3$-treated skin fibroblasts required the participation of a functional $1,25(OH)_2D_3$ receptor, suggesting that both genomic and rapid actions of $1,25(OH)_2D_3$ are receptor mediated (156). The relative importance of these two mechanisms of action of $1,25(OH)_2D_3$ in the *in vivo* situation clearly requires further investigation.

Role of 1,25-Dihydroxyvitamin D_3 in Regulation of Cell Growth and Differentiation

The widespread distribution of high-affinity receptors for $1,25(OH)_2D_3$ in tissues not believed to participate in mineral metabolism suggests that the vitamin D hormone may play a wider biological role than was previously realized (2, 4). It has been shown by several groups that $1,25(OH)_2D_3$ can suppress the proliferation and induce the differentiation of a wide variety of neoplastic cells, and the importance of the receptor in mediating this action of $1,25(OH)_2D_3$ has been demonstrated. Cultured myeloid leukemia cells derived from mouse and man (HL-60) assume many of the morphological features of monocytes and macrophages after treatment of cultures with $1,25(OH)_2D_3$ (157). The $1,25(OH)_2D_3$-induced phenotypic changes in HL-60 cells is associated in a dose-dependent fashion with a decrease in the expression of the *c-myc* oncogene (158). In addition, $1,25(OH)_2D_3$ prolonged survival time of mice inoculated with myeloid leukemia cells (159). These results suggest the possible use of $1,25(OH)_2D_3$ in the treatment of human leukemias.

Recent studies have suggested that $1,25(OH)_2D_3$ may also play a role in the regulation of the immune system (160). Receptors for $1,25(OH)_2D_3$ were demonstrated in human T-lymphocytes 24 h after mitogen activation. Moreover, $1,25(OH)_2D_3$ inhibited the proliferation of and suppressed interleukin-2 activity of mitogen-activated T lymphocytes (160). In addition, $1,25(OH)_2D_3$ inhibited antigen-induced production of IL-2 by cloned T cell hybridomas (161). The physiological significance of an immunoregulatory role for $1,25(OH)_2D_3$ must await further investigation.

Because $1,25(OH)_2D_3$ has potent bone-resorbing activity, it was of interest to establish whether the vitamin D hormone was important in the formation of osteoclasts, which participate exclusively in bone resorption. It has been demonstrated that $1,25(OH)_2D_3$ inhibits proliferation and promotes monocytic differentiation of authentic bone marrow-derived mononuclear phagocytes (162). In addition, $1,25(OH)_2D_3$, added to cultured normal primate marrow mononuclear cells, stimulated the formation of large multinucleated cells that closely resemble osteoclasts

(163). Because osteoclasts are derived from circulating monocyte precursors, these results are consistent with a role for $1,25(OH)_2D_3$ in the formation of osteoclasts.

BIOLOGICAL ACTION OF 24,25-DIHYDROXYVITAMIN D_3

Although $24,25(OH)_2D_3$ is the major vitamin D metabolite produced in the kidney of vitamin D-replete animals with normal calcium and phosphate intake, its precise biological function is poorly understood. The evidence for and against a physiologically significant role of $24,25(OH)_2D_3$ was recently reviewed in detail (4, 10), and a brief summary of these findings will be presented below.

To evaluate the importance of 24-hydroxylation for the function of vitamin D metabolites, DeLuca and co-workers assessed the biological activity of synthetic 24,24-difluoro derivatives of vitamin D in which 24-hydroxylation would presumably be blocked by the presence of the fluorine atoms and in which fluorine atoms would presumably behave chemically more like hydrogen atoms than hydroxyl moieties (13). These investigations demonstrated that the biological potency of 24,24-difluoro-25-OH-D_3 was equivalent to that of 25-OH-D_3 in all assay systems studied, implying that 24-hydroxylation is not a prerequisite for expression of biological activity. On the basis of these and other results, DeLuca *et al.* suggest that $24,25(OH)_2D_3$ simply leads to a catabolic pathway and has no intrinsic physiological significance.

Evidence supporting a biological role for $24,25(OH)_2D_3$ has been obtained independently in several laboratories (4, 10). Receptorlike binding proteins for $24,25(OH)_2D_3$ have been identified in parathyroid gland, chondrocytes, endochondrial bone, and limb bud mesenchymal cells. 24,25-Dihydroxyvitamin D_3 and not $1,25(OH)_2D_3$ can normalize parotid gland function in vitamin D deficient rats (164). 24,25-Dihydroxyvitamin D_3 stimulates DNA and proteoglycan synthesis in cultured rat and rabbit chondrocytes, increases ornithine decarboxylase activity and DNA synthesis in the epiphyses but not diaphyses of rat bone, and suppresses bone resorption in uremic humans and rats. Furthermore, in combination with $1,25(OH)_2D_3$, $24,25(OH)_2D_3$ is essential for hatchability of fertile eggs in both chick and quail and for regression of hyperplastic parathyroid glands in vitamin D-deficient chicks. Clearly, it will be necessary to establish whether $24,25(OH)_2D_3$ or a metabolic thereof is responsible for these biological actions.

MEASUREMENT OF VITAMIN D METABOLITES

The ability to quantitate vitamin D and its metabolites accurately in plasma and other biological samples is crucial to our understanding of vitamin D metabolism and its regulation in normal and abnormal states. The development of suitable methods for the assay of vitamin D metabolites presented a formidable challenge because of their low plasma concentration, the existence of several different but chemically similar metabolites, and the lability of these secosteroids to UV light and heat. Although there are a number of physicochemical and colorimetric methods available for measuring vitamin D, none had the sensitivity and/or specificity for use in the analysis of biological samples. To overcome these limitations, bioassay methods were developed. These methods, which are based on comparing the biological response of the test sample with that of measured doses of vitamin D standards, proved to be extremely tedious and often generated variable results (165).

More recently, competitive protein-binding assays were adapted to quantitate vitamin D metabolites in lipid extracts of plasma and other biological samples (165). These procedures make use of either DBP or the high-affinity cytosolic receptor for $1,25(OH)_2D_3$ and have the following advantages: high sensitivity, ease of execution, small sample volume required, and large number of samples which can be assayed simultaneously. The major disadvantage is interference from related vitamin D metabolites, which compete with the metabolite to be quantitated for the binding protein. For this reason, competitive binding assays must be preceded by a fractionation procedure in order to purify the vitamin D metabolite to be assayed. The recent development of HPLC technology has permitted the efficient and rapid separation of vitamin D metabolites (165). Rapid batch elution preparative chromatographic techniques using disposable SEP-PAK silica cartridges have also been used to achieve separation and purification of vitamin D metabolites from lipid extracts of plasma or serum (166).

The vitamin D parent compound purified by procedures described above is generally quantitated by direct spectrophotometric analysis. The vitamin D hormone $1,25(OH)_2D_3$ is quantitated by competitive binding assay using either chick intestine or calf thymus cytosol as a source of receptor-binding protein. Following initial purification, $25\text{-}OH\text{-}D_3$ and $24,25(OH)_2D_3$, which bind DBP with similar affinity and are present in plasma at concentrations greatly exceeding that of $1,25(OH)_2D_3$ (see Table 8-1), are quantitated by competitive binding assay using DBP.

Several laboratories have developed protocols for the simultaneous determination of $25\text{-}OH\text{-}D_3$, $24,25(OH)_2D_3$, and $1,25(OH)_2D_3$ in plasma or serum (167). These multicomponent analyses exploit a combination of the procedures described above. Other protocols permit the extraction, separation, and reliable assay of vitamin D_2 as well as vitamin D_3 metabolites in human plasma (168). Finally, several commercial competitive protein-binding assay kits for the quantitation of vitamin D metabolites are now available from INCSTAR Corporation and Amersham.

The development of radioimmunoassays for the quantitation of vitamin D metabolites has also received much attention. However, prior purification of the metabolites is required because the antibodies generated cross-react with more than one vitamin D metabolite. For example, the monoclonal antibody raised against calcitroic acid, conjugated to bovine serum albumin, with high affinity for $1,25(OH)_2D_3$, also recognizes $24,25(OH)_2D_3$ and $25\text{-}OH\text{-}D_3$ (169). Another antibody, generated in rabbits immunized with a new vitamin D analog lacking the C-23 side chain and coupled directly to bovine serum albumin, cross-reacted equally with all vitamin D_2 and vitamin D_3 metabolites tested except for $1,25(OH)_2D_2$, $1,25(OH)_2D_3$, and the parent vitamin D_2 and vitamin D_3 compounds (170). Clearly, antibody specificity must be carefully established before it can be reliably adapted to radioimmunoassay of vitamin D metabolites.

VITAMIN D TOXICITY

Hypervitaminosis D, which occurs most frequently after ingestion of pharmacological doses of vitamin D, is associated with markedly elevated circulating levels of vitamin D and 25-OH-D$_3$ and a normal plasma concentration of 1,25(OH)$_2$D$_3$. The hypercalcemia and hypercalciuria that occur in such patients are due to the interaction of the large amounts of 25-OH-D$_3$ with the receptor for 1,25(OH)$_2$D$_3$ in target tissues. The clinical symptoms associated with vitamin D toxicity include nausea, headache, fatigue, and restlessness. Kidney and cardiovascular damage may result form cellular and interstitial calcification (171).

Patients with hyperparathyroidism (172), sarcoidosis (173), and adsorptive hypercalciuria (72) present with elevated plasma levels of 1,25(OH)$_2$D$_3$ and may exhibit some of the clinical manifestations of vitamin D toxicity. In patients with Williams syndrome, excessive production of 25-OH-D$_3$ was reported after administration of exogenous vitamin D (174).

VITAMIN D DEFICIENCY SYNDROMES
(see Table 8-4)

Nutritional Deficiency

Nutritional rickets is not a significant problem in countries where foods have been fortified with vitamin D. Furthermore, in many geographical areas, endogenous production of vitamin D in the skin under the influence of UV irradiation usually satisfies vitamin D needs. The minimal requirement for vitamin D is approximately 10 μg/day (400 IU/day) for infants, 5 μg/day for children of 2–6 years, and 2.5 μg/day for individuals over 6 years of age (175). Endogenous production of vitamin D can vary from 10 to 100 μg/day. Factors predisposing to nutritional

Table 8-4 Causes of Vitamin D Deficiency

Nutritional deficiency
    Inadequate intake
    Malabsorption
Failure of formation of 25-OH-D$_3$
    Liver disease
    Drugs
Failure of formation of 1,25(OH)$_2$D$_3$
    Renal disease
    Hypoparathyroidism
    Genetic disorders
        Vitamin D dependency rickets Type I
        Pseudohypoparathyroidism
        X-linked hypophosphatemia
    Osteoporosis
End organ resistance to 1,25(OH)$_2$D$_3$
        Vitamin D dependency rickets Type II

vitamin D deficiency include prematurity; rapid growth, with a consequent increased need for calcium and phosphate; inadequate exposure to sunlight; and avoidance of vitamin D-supplemented foods.

The characteristic skeletal disturbance in vitamin D deficiency is osteomalacia, which can lead to bone deformity and rickets during infancy and childhood. In adults, osteomalacia rising from vitamin D deficiency is less severe. In fact, a mineralization defect in adults must be present for several years to produce clinical manifestations.

Vitamin D deficiency is associated with deficient intestinal calcium absorption and mild hypocalcemia. This promotes secondary hyperparathyroidism, consequent bone resorption, and restoration of serum calcium to the normal range. Secondary hyperparathyroidism also induces a phosphaturia and attendant hypophosphatemia. In vitamin D deficiency, the circulating concentrations of vitamin D and 25-OH-D$_3$ are low. The level of 1,25(OH)$_2$D$_3$ may also be low. However, in partial deficiency states, 1,25(OH)$_2$D$_3$ levels may be high because of the presence of severe secondary hyperparathyroidism and reduced, but not totally absent, amounts of 25-OH-D$_3$.

An inadequate intake of vitamin D can arise in disorders of fat absorption. As discussed earlier (see Intestinal Absorption and Enterohepatic Circulation of Vitamin D), vitamin D is absorbed from the small intestine through the mesenteric lymph. Bile acids are crucial for optimal absorption, and 80 percent of absorbed vitamin D is associated with chylomicrons (24, 25). Therefore, any disorder that interferes with the absorption of fat will necessarily result in malabsorption of vitamin D.

Failure of Formation of 25-Hydroxyvitamin D$_3$

Certain drugs interfere with the hydroxylation of vitamin D in the liver, and the effects of some of these drugs on the production of hepatic 25-OH-D$_3$ have been discussed (see Hepatic Metabolism of Vitamin D and Effect of Xenobiotics). In addition, in certain liver diseases such as cirrhosis, some (but not all) patients have low plasma levels of 25-OH-D$_3$.

Decreased Formation of 1,25-Dihydroxyvitamin D$_3$

In a number of renal disorders, the production of 1,25(OH)$_2$D$_3$ by the kidney is perturbed, and distinctive skeletal disturbances become apparent (e.g., renal osteodystrophy). The mechanism for reduced renal 1,25(OH)$_2$D$_3$ synthesis in these disorders is not clear but may be attributed to loss of nephrons, phosphate retention, or metabolic acidosis.

A genetic disorder known as autosomal-recessive vitamin D dependency rickets Type I, which interferes with renal 1-hydroxylase, has been described (176). Patients with this disorder develop early-onset vitamin D deficiency and rickets and are unresponsive to physiological doses of either vitamin D or 25-OH-D$_3$. The demonstration of a complete cure with physiological doses of 1,25(OH)$_2$D$_3$ suggested an abnormality of the renal 1-hydroxylase.

An animal model for autosomal-recessive vitamin D dependency rickets Type I has been reported in pigs (177, 178). Affected homozygotes develop profound hypocalcemia with severe secondary hyperparathyroidism and hypophosphatemia by 8 weeks of age. The plasma concentration of $1,25(OH)_2D_3$ is markedly reduced despite an elevated plasma concentration of 25-OH-D_3. Physiological doses of $1,25(OH)_2D_3$, but not of vitamin D_3 or 25-OH-D_3, could reverse the hypocalcemia, hypophosphatemia, hyperparathyroidism, and bone disease in rachitic pigs. Renal homogenates from affected animals failed to synthesize either $1,25(OH)_2D_3$ or $24,25(OH)_2D_3$ from 25-OH-D_3, thereby providing direct evidence for a disturbance in the renal hydroxylases. The rachitic pigs will serve as a useful animal model to study the mechanism for the 1-hydroxylase defect in this disorder and to elucidate the nature of the primary mutation.

PTH is a major regulator of renal $1,25(OH)_2D_3$ synthesis and, as described above (see Renal Metabolism of 25-Hydroxyvitamin D_3 and Its Regulation), PTH stimulates renal mitochondrial 1-hydroxylase activity. Accordingly, patients with hypoparathyroidism and pseudohypoparathyroidism have low levels of circulating $1,25(OH)_2D_3$ in the face of a normal plasma concentration of 25-OH-D_3 and manifest bony abnormalities. Individuals with hypoparathyroidism demonstrate a normal increase in circulating levels of $1,25(OH)_2D_3$ after PTH infusion (179). However, because of the end organ resistance to PTH characteristic of pseudohypoparathyroidism, patients with this disorder fail to show a plasma $1,25(OH)_2D_3$ response when challenged with PTH (179). Effective treatment of both these disorders can be achieved with physiological concentrations of vitamin D hormone.

The regulation of $1,25(OH)_2D_3$ synthesis is also disturbed in X-linked hypophosphatemia, an inherited disorder of phosphate homeostasis characterized by hypophosphatemia, normocalcemia, reduced growth rate, shortened stature, rickets, and a normal circulating concentration of parathyroid hormone (176). Patients with this disorder have a renal defect in phosphate reabsorption as well as an abnormality in renal $1,25(OH)_2D_3$ production, as judged by the inappropriately low plasma concentration of $1,25(OH)_2D_3$ for the degree of hypophosphatemia present. Both renal abnormalities contribute to the clinical phenotype, although the nature of the primary defect is still unclear. Treatment of X-linked hypophosphatemic patients with phosphate supplements in combination with physiological doses of $1,25(OH)_2D_3$ improves growth rate, partially restores serum phosphate, and corrects the rickets (176).

In 1976, Eva Eicher at the Jackson Laboratory discovered a murine model (*Hyp*) for X-linked hypophosphatemia in man (180). The mode of inheritance in the mouse is also X-linked dominant. Because genes on the X chromosome have been highly conserved during mammalian evolution, it is highly likely that X-linked hypophosphatemia of mouse and man involves a mutation of homologous genes and that the same gene product is involved. Studies with *Hyp* mice have demonstrated a specific defect in Na^+-dependent phosphate transport at the renal brush border membrane (181) as well as an abnormality in the regulation of renal 25-OH-D_3 metabolism (66, 73, 182, 183). The relationship between these two renal disorders and the elucidation of the primary gene product will require further study.

End Organ Resistance to 1,25-Dihydroxyvitamin D_3

Vitamin D dependency rickets type II is another genetic disorder characterized by hypocalcemia, secondary hyperparathyroidism, and rickets (184). The report of elevated plasma levels of $1,25(OH)_2D_3$ in patients with this disorder suggested that end organ resistance to the vitamin D hormone is responsible for the clinical phenotype. An analysis of high-affinity cytosolic receptors for $1,25(OH)_2D_3$ in skin fibroblasts of these patients confirmed the presence of a receptor defect and demonstrated marked heterogeneity in the pedigrees examined (184). The defects included absence of receptor, decreased receptor capacity, unmeasurable nuclear uptake of receptor, and decreased receptor affinity for either $1,25(OH)_2D_3$ or DNA. In all pedigrees examined, $1,25(OH)_2D_3$-inducible 24-hydroxylase was absent or markedly deficient in skin fibroblasts (185). Furthermore, using a monoclonal antibody raised against purified intestinal chick receptor, it was established that fibroblasts from all patients were CRM-positive, indicating that the genetic defect cannot be accounted for by gene deletion (186).

Patients with target tissue resistance to $1,25(OH)_2D_3$ are difficult to manage clinically, since many show no response to pharmacological doses of $1,25(OH)_2D_3$ (185). The clinical consequences of mutations involving the gene for the $1,25(OH)_2D_3$ receptor protein point to the physiological importance of receptor-mediated responses to $1,25(OH)_2D_3$ in target tissues.

Osteoporosis

Osteoporosis (187) is a metabolic bone disease characterized by a decrease in total bone to the extent that structural integrity of the skeleton is no longer maintained. The bone loss is associated with pain, compression fractures, kyphosis, and progressive loss of height. Osteoporosis is the most common skeletal disorder worldwide and can be classified into two main groups: postmenopausal and senile. In both types an impairment in intestinal calcium absorption has been demonstrated. However, it is not clear whether the defect in calcium absorption is secondary to an age-related decrease in renal $1,25(OH)_2D_3$ production or whether it arises from an intrinsic age-related defect of intestinal calcium transport.

Postmenopausal osteoporosis occurs in women and is associated with a disproportionate loss of trabecular bone and fractures of vertebrae and distal radius. The decreased plasma levels of $1,25(OH)_2D_3$ in postmenopausal osteoporosis are believed to be a consequence of accelerated bone loss due to estrogen deficiency. The ability of subphysiological doses of the vitamin D hormone to restore calcium balance provided convincing evidence that intestinal calcium malabsorption in postmenopausal osteoporosis is secondary to impaired renal production of $1,25(OH)_2D_3$.

Senile osteoporosis occurs in both men and women and involves a loss of both cortical and trabecular bone. In this disorder it is postulated that the increase in bone loss is associated with an age-related decrease in renal 1-hydroxylase activity and subsequent decrease in $1,25(OH)_2D_3$ production leading to impaired intestinal calcium absorption and secondary hyperparathyroidism. In this group of patients, a blunted 1-hydroxylase response to PTH infusion has also been reported.

Therapeutic agents for the treatment of osteoporosis fall into two general classes: those that decrease bone resorption and those that increase bone formation. Treatment programs that attempt to reduce the rate of bone resorption have included estrogens, calcitonin, calcium, diphosphonates, and vitamin D or its metabolites. The only therapeutic agent known to enhance bone formation is sodium fluoride, and several clinical trials using this agent, alone or in combination with other drugs, have been initiated. These studies should provide a basis for the development of improved protocols for the treatment of osteoporosis (see Slemenda and Johnston, Chapter 6).

SUMMARY

It is well established that vitamin D, a fat-soluble secosteroid, must undergo two hydroxylation reactions before it can exert its physiological actions on calcium and phosphate homeostasis. The first of these activation steps occurs in the microsomal and mitochondrial fractions of the liver. The 25-OH-D_3 thus produced is further hydroxylated in renal mitochondria to $1,25(OH)_2D_3$, the active hormonal form of vitamin D, and $24,25(OH)_2D_3$, a major renal metabolite of vitamin D with little apparent biological activity. In contrast to the hepatic synthesis of 25-OH-D_3, the renal production of $1,25(OH)_2D_3$ is subject to tight homeostatic regulation, although the molecular mechanisms involved have not been clearly elucidated.

The small intestine and bone are the major target tissues for $1,25(OH)_2D_3$, which stimulates the absorption of calcium and phosphate and accelerates the resorption of mineral from bone. Both these actions of $1,25(OH)_2D_3$ serve to maintain the extracellular calcium and phosphate concentrations. The demonstration of specific, high affinity, intracellular receptors for $1,25(OH)_2D_3$ in tissues not previously regarded as targets for $1,25(OH)_2D_3$ has led to the suggestion that the vitamin D endocrine system may play a role in cellular calcium and, perhaps, phosphate metabolism. Furthermore, the recently described action of $1,25(OH)_2D_3$ on the regulation of cell growth and differentiation has provided exciting new concepts and raised many important questions regarding the role of the vitamin D endocrine system in physiological functions other than mineral metabolism.

Genetic disorders involving the metabolism and action of vitamin D metabolites have been described. These "experiments of nature" will provide valuable models to elucidate the molecular and cellular mechanisms involved in the regulation of vitamin D hormone biosynthesis and its precise function in target tissues.

Acknowledgments: I would like to express sincere thanks to Lynne Prevost and Huguette Rizziéro for their expertise in the preparation of this manuscript and to Suzan Mandla for her critical review.

REFERENCES

1. Fraser, D. (1980) Physiol. Rev. 60:551.
2. Reichel, H., Koeffler, P., Norman, A. W. (1989) N. Engl. J. Med. 320:980.
3. DeLuca H. F. (1981) Clin. Biochem. 5:213.
4. Norman, A. W., Roth, J., Orci, L. (1982) Endocr. Rev. 3:331.
5. Kawashima, H., Kurokawa, K. (1986) Kidney Intl. 29:98.
6. Holick, M. (1987) Kidney Intl. 32:912.
7. Norman, A. W., Schaefer, K., Grigoleit, H. G., Herrath, D. V. (eds.), *Vitamin D: Molecular, Cellular and Clinical Endocrinology* Berlin, New York: Walter de Gruyter, 1988.
8. Marx, S. J., Liberman, U. A., Eil, C. (1983) Vitamins and Hormones 40:235.
9. Kumar, R. (1984) Physiol. Rev. 64:478.
10. Henry, H. L., Norman, A. W. (1984) Ann. Rev. Nutr. 4:493.
11. Bell, N. H. (1985) J. Clin. Invest. 76:1.
12. Audran, M., Kumar, R. (1985) Mayo Clin. Proc. 60:851.
13. Brommage, R., DeLuca, H. F. (1985) Endocr. Rev. 6:491.
14. Holick, M. (1985) Ann. New York Acad. Sci. 453:1.
15. Holick, M. F., MacLaughlin, J. A., Doppelt, S. H. (1981) Science 211:590.
16. MacLaughlin, J., Holick, M. F. (1985) J. Clin. Invest. 76:1536.
17. Holick, S. A., St. Lezin, M., Young, D., Malaikal, S., Holick, M. F. (1985) J. Biol. Chem. 260:12181.
18. Esvelt, R. P., Deluca, H. F., Wichmann, J. K., Yoshizawa, S., Zurcher, J., Sar, M. (1980) Biochemistry 19:6158.
19. Clemens, T. L., Adams, J. S., Horiuchi, N., Gilchrest, B. A., Cho, H., Tsuchiya, Y., Matsuo, N., Suda, T., Holick, M. F. (1983) J. Clin. Endocrinol. Metab. 56:824.
20. Cleve, H., Constans, J. (1988) Vox Sang 54:215.
21. Harper, K. D., McLeod, J. B., Kowalski, M. A., Haddad, J. G. (1987) J. Clin. Invest. 79:1365.
22. Bouillon, R., Van Baelen, H. (1981) Calcif. Tissue Int. 33:451.
23. Cooke, N. E. (1986) J. Biol. Chem. 261:3441.
24. Sitrin, M. D., Pollack, K. L., Bolt, M. J. G., Rosenberg, I. H. (1982) Am. J. Physiol. 242:G326.
25. Dueland, S., Pedersen, J. I., Helgerud, P., Drevon, C. A. (1983) Am. J. Physiol. 245:E463.
26. Sitrin, M. D., Pollack, K. L., Bolt, M. J. G. (1985) Am. J. Physiol. 248:G718.
27. Arnaud, S. B., Goldsmith, R. S., Lambert, P. W., Go, V. L. W. (1975) Proc. Soc. Exp. Biol. Med. 149:570.
28. Clements, M. R., Chalmers, T. M., Fraser, D. R. (1984) Lancet I:1376.
29. Gascon-Barre, M. (1982) Am. J. Physiol. 242:G522.
30. Ichikawa, Y., Hiwatashi, A., Nishii, Y. (1983) Comp. Biochem. Physiol. 75B:479.
31. Dueland, S., Holmberg, I., Berg, T., Pedersen, J. I. (1981) J. Biol. Chem. 256:10430.
32. Andersson, S., Holmberg, I. Wikvall, K. (1983) J. Biol. Chem. 258:6777.
33. Saarem, K., Bergseth, S., Oftebro, T., Pedersen, J. (1984) J. Biol. Chem. 259:10936.
34. Dahlback, H., Wikvall, K. (1987) Biochem Biophys. Res. Comm. 142:999.
35. Delvin, E. E., Arabian, A., Glorieux, F. H. (1978) Biochem. J. 172:417.
36. Smith, B. S. W., Wright, H. (1985) Res. Vet. Science 39:59.
37. Bell, N. H., Shaw, S., Turner, R. T. (1984) J. Clin. Invest. 74:1540.

38. Baran, D. T., Milne, M. L. (1983) Calcif. Tissue Int. 35:461.
39. Halloran, B. P., Bikle, D. D., Levens, M. J., Castro, M. E., Globus, R. K., Holton, E. (1986) J. Clin. Invest. 78:622.
40. Clements, M. R., Johnson, L., Fraser, D. R. (1987) Nature 325:62.
41. Baran, D. T. (1983) Am. J. Physiol. 245:E55.
42. Bengoa, J. M., Bolt, M. J. G., Rosenberg, I. H. (1984) J. Lab. Clin. Med. 104:546.
43. Brodie, M. J., Boobis, A. R., Hillyard, C. J., Abeyasekera, G., MacIntyre, I., Park, B. K. (1981) Clin. Pharmacol. Ther. 30:363.
44. Brodie, M. J., Boobis, A. R., Dollery, C. T., Hillyard, C. J., Brown, D. J., MacIntyre, I., Park, B. K. (1980) Clin. Pharmacol. Ther. 27:810.
45. Brunette, M. G., Chan, M., Ferriere, C., Roberts, K. D. (1978) Nature 276:287.
46. Kawashima, H., Torikai, S., Kurokawa, K. (1981) Proc. Natl. Acad. Sci. USA. 78:1199.
47. Rosenthal, A. M., Jones, G., Kooh, S. W., Fraser, D. (1980) Am. J. Physiol. 239:E12.
48. Kawashima, H., Kurokawa, K. (1983) Mineral Electrolyte Metab. 9:227.
49. Henry, H. L. (1979) J. Biol. Chem. 254:2722.
50. Armbrecht, H. J., Zenser, T. V., Davis, B. B. (1981) Endocrinology 109:218.
51. Tanaka, Y., DeLuca, H. F. (1981) Anal. Biochem. 110:102.
52. Vieth, R., Fraser, D. (1979) J. Biol. Chem. 254:12455.
53. Hiwatashi, A., Nishii, Y., Ichikawa, Y. (1982) Biochem. Biophys. Res. Commun. 105:320.
54. Warner, M. (1982) J. Biol. Chem. 257:12995.
55. Warner, M. (1983) J. Biol. Chem. 258:11590.
56. Brown, A. J., DeLuca, H. F. (1985) J. Biol. Chem. 260:14132.
57. Hughes, M. R., Haussler, M. R., Wergedal, J., Baylink, D. J. (1975) Science 190:578.
58. Kremer, R., Goltzman, D. (1982) Endocrinol. 110:294.
59. Armbrecht, H. J., Wongsurawat, N., Zenser, T. V., Davis, B. B. (1982) Endocrinology 111:1339.
60. Matsumoto, T., Ikeda, K., Morita, K., Fukumoto, S., Takahashi, H., Ogata, E. (1987) Am. J. Physiol. 253:E503.
61. Hove, K., Horst, R. L., Littledike, E. T., Beitz, D. (1984) Endocrinology 114:897.
62. Horiuchi, N., Suda, T., Takahashi, H., Shimazawa, E., Ogata, E. (1977) Endocrinology 101:969.
63. Shigematsu, T., Horiuchi, N., Ogura, Y., Miyahara, T., Suda, T. (1986) Endocrinology 118:1583.
64. Armbrecht, H. J., Forte, L. R., Wongsurawat, N., Zenser, T., Davis, B. B. (1984) Endocrinology 114:644.
65. Henry, H. L. (1985) Endocrinology 116:503.
66. Tenenhouse, H. S., Jones, G. (1987) Endocrinology 120:609.
67. Fukase, M., Birge, S. J., Rifas, L., Avioli, L. V., Chase, L. R. (1982) Endocrinology 110:1073.
68. Trechsel, U., Eisman, J. A., Fischer, J. A., Bonjour, J. P., Fleisch, H. (1980) Am. J. Physiol. 239:E119.
69. Hulter, H. N., Halloran, B. P., Toto, R. D., Peterson, J. C. (1985) J. Clin. Invest. 76:695.
70. Fukase, M., Avioli, L. V., Birge, S. J., Chase, L. R. (1984) Endocrinology 114:1203.
71. Trechsel, U., Bonjour, J. P., Fleisch, H. (1979) J. Clin. Invest. 64:206.

72. Gray, R. W., Wilz, D. R., Caldas, A. E., Lemann, J. (1977) J. Clin. Endocrinol. Metab. 45:299.

73. Lobaugh, B., Drezner, M. K. (1983) J. Clin. Invest. 71:400.

74. Gray, R. W., Napoli, J. L. (1983) J. Biol. Chem. 258:1152.

75. Engstrom, G. W., Horst, R. L., Reinhardt, T. A., Littledike, E. T. (1985) J. Animal Sci. 60:85.

76. Gray, R. W. (1981) Calcif. Tissue Int. 33:477.

77. Portale, A. A., Holloran, B. P., Morris, R. C. (1987) J. Clin. Invest. 80:1147.

78. Gray, R. W., Haasch, M. L., Brown, C. E. (1983) Calcif. Tissue Int. 35:773.

79. Ikeda, K., Matsumoto, T., Morita, K., Kawanobe, Y., Ezawa, I., Ogata, E. (1987) Metabolism 36:555.

80. Gray, R. W. (1981) Calcif. Tissue Int. 33:485.

81. Kawashima, H., Kurokawa, K. (1983) Mineral Electrolyte Metab. 9:227.

82. Henry, H. L., Noland, T. A., Alabdaly, F., Cunningham, N. S., Luntao, E. (1982) In: Norman, A. W., Schaefer, K., Herrath, D. V., Grigoleit, H. G. (eds.), *Vitamin D: Chemical, Biochemical, and Clinical Endocrinology of Calcium Metabolism* Berlin, New York: Walter de Gruyter, p. 533.

83. Kawashima, H., Torikai, S., Kurokawa, K. (1981) Nature 291:327.

84. Nishioka, T., Yasuda, T., Niimi, H., Nakajima, H. (1988) Eur. J. Pediatr. 147:148.

85. Jaeger, P., Jones, W., Clemens, T. L., Hayslett, J. P. (1986) J. Clin. Invest. 78:456.

86. Tanaka, Y., Castillo, L., Wineland, M. J., DeLuca, H. F. (1978) Endocrinology 103:2035.

87. Gray, T. K., McAdoo, T., Hatley, L., Lester, G. E., Thierry, M. (1982) Am. J. Obstet. Gynecol. 144:880.

88. Henry, H. L. (1981) Am. J. Physiol. 240:E119.

89. Forte, L. R., Langeluttig, S. G., Biellier, H. V., Peolling, R. E., Magliola, L., Thomas, M. L. (1983) Am. J. Physiol. 245:E273.

90. Frazer, T. E., White, N. H., Hough, S., Santiago, J. V., McGee, B. R., Bryce, G., Mallon, J., Avioli, L. V. (1981) J. Clin. Endocrinol. Metab. 53:1154.

91. Wilson, H. D., Horst, R. L., Schedl, H. P. (1982) Diabetes 31:401.

92. Wongsurawat, N., Armbrecht, H. J., Zenser, T. V., Davis, B. B., Thomas, M. L., Forte, L. R., (1983) Diabetes 32:302.

93. Hough, S., Fausto, A., Sonn, Y., Jo, K. D., Birge, S. J., Aviolo, L. V. (1983) Endocrinology 113:790.

94. Henry, H. L. (1981) Endocrinology 108:733.

95. Wongsurawat, N., Armbrecht, H. J. (1985) Acta. Endocrinol. 109:243.

96. Wongsurawat, N., Armbrecht, H. J., Zenser, T. V., Forte, L. R., Davis, B. B. (1984) J. Endocrinol. 101:333.

97. Gertner, J. M., Horst, R. L., Broadus, A. E., Rasmussen, H., Genel, M. (1979) J. Clin. Endocrinol. Metab. 49:185.

98. Eskildsen, P. C., Lund, B. J., Sorensen, O. H., Lund, B. I., Bishop, J. E., Norman, A. W. (1979) J. Clin. Endocrinol. Metab. 49:484.

99. Carlson, H. E., Lamberts, S. W. J., Brickman, A. S., Deftos, L. J., Horst, R. L., Forte, L. R. (1985) Endocrinology 117:1602.

100. Gray, R. W., Garthwaite, T. L. (1985) Endocrinology 116:189.

101. Tenenhouse, H. S., Klugerman, A. H., Gurd, W., Lapointe, M., Tannenbaum, G. S. (1988) Am. J. Physiol. 255:R373.

102. Gray, R. W., Garthwaite, T. L., Phillips, L. S. (1983) Calcif. Tissue Int. 35:100–106.

103. Spencer, E. M., Tobiassen, O. (1981) Endocrinology 108:1064.

104. Spanos, E., Brown, D. J., Stevenson, J. C., MacIntyre, I. (1981) Biochim Biophys Acta 672:7.

105. Kumar, R., Abdoud, C. F., Riggs, B. L. (1980) Mayo Clin. Proc. 55:51.

106. Kawashima, H., Kraut, J. A., Kurokawa, K. (1982) J. Clin. Invest. 70:135.

107. Reddy, G. S., Jones, G., Kooh, S. W., Fraser, D. (1982) Am. J. Physiol. 243:E265.

108. Gafter, U., Edelstein, S., Levi, J. (1985) Clin. Sci. 68:97.

109. Markestad, T. (1983) J. Clin. Endocrinol. Metab. 57:755.

110. Fujisawa, Y., Kida, K., Matsuda, H. (1984) J. Clin. Endocrinol. Metab. 59:719.

111. Halloran, B. P., Portale, A. A., Castro, M., Morris, R. C., Goldsmith, R. S. (1985) J. Clin. Endocrinol. Metab. 60:1104.

112. Armbrecht, H. J., Zenser, T. V., Davis, B. B. (1982) Endocrinology 110:1983.

113. Tenenhouse, H. S. (1985) Comp. Biochem. Physiol. 81A:367.

114. Ishida, M., Bulos, B., Sacktor, B. (1985) Fed. Proc. 44:1153.

115. Tanaka, Y., Halloran, B., Schnoes, H. K., DeLuca, H. F. (1979) Proc. Natl. Acad. Sci. USA. 76:5033.

116. Delvin, E. E., Arabian, A. (1987) Eur. J. Biochem. 163:659.

117. Barbour, G. L., Coburn, J. W., Slatopolsky, E., Norman, A. W., Horst, R. L. (1981) N. Engl. J. Med. 305:440.

118. Adams, J. S., Singer, F. R., Gacad, M. A., Sharma, O. P., Hayes, M. J., Vouros, P., Holick, M. F. (1985) J. Clin. Endocrinol. Metab. 60:960.

119. Reichel, H., Koeffler, H. P., Norman, A. W. (1987) J. Biol. Chem. 262:10931.

120. Turner, R. T., Puzas, J. E., Forte, M. D., Lester, G. E., Gray, T. K., Howard, G. A., Baylink, D. (1980) Proc. Natl. Acad. Sci. USA. 77:5720.

121. Puzas, J. E., Turner, R. T., Howard, G. A., Brand, J. S., Baylink, D. J. (1987) Biochem. J. 245:333.

122. Bikle, D. D., Nemanic, M. K., Gee, E., Elias, P. (1986) J. Clin. Invest. 78:557.

123. Puzas, J. E., Turner, R. T., Howard, G. A., Baylink, D. J. (1983) Endocrinology 112:378.

124. Shultz, T. D., Fox, J., Heath III, H., Kumar, R. (1983) Proc. Natl. Acad. Sci. USA. 80:1746.

125. Reeve, L., Tanaka, Y., DeLuca, H. F. (1983) J. Biol. Chem. 258:3615.

126. Napoli, J. L., Horst, R. (1983) Biochemistry 22:5848.

127. Mayer, E., Bishop, J. E., Chandraratna, R. A. S., Okamura, W. H., Kruse, J. R., Popiak, G., Ohnuma, N., Norman, A. W. (1983) J. Biol. Chem. 258:13458.

128. Jones, G., Kung, M., Kano, K. (1983) J. Biol. Chem. 258:12920.

129. Napoli, J. L., Martin, C. A. (1984) Biochem. J. 219:713.

130. Lohnes, D., Jones, G. (1987) J. Biol. Chem. 262:14394.

131. Yamada, S., Ino, E., Takayama, H., Horiuchi, N., Shinki, T., Suda, T., Jones, G., DeLuca, H. F. (1985) Proc. Nat. Acad. Sci. USA. 82:7485.

132. Kumar, R., Harnden, D. H., DeLuca, H. F. (1976) Biochemistry 15:2420.

133. Reddy, G. S., Tserng, K., Thomas, B. R., Dayal, R., Norman, A. W. (1987) Biochemistry 26:324.

134. Esvelt, R. E., DeLuca, H. F. (1981) Arch. Biochem. Biophys. 206:403.

135. Bikle, D. D., Munson, S. (1985) J. Clin. Invest. 76:2312.

136. Raisz, L. G., Kream, B. E. (1983) N. Engl. J. Med. 309:29.

137. Clark, S. A., Boass, A., Toverud, S. V. (1987) Bone and Mineral 2:257.

138. Stern, P. H. (1981) Calcif. Tissue Int. 33:1.

139. Liang, C. T., Barnes, J., Balakir, R., Cheng, L., Sacktor, B. (1982) Proc. Natl. Acad. Sci. USA. 79:3532.

140. Kurnik, B. R. C., Hruska, K. (1984) Am. J. Physiol. 247:F177.

141. Yamamota, M., Kawanobe, Y., Takahashi, H., Shimazawa, E., Kimura, S., Ogata, E. (1984) J. Clin. Invest. 74:507.

142. O'Malley, B. W. (1984) J. Clin. Invest. 74:307.

143. Boland, R., Norman, A., Ritz, E., Hasselbach, W. (1985) Biochem. Biophys. Res. Commun. 128:305.

144. Haussler, M. R. (1986) Ann. Rev. Nutr. 6:527.

145. Allegretto, E. A., Pike, J. W., Haussler, M. R. (1987) J. Biol. Chem. 262:1312.

146. McDonnell, D. P., Mangelsdorf, D. J., Pike, J. W., Haussler, M. R., O'Malley, B. W. (1987) Science 235:1214.

147. Baker, A. R., McDonnell, D. P., Hughes, M. Crisp, T. M., Mangelsdorf, D. J., Haussler, M. R., Pike, J. W., Shine, J., O'Malley, B. W. (1988) Proc. Natl. Acad. Sci. USA. 85:3294.

148. Theofan, G., Hall, A. K., King, M., Norman, A. W. (1985) In: Norman, A. W., Schaefer, K., Grigoleit, H. G., Herrath, D. V. (eds.) *Vitamin D. A Chemical, Biochemical and Clinical Update.* Berlin, New York: Walter de Gruyter, p. 333.

149. Thomasset, M., Desplan, C., Warembourg, M., Perret, C. (1986) Biochimie. 68:935.

150. Mayel-Afshar, S., Lane, S. M., Lawson, D. E. M. (1988) J. Biol. Chem. 263:4355.

151. Clemens, T. L., McGlade, S. A., Garrett, K. P., Horiuchi, N., Hendy, G. N. (1988) J. Biol. Chem. 263:13112.

152. (1984) Nutrition Reviews 42:230.

153. Nemere, I., Norman, A. W. (1982) Biochim. Biophys. Acta. 694:307.

154. Rasmussen, H., Matsumoto, T., Fontaine, O., Goodman, D. B. P. (1982) Fed. Proc. 41:72.

155. Kurnik, B. R. C., Hruska, K. A. (1985) Biochim. Biophys. Acta. 817:42.

156. Barsony, J., Marx, S. J. (1988) Proc. Natl. Acad. Sci. USA. 85:1223.

157. Abe, E., Miyaura, C., Sakagami, H., Takeda, M., Konno, K., Yamazaki, T., Yoshiki, S., Suda, T. (1981) Proc. Natl. Acad. Sci. USA. 78:4990.

158. Reitsma, P. H., Rothberg, P. G., Astrin, S. M., Trial, J., Bar-Shavit, Z., Hall, A., Teitelbaum, S. L., Kahn, A. J. (1983) Nature 306:492.

159. Homma, Y., Hozumi, M., Abe, E., Konno, K., Fukushima, M., Hata, S., Nishii, Y., DeLuca, H. F., Suda, T. (1983) Proc. Natl. Acad. Sci. USA. 80:201.

160. Tsoukas, C. D., Provuedini, D. M., Manolagas, S. C. (1984) Science 224:1438.

161. Bhalla, A. K., Amento, E. P., Serog, B., Glimcher, L. H. (1984) J. Immunol. 113:1748.

162. Clohisy, D. R., Bar-Shavit, Z., Chappel, J. C., Teitelbaum, S. L. (1987) J. Biol. Chem. 262:15922.

163. Roodman, G. D., Ibbotson, K. J., MacDonald, B. R., Kuehl, T. J., Mundy, G. R. (1985) Proc. Natl. Acad. Sci. USA. 82:8213.

164. Peterfy, C., Tenenhouse, A., Yu, E. (1988) J. Physiol. 398:1.

165. Seamark, D. A., Trafford, J. H., Makin, H. L. J. (1981) J. Steroid. Biochem. 14:111.

166. Adams, J. S., Clemens, J. L., Holick, M. F. (1981) J. Chromatog 226:198.

167. Jongen, M. J. M., Van der Vijgh, J. F., Willems, H. J. J., Netelenbos, J. C., Lips, P. (1981) Clin. Chem. 27:1757.

168. Jones, G. (1978) Clin. Chem. 24:287.

169. Perry III, H. M., Chappel, J. C., Clevinger, B. L., Haddad, J. G., Teitelbaum, S. L. (1983) Biochem. Biophys. Res. Commun. 112:431.

170. Hollis, B. W., Napoli, J. L. (1985) Clin. Chem. 31:1815.

171. Holmes, R. P., Kummerow, F. A. (1983) J. Amer. Coll. Nut. 2:173.

172. Broadus, A. E., Horst, R. L., Lang, R., Littledike, E. T., Rasmussen, H. (1980) N. Eng. J. Med. 302:421.

173. Bell, N. H., Stern, P. H., Pantzer, E., Sinha, T. K., DeLuca, H. F. (1979) J. Clin. Invest. 64:218.

174. Taylor, A. B., Stern, P. H., Bell, N. H. (1982) N. Engl. J. Med. 306:972.

175. Recommended Nutrient Intake for Canadians. Health and Welfare Canada 1983.

176. Rasmussen, H., Anast, C. (1983) In: Stanbury, J. B., Wyngaarden, J. B., Fredrickson, D. S., Goldstein, J. L., Brown, M. S. (eds.) *The Metabolic Basis of Inherited Disease*. New York: McGraw Hill, p. 1743.

177. Harmeyer, J., Grabe, C., Winkler, I. (1982) Expl. Biol. Med. 7:117.

178. Fox, J., Maunder, E. M. W., Randall, V. A., Care, A. D. (1985) Clin. Sci. 69:541.

179. Lambert, P. W., Hollis, B. W., Bell, N. H., Epstein, S. (1980) J. Clin. Invest. 66:782.

180. Eicher, E. M., Southard, J. L., Scriver, C. R., Glorieux, F. H. (1976) Proc. Natl. Acad. Sci. USA. 73:4667.

181. Tenenhouse, H. S., Scriver, C. R. (1978) Can. J. Biochem. 56:640.

182. Tenenhouse, H. S. (1984) Endocrinology 115:634.

183. Tenenhouse, H. S., Yip, A., Jones, G. (1988) J. Clin. Invest. 81:461.

184. Liberman, U. A., Eil, C., Marx, S. J. (1983) J. Clin. Invest. 71:192.

185. Gamblin, G. T., Liberman, U. A., Eil, C., Downs, R. W., DeGrange, D. A., Marx, S. J. (1985) J. Clin. Invest. 75:954.

186. Pike, J. W., Dokoh, S., Haussler, M. R., Liberman, U. A., Marx, S. J. (1984) Science 224:879.

187. Osteoporosis (1984) Proceedings of the Copenhagen International Symposium on Osteoporosis. Printed by Aalborg Stiftsbogtrykkeri. Christiansen, C., Arnaud, C. D., Nordin, B. E. C., Parfitt, A. M., Peck, W. A., Riggs, B. L. (eds.) Vol I and II.

9
Vitamin C

G. C. CHATTERJEE

Vitamin C (L-ascorbic acid) is unique among the vitamins. Not only does it have a simple structure and multiple structural and functional roles in various forms of life processes, but it is also unique, because most vertebrates, with the exception of man, monkey, guinea pigs, fruit-eating bats, and the bird *Pycnonotus cafer,* can synthesize it through the glucuronic acid pathway (1–5). Hence, these forms are not dependent upon a supply from external sources. Although the vitamin's exact molecular mechanism of action is not precisely known, we are beginning to understand how it functions in several biochemical unit processes and to understand the reasons for its efficacy as a therapeutic or prophylactic agent in a few pathological disorders of man.

Among the important roles of Vitamin C, we especially appreciate its role as a cofactor for mixed-function oxidases: prolyl hydroxylase, butyrobetaine hydroxylase, trimethyl lysine hydroxylase, cytochrome P = 450 function, cholesterol hydroxylase in the formation of bile acids, and a few other hydroxylation reactions in living systems. Moreover, it participates importantly in copper metabolism and in iron transport and mobilization. The vitamin has also been found to be effective in eliminating the toxicity caused by the intake of several xenobiotics. For a few of these elements, its efficacy is due to its ability to operate as a free-radical scavenger, interracting to form free radicals or peroxyl radicals under normal conditions and toxicant-induced stress (6–8). The vitamin is known for its oxidant reductant properties, which are also of major importance for its metabolic role (9).

Vitamin C is unlike most other vitamins in one important respect. No cofactor derivative for vitamin C has been isolated, nor its activity established. However, the discovery of a vitamin C metabolite such as 5-ketoascorbate in the urine of primates, has kindled new interest about the issue of the formation of a cofactor molecule from the parent vitamin (6). In addition to this metabolic product, two other substances have been found to form in animal systems—ascorbic acid 2-sulfate and methyl ascorbate. The former is eliminated mostly through the kidneys in primates, but it is accumulated and stored in fish (10).

The involvement of vitamin C in biochemical unit processes has been demonstrated classically by indirect methods, for example, estimating the metabolic pathways under conditions of experimental vitamin-deficiency. Recently, tissue culture techniques have been used, particularly to study how the vitamin functions in relation to collagen synthesis and immunological responses.

In this review, we briefly summarize the current information about vitamin C, with special reference to its involvement in certain specific areas. We will discuss its role in the formation and development of bone and other connective tissues, cholesterol and fat metabolism, immunological responsiveness, pathological conditions such as viral infections and carcinogenesis, the metabolism of drugs and other toxic chemicals, and the pathophysiology of the aging process. Again, we emphasize that the exact molecular mechanism of its action has yet to be determined.

FORMATION AND DEVELOPMENT OF BONE AND OTHER CONNECTIVE TISSUES

It has long been recognized that a hallmark of vitamin C deficiency is the structural degeneration of connective tissue in different organs and glands, muscle, and the vascular system (see for reviews 11, 12). In the skeleton, we note a variety of changes such as hemorrhage, loss of "original red color," and a deficit in the production of collagen and ground substance. Cartilage cells cease to form matrix; they become irregularly shaped, with pyknotic nuclei. This condition is normalized by vitamin C administration (13–18).

Scurvy is known to induce pathologic alterations in dental tissues, such as the odontoblasts and ameloblasts, and these cells fail to form normal dentin and enamel matrices. There is fibroid degeneration of the pulp and subsequent hemorrhage. Periodontal membranes in acutely scorbutic guinea pigs appear "less dense" than normal, indicating destruction of collagen (19–21). The oxitalan fibers of these connective tissues are also found to be partially degraded (22). Severe microscopical changes are seen in the jaw bones of scorbutic guinea pigs, and the changes are associated with a greater than normal incorporation of parenterally administered ascorbic acid-1-^{14}C into periodontal membrane, alveolar bone, and tooth pulp (23).

In experiments on fish, it has been reported (24) that a scorbutic diet produces gross clinical symptoms such as acute scoliosis and lordosis, leading to atrophy of the spinal cord and fracture dislocation of the vertebral column. The supporting gill cartilages become distorted or twisted, and this is perhaps the first visible sign of hypovitaminosis C. The changes lead to distortion of the eyeball. Petechial hemorrhage occurs in the lips, on the roof of the mouth, on the tongue, and on the internal and external opercular surfaces (25).

In scurvy, intramuscular hemorrhage is noted along with muscle atrophy, necrosis, and fatty degeneration. Chronic scurvy produces some hyaline changes in skeletal muscles, neuromuscular degeneration, and fatty degeneration as well as aberrant calcium deposits in heart muscle. In general, vitamin C is involved in the metabolism of skeletal connective tissues and their associations with calcium and phosphorus during calcification. Thus, it is essential for normal skeletal development. In terms of hard-tissue matrix formation, vitamin C deprivation leads to decreased synthesis of the glycosaminoglycans. Radiosulfur (^{35}S-sulfate) incorporation into chondroitin sulfate of various tissues, rib cartilage, sclera, and cornea is diminished. Thus, the vitamin promotes the formation of normal connective tissue matrices and bone mineral (e.g., ^{32}P into bone and tooth apatite) and enhances the storage of fluoride in the skeleton and soft tissues. The interrelationship between mineral nutrition and vitamin C has been reviewed by Chatterjee (11, 12).

Increased capillary fragility is common in scorbutic conditions; hemorrhage is common due to the thinning of arterial and capillary walls. Chronically vitamin C-deficient animals show many histologic alterations in the walls of the aorta. These include the presence of large intimal plaques of the musculofibrotic type (e.g., collagen in the aortic walls), marked endothelial proliferation, and a consistent high degree of ground substance metachromasia in the walls, and, in some cases, a variably thick layer of amorphous fibrous material underlies the endothelium (12).

In recent years, a large number of studies have been carried out to identify the exact role vitamin C plays in processes involving the synthesis, storage, and modification of connective tissue proteins—collagen, elastin, and proteoglycans (26–28). Vitamin C is regarded as a cofactor in prolyl and lysyl hydroxylation reactions (29), and it probably also functions in this way in certain glycosylation and sulfation reactions (30–33). If the vitamin is either absent or present in very low concentrations, collagen synthesis is decreased (34), bone formation is impaired, and the integrity of basement membrane is lost—and wound healing processes suffer (11, 12, 34). Vitamin C also exerts a major influence on the composition of the extracellular matrices formed by cultured smooth muscle cells and fibroblasts. In vitro, a (vitamin) deficiency promotes elastin formation and inhibits collagen formation (35–54); in the presence of the vitamin, the amount of elasin synthetized is decreased, and collagen synthesis is increased. Furthermore, it has been reported that rabbit pulmonary artery smooth muscle cells cultured in the presence of vitamin C accumulate less insoluble elastin with lower amounts of cross-links (41). The effect of vitamin C on elastin and collagen metabolism varies a great deal, depending on the source and species of cells used for culture experiments (40, 55–59). Excessive vitamin C supplementation, particularly in the postnatal rat pup, has little effect on elastin and collagen synthesis (36).

The role of vitamin C in the hydroxylation of proline and lysine, and in sulfation reactions, has not been clearly defined. Recently, it has been suggested that the vitamin functions through the stimulation of prolyl hydroxylase by maintaining the iron molecule of the enzyme in a reduced state at its active site. During the development of scurvy, the extracellular matrix becomes increasingly richer in glycosaminoglycans and contains dispersed and underhydroxylated collagen fibers. The tensile properties of the collagen-rich tissues is also reduced, because the molecules are underhydroxylated (26).

The role of vitamin C in elastin metabolism is not clear, since elastin does not contain hydroxylysine—but it does contain hydroxyproline, the synthesis of which is dependent upon vitamin C. However, extreme proline hydroxylation leads to an inhibition of formation of insoluble elastic fibers, and abundantly hydroxylated elastin fibers are unstable in vitro (60).

In scurvy, it is notable that prolyl hydroxylase activity is lowest in the tissues that contain the highest proportions of collagen. In other tissues, such as liver and kidney, the scorbutic state is not always associated with diminished enzyme activity. In fact, enzyme concentrations are increased during the later stages of an avitaminosis condition (44).

Lysyl hydroxylase activity appears to be modulated by dietary vitamin C status. Individuals with lysyl hydroxylase deficiency (an inborn error of metabolism) suffer pathologies such as lax joints, friable skin, and hemorrhagic scarring, conditions that could be reversed by the administration of vitamin C. Moreover, in addition to its cofactor role, the vitamin appears to stimulate both the synthesis and secretion of collagen (61).

Vuust et al. (62) have shown the modulatory effect of the vitamin on the synthesis of Type I collagen at the level of transcription. Spanheimer and Peterkofsky (63) have observed that acute fasting is associated with decreased proline incorporation into collagen, without affecting the synthesis of noncollagen protein. This occurs as a result of the decrease of the mRNA species for the procollagen molecule alone. Sodek et al. (64) have demonstrated the effect of vitamin C on collagenous and noncollagenous protein synthesis and collagen hydroxylation (^{3}H-proline incorporation) in adult mouse periodontal tissues maintained in a continuous-flow organ culture system. With suboptimal vitamin C concentration in the medium, the collagen synthesized was found to be highly unhydroxylated. Increasing the amount of vitamin C stimulated collagen and noncollagenous protein synthesis. In this system, the proportion of the radioactivity incorporated into the collagenous and noncollagenous proteins, the percent of Type III collagen synthesized (e.g., alveolar bone and periodontal ligament), and the pattern of collagen hydroxylation were similar to the *in vivo* state.

Less is known about the role of vitamin C in terms of influencing bone turnover. However, Basu (65) reported a very significant observation about the efficacy of the vitamin to relieve certain symptoms associated with bone metastasis from carcinoma. Such patients experience increased urinary excretion of hydroxyproline, presumably due to collagen degradation during bone resorption. The administration of vitamin C to these patients effectively eliminated this symptom.

The glycosaminoglycans of the ground substance appear to be another important component of connective tissues. These are extremely heterogeneous in origin and structure, and they have varying metabolic turnover rates. This property makes it difficult to identify correctly how vitamin C influences their metabolic turnover, and not unexpectedly, the results obtained in different studies often appear contradictory. In scurvy, there is a decrease in the amount of the sulfated glycosaminoglycans such as chondroitin-4-6-sulfate, dermatan sulfate, and hyaluronic acid, and this probably reflects an increase in the catabolic rate (66). In aortic tissue, most of the lysosomal enzymes responsible for the breakdown of these compounds appear to be stimulated (27). High doses of vitamin C are able to lower the rate of degradation in other connective tissues and, at the same time, stimulate the enzymes concerned with biological sulfation (67, 68). It is not yet clear whether ascorbate-2-sulfate plays any role in this process (69, 70).

Using cultured human cartilage chondrocytes, increasing levels of medium vitamin C lead to decreases in the activities of the aryl sulfatases A and B. This indicates that the vitamin acts to protect skeletal tissue glycosaminoglycans (28).

It also appears that the vitamin influences the biosynthesis and distribution of newly synthesized sulfated proteoglycans (s-PG) between the medium and the cell layers. It appears to stimulate the net s-PG synthesis per unit DNA and to increase the deposition of the newly synthesized molecules into the cell layers, in both cell and organ cultures (71). Meier and Solursh (71) have studied the effect of ascorbic acid on the secretion and assembly of the extracellular matrix by cultured chick embryo sternal chondrocytes. They reported that although ascorbate reduced the cysternal swelling of cells, the tissue formed by the cells was similar to that of normal cartilage in terms of the morphology of the matrix, the synthesis and deposition of the extracellular matrix (predominantly a1 chains), and the resistance of the matrix to hyaluronidase digestion. Thus, we can conclude that vitamin C is necessary both for collagen secretion and for the proper deposition of extracellular matrix. Under its aegis, collagen deposition is increased, and a stable environment is maintained for the deposition of newly synthesized proteoglycans. Since cysteine residues are the known components of the proteoglycan protein core, the vitamin probably helps to favor the conversion of cystine to cysteine. Peterkofsky et al. (72) have provided another approach; they have studied proline hydroxylation reactions in cultures of L-929 cells. These cells elaborate a factor that can replace vitamin C *in vitro* as a reductant for prolyl hydroxylase. This factor can account for the ascorbate-independent proline hydroxylation recorded in such cultures.

Multiple roles, therefore, have been identified for the participation of vitamin C in connective tissue metabolism. The vitamin is required for the biosynthesis of most of the components of connective tissues, and it is responsible for the structural integrity and stability of the components. When vitamin C is present suboptimally or is absent, the lytic enzymes responsible for the breakdown of these components become abundant. This is an interesting area for research, since the vitamin is known to modulate enzyme activity.

CHOLESTEROL AND FAT METABOLISM

In recent years, there has been increasing concern about the interaction of vitamin C with cholesterol and fat metabolism. This topic, and particularly its early literature, has been reviewed extensively by Chatterjee (12). A general picture about these interactions has emerged from work with the scorbutic guinea pig. The data indicate that the effects of the vitamin are expressed by altered serum and tissue levels of cholesterol lipids, lipoproteins, and phospholipids (73–88).

In the livers from scorbutic guinea pigs, the tricarboxylic acid cycle is impaired, and this leads to an accelerated utilization of the acetate pool for increased cholesterologenesis (89, 90). However, in this animal model, Guchait et al. (91) noted that there was a significant decrease in the incorporation of cholesterol-4-^{14}C into liver bile acids and gallbladder *in vivo* and into liver mitochondria *in vitro*. On the other hand, in species that can synthesize the vitamin, the vitamin C–cholesterol relationship has been studied in terms of the (complicated) alteration of cholesterol metabolism under the influences of high doses of vitamin C (92–95).

Ginter et al. (96) have designed an interesting approach to this problem in the guinea pig, and their model entails a study of latent vitamin C deficiency. Here, animals are maintained in a hypovitaminosis C state for some 3 months or more. They develop hypercholesterolemia, an accumulation of cholesterol in the liver, and demonstrate a significant reduction in total cholesterol turnover (re: 4-^{14}C-cholesterol) (97, 98). Serum cholesterol has been found to be elevated in acutely vitamin C-deficient patients. Ginter's laboratory (99) suggests that the impaired transformation of cholesterol to bile acids in vitamin C deprivation takes place through a 7α-hydroxylation of the cholesterol nucleus and that the vitamin probably has an effect on this hydroxylation step. The transformation of cholesterol into the principal bile acids in guinea pigs involves two hydroxylations—one at position 7 in the cholesterol nucleus, and another at position 26 on the side chain. In contrast to the adrenal and ovarian tissue (100, 101), ascorbic acid does not have any effect on 26-hydroxylation of cholesterol in liver mitochondria (102). It has further been noted that ascorbate stimulates the 7α-hydroxylation of cholesterol in the normal guinea pig liver microsomes. The enzyme cholesterol 7α-hydroxylase behaves like a mixed-function oxidase, and cytochrome P-450 probably has a role in this hydroxylating step (103, 104). The concentration of cytochrome P-450 in liver microsomes is decreased in vitamin C deficiency (105), and it is increased by administering the vitamin to such animals (106, 107). It is likely, then, that the ability of vitamin C to stimulate the 7-hydroxylation step is mediated through its actions on cytochrome P-450 levels.

It is, therefore, apparent that vitamin C has a role in the transformation of cholesterol into bile acids. Bjorkhum and Kallner (108) showed that vitamin C deficiency influences the turnover of a specific type of cytochrome P = 450 involved in several α = hydroxylations of cholesterol, resulting in the development of permanent hypercholesterolaemia. This disorder can induce focal desquamation in the vascular endothelium. The secondary effect of hypercholesterolemia is more important, since it involves the permanently raised concentrations of LDL in plasma. This results in increased LDL transport across the damaged endothelial barrier and enhanced cholesterol deposition in the area of a lesion. In vitamin C-deficient guinea pigs, significant cholesterol accumulates in the aorta (109–111). These accumulations can be exaggerated when guinea pigs are made marginally C-deficient and subsequently fed an atherogenic diet.

However, chronic vitamin C deficiency causes a significantly lower cholesterol turnover rate in the guinea pig (112). Hanck and Weiser have systematically studied the influence of vitamin C on lipid metabolism in man and animals (113). Latent vitamin C deficiency appeared to be responsible for raising the levels of blood lipids. When animals were maintained on low dietary vitamin C levels (with or without a cholesterol load), there was an increase in free and total cholesterol, triglycerides, and also uric acid, with subsequent lowering of plasma and leukocyte vitamin C and of lecithin cholestrerol acyl transferase (LCAT) activity.

The cholesterol content of aorta was negatively correlated to the vitamin C intake. High vitamin C administration to animals is known to depress cholesterol levels significantly. It should be noted that this effect is not significant when the diet also contains cholesterol; under this circumstance, the vitamin C level has to be much increased to elicit a depression in cholesterol. It is likely that vitamin C exerts this effect by increasing LCAT activity. In the presence of LCAT. the concentration of esterified cholesterol increases rapidly, with a decrease in the free cholesterol content (114). A significant increase of HDL cholesterol by the administration of vitamin C has also been reported for man (115).

Vitamin C can act as a cofactor for the metabolism of iodine, carbohydrates, and nucleic acids. In hypothyroidism, cholesterol degradation and excretion are diminished. In the case of hypercholesterolemia, the vitamin is shown to have a lowering effect (116). When administered with thyroid-stimulating hormone (TSH), vitamin C enhances the incorporation of ^{131}I to form the active hormone. It has been reported that gout is associated with hypercholesterolemia and atherosclerosis (which lead to the development of hyperuricaemia) and that vitamin C administration decreases the severity of these conditions (117). The uricosuric effect of the vitamin is dose-dependent and effective only at very high doses (118). Vitamin C, then, is effective in lowering both elevated uric acid levels and hyperlipoproteinemia. Although the concentration of the vitamin is negatively correlated with the levels of free fatty acid, triglyceride, cholesterol, and beta-lipoprotein in plasma and with aortic cholesterol, it is positively correlated with the plasma α-lipoprotein level. As such, extremely high levels of vitamin C intake could be a useful modality to control blood lipid levels, particularly so among the aged population (see below).

As noted above with regard to the effect of low vitamin C intake levels, scurvy induces hypertriglyceridemia [in guinea pigs (119, 120)]. This is associated with a decrease in lipolytic activity in certain tissues (121). Subsequently, there is an increase in certain tissue lipids and serum lipids (122–124). Although there is a decrease in the synthesis of cholesterol in chronic scurvy, the increase in the level of cholesterol occurs because its conversion into the bile acids and its turnover are slower than normal (125, 126). Chronic vitamin C deficiency in guinea pigs *in vivo* leads to a decrease in the activity of hepatic hMG Co-A reductase, a rate-limiting enzyme in the cholesterol biosynthesis pathway (126, 127). Vitamin C also operates to regulate plasma cholesterol levels by influencing the LDL receptor number. It enhances lipoprotein catabolism by increasing the number of receptors in cultured bovine aorta (128). In normocholesterolemic human subjects, it has been shown that vitamin C administration "in excess" has no effect on the serum and tissue lipids (129, 130).

IMMUNOLOGICAL RESPONSIVENESS

The nutritional standards recommended for animals have a very important role to play in controlling immunologic responses. Vitamin C is very important in this regard. It enhances host resistance through stimulation of immunocompetent cells and by promoting the elaboration of several nonspecific immunological factors (131–142). These interrelationships have been reviewed (12). Recent reports also signal that vitamin C may protect against the common cold (143, 144) and prolong the survival of (?immunologically compromised) terminal cancer patients (132). The vitamin improves (scorbutic guinea pig-derived) macrophage migration *in vitro* (135), and it enhances the production of interferon by human embryonic fibroblasts (140). Other effects include the stimulation of chemotactic responses via amplifying the hexose monophosphate shunt in human neutrophils (134, 136, 137, 145). Bacteriocidal activity via phagocytosis by neutrophils is also modulated by the vitamin C status (141, 142). Recent studies have shown that the vitamin can augment immunological responses through lymphocyte stimulation in cell cultures (146, 147); the effect is associated with the enhancement of DNA and protein synthesis *in vitro,* and it is independent of a change in the macrophage population.

As noted above, vitamin C is engaged in a number of immunological responses such as chemotaxis and phagocytosis via mechanisms that involve stimulation of pathways such as the hexose monophosphate shunt, or by a myeloperoxidase function or changes in cGMP levels (148). Moreover, vitamin C is linked with both the delayed and the immediate type of hypersensitivity reactions as well as with monocyte–macrophage reactivity. The modulating effect of vitamin C on the immune responses occurs through mediation of interferon production and T-cell function (149). Migliozzi (150) demonstrated that animals receiving a low dose of vitamin C show degradation/regression of methylcholanthrene-induced tumors; animals maintained on a high-dose vitamin C regimen showed no evidence of tumor degradation. These data infer that vitamin C (1) modulates T-lymphocyte function through the release of lymphokines and (2) balances the production of the macrophage inhibitory and activating factors while simultaneously effecting interferon production. B-cell activity was not altered (149, 151, 152). Finally, it has been suggested (153) that PGE_2 synthesis is required for the cytolytic activities of natural killer T-cells. The argument is that the "balance" that exists between interferon—the "activator" of– and prostaglandin—the "inhibitor of"—macrophage products is probably the determinant for the actual census of cytolytic killer cells. When vitamin C is administered to animals, the level of PGE_2 is increased, bringing about a change in natural killer cell activity.

Because it appears to be a very effective immunopotentiator in man, a combination of vitamin C and human cell culture rabies vaccine has been recommended for the treatment of rabies (154–156). Banic and Kossack (157) also recommend the vitamin be used to prevent the occurrence of posttransfusion hepatitis that is caused by the hepatitis virus B.

PATHOLOGICAL CONDITIONS INCLUDING VIRAL INFECTIONS AND CARCINOGENESIS

Although there is a controversy regarding the therapeutic and/or prophylactic efficacy of vitamin C treatment for a number of human diseases, these parameters continue to be tested. As stated earlier, the vitamin is intimately involved in the metabolism of collagen, the glycosaminoglycans, cholesterol, and lipids. Deficiency leads to vascular degeneration and development of atherosclerosis (158). Since there is reason to believe that a relative deficit in vitamin C stores develops during aging, there is interest in the benefit that might be derived by increasing the intake of the vitamin, especially in combating atherosclerosis. Vitamin C appears to be useful therapeutically in hyperlipoproteinaemia (159). Hanck and Weiser (113) also indicate the importance of the vitamin in controlling the symptoms of gout, diabetes mellitus, hypothyroidism, and hyperlipidemia (113). Ginter and Minkus (160) have shown that vitamin C administration reduces gallstone formation in hamsters.

The concept that vitamin C therapy could be helpful in controlling cancer (132, 161, 162) is based on the observation that cancer patients have subnormal levels of leukocytic ascorbate. The putative effect of vitamin C has been confirmed using tumor cell lines in culture (164). An interesting relationship has been inferred between the vitamin, trace elements, and malignancy. For example, zinc concentrations are elevated severalfold in patients suffering from breast cancer (165, 166). Experimental studies have demonstrated that tumor growth can be retarded by a low-zinc diet (167). This has led to the postulate that the administration of vitamin C could benefit such patients by lowering their tissue zinc concentrations. The beneficial role of the vitamin in cancer treatment may also involve its ability to stimulate cAMP formation. It was early observed that polyoma virus-transformed cells have diminished adenyl cyclase activity (168) and that tumor growth is inhibited bt cAMP (169). Prasad et al. (170) have shown that vitamin C potentiates the growth inhibitory effects of 5-fluorouracil, bleomycin sulfate, sodium buyrate, cAMP-stimulating agents, and X-irradiation on mouse neuroblastoma cells. However, this effect is not produced in rat glioma cell cultures.

The efficacy of vitamin C in combating the common cold is also not without controversy (171–173). There is a significant reduction in leukocyte ascorbate levels during the symptomatic phase (174). Most of the effects of the vitamin seem to be dependent upon its role in immunopotentiation (175, 176).

METABOLISM OF DRUGS AND OTHER TOXIC CHEMICALS

Vitamin C has long been known to be involved in the metabolism of pharmacological agents. In scorbutic guinea pigs, the metabolism of drugs such as pentobarbital, acetanilide, aniline, or antipyrine is reduced (177, 178). In that species, vitamin C deprivation also decreases the microsomal oxidation rates of coumarin, diphenylhydramine, and zoxazolamine. This deficit in drug-metabolizing processes like O-demethylation, N-demethylation, and hydroxylation is linked to microsomal electron transport components such as cytochrome P-450, NADPH cytochrome P-450 reductase; the levels of these components are also decreased under the conditions of vitamin C deprivation (180, 181). Administration of the vitamin leads to an increase in the microsomal drug oxidation system (182–185). Moreover, the quality as well as the quantity of microsomal cytochrome P-450 is altered in scorbutic guinea pigs.

Most of the drugs and foreign compounds, as well as endogenous substrates like cholesterol, are metabolized through the mixed-function oxidase system, and vitamin C status is related to the maintenance of the levels of the various components and enzymes of this system (185–189). Vitamin C deficiency in animals leads to depression in the mixed-function oxidase system and lipoperoxidation, resulting, in a reduced capacity to catabolize xenobiotics and to transform cholesterol to bile acids. A disturbance in this mechanism would promote the formation of cholesterol gallstones and atherosclerosis (187–193). Enhanced intake of the vitamin brings about a dose-related increase of the components and enzymes of the mixed-function oxidases and of cholesterol 7α-hydroxylase (189, 192). Hence, animals on a high vitamin C intake appear to be more resistant to the toxic effects caused by xenobiotics and to the hypercholesterolaemic condition.

This effect of vitamin C appears to be dose-dependent in a biphasic manner, since beyond a certain level, extremely high vitamin C intake could lower the mixed-function oxidase activity (126, 193–199). This effect of very high vitamin C intake is probably associated with an increased requirement for vitamin E, depressing the overall tissue antioxidant potential (200, 201).

It has been shown that the hemolytic and perioxidative effects of vitamin C can be countered by increased tocopherol supplements. With an extremely high vitamin C intake, two events occur: *in vitro*, the mixed-function oxidase activity decreased (189, 194, 195), and an antiperoxidating effect was noted (202–205). These observations indicate that in the presence of peroxidases, the cytochrome P-450 cycle is stimulated through the oxidating properties of vitamin C (206, 207). Extremely high dietary levels of vitamin C also lead to a depression of blood and liver copper levels (guinea pigs) and an alteration of ceruloplasmin levels (208, 209), effects that interfere with the transport and availability of iron for cytochrome biosynthesis (192) and that affect the formation of oxygen radicals. An interaction is assumed between vitamin C and heme iron of cytochrome P-450 (210). High vitamin C levels enhance iron incorporation into heme (211).

The vitamin is known to act both as a superoxide scavenger (212) and as a suppressor of peroxidation. But, simultaneously, the system ascorbate-Fe^{2+} may induce lipid peroxidation in biological membranes, because it generates superoxide anion radicals (213). Hence, under certain conditions, high vitamin C doses may exert an adverse effect on membrane enzymes. The same type of effect occurs in the case of cholesterol 7α-hydroxylase (189).

Several xenobiotics such as the organochlorine and organophosphorus compounds, various toxic metals, and certain industrial chemicals have an interesting interrelationship with vitamin C in living systems (see 12 for review). The gross effects of these agents include alteration of tissue morphology and alterations in tissue levels of vitamin C by changes in its biosynthesis and metabolism and in its urinary excretion, and they impair the induction of hepatic microsomal hydroxylating enzymes and certain other marker enzymes in different tissues (12, 142, 214–222).

An interesting aspect of vitamin C function that has been investigated in detail regards its role in alleviating the toxicity of several xenobiotics; these effects occur when the vitamin is administered in high doses (12). Vitamin C supplementation reverses the toxicities of nickel (223), rubidium (224), vanadium (225), lead (216), mercury (215, 226), cadmium (214), dieldrin (227, 228), lindane (229, 230), monocrotophos (231), chlordane (232), parathion and malathion (223), and the polychlorinated biphenyls (234). The major parameters that have been used to monitor xenobiotic toxicity include the growth rate, organ weight, mortality, tissue vitamin C levels, and the tissue and organ concentrations of several marker enzymes and their histologies. The precise mechanism(s) by which vitamin C functions to reverse many of the expressions of toxicity have not been established. But it has been suggested that under the stressful conditions caused by the intake of different toxicants, the vitamin exerts its effect through its oxidant-reductant property and through its interaction as a free-radical scavenger.

PATHOPHYSIOLOGY OF THE AGING PROCESS

Aging individuals are usually prone to develop certain specific pathologies such as hyperlipidemia and hypercholesterolemia, and their vascular walls are likely to show damage due, in part, to defects of connective tissue synthesis and impairment of repair processes. Cardiovascular disorders, a high incidence of sublingual venular dilatations and varicosities, increased capillary fragility, a lowered immunological competence, increased susceptibility to infection, arthritic changes, gout, hypothyroidism, diabetes mellitus, and increased skeletal fragility are all part of the aging process. Almost all of these disorders in man and other animals can be linked to the nutritional status of vitamin C. The involvement of the vitamin on the biochemical unit processes associated with these conditions has been verified in experimentally produced avitaminotic states, using animals that, like man, cannot synthesize vitamin C—that is, they are dependent upon an exogenous supply of the vitamin. The development of a marginal deficiency of vitamin C is sufficient to produce the discrete disorders noted above.

Extensive studies have been conducted in man to determine if aging involves a change in tissue vitamin C concentrations. These investigations have signaled significant decreases of the vitamin in plasma, leukocytes, and platelets (235–241). There is comparatively little information available about the status of the vitamin in other tissues, but there are trends that indicate that these decline as well (242). Hughes and Jones (243) observed that older guinea pigs showed reduced concentrations of vitamin C in their spleen, adrenal, and lens of the eye but increased levels in brain. However, the capacity of these tissues to "retain" vitamin C also appeared low. Vitamin C levels in tissues from inbred mouse strains also appear to correlate negatively with age (244).

Schorah (245) compared the vitamin C status of geriatric patients and elderly outpatients with that in young control subjects, all of whom received dietary vitamin C supplements. He reported that the regimen raised the initially low plasma levels in the elderly population and that these individuals also gained weight. Nearly identical studies have been pursued by other workers (246, 247). There are also reports (248) that diets supplemented with vitamin C cause young people to "replete" more rapidly than the elderly, and this suggests that the group differences might obtain in terms of their respective patterns of leukocyte metabolism. When Eddy (248) examined this issue in elderly patients, it was observed that the patients who had attained high leukocyte ascorbic acid levels were those who had a high capillary resistance. Elderly vegetarian subjects who enjoyed a high dietary intake of vitamin C had higher levels of plasma and leukocyte vitamin C and a negligible incidence of the sublingual venular dilatations and varicosities that are commonly found among the elderly who are compromised by a low-vitamin status (250).

Permanent chronic vitamin C deficiency, then, is common among aged individuals and those suffering from the age-related disorders (see above) and certain pathologies caused by infective agents. It may be that the immunological mechanisms that have been invoked in the etiology of some joint disease problems and that appear to be particularly involved in osteoporotic bone resorption could be amenable to treatment with vitamin C because of the immunopotentiation it evokes. Its cofactor activity in modulating enzymes, its oxidation–reduction properties, and its capacity to scavenge free radicals under normal and stressful states also increases the utility of the vitamin to alleviate many of these conditions.

REFERENCES

1. Chatterjee, I. B., Chatterjee G. C., Ghosh N. C., Ghosh J. J., Guha B. C. (1960) Biochem. J. 76:279.

2. Chatterjee, I. B., Chatterjee G. C., Ghosh N. C., Ghosh J. J., Guha B. C. (1960) Biochem. J. 74:193.

3. Roy, R. N., Guha B. C. (1958) Nature 182:319.

4. Roy, R. N., Guha B. C. (1958) Nature 182:1689.

5. Chatterjee, I., Chatterjee G. C. (1968) Indian J. Exp. Biol. 6:103.

6. Tolbert, B. M. (1985) Int J. Vit. Nutr. Res. Suppl. 27:121.

7. Tolbert, B. M., Downing M., Carlson R. W., Knight M. K., Baker E. M. (1975) Ann. N. Y. Acad. Sci. 258:48.

8. Bates, C. J. (1982) In: Counsell G., Hornig D. (eds) *Vitamin C*. London: Applied Science, p 1.

9. Weis, W. (1975) Ann. N. Y. Acad. Sci. 258:190.

10. Tucker, B., Halver J. (1984) J. Nutr. 114:991.

11. Chatterjee, G. C. (1967) In: Sebrell W. H., Harris R. S. (eds) *The Vitamins*. New York: Academic Press, p. 407.

12. Chatterjee, G. C. (1978) In: Rechcigl M. Jr. (ed) *Handbook Series in Nutrition and Food*. Florida: CRC Press, p. 149.

13. King, C. G. (1975) Ann. N. Y. Acad. Sci. 258:540.

14. Maclean, D. L., Sheppard M., McHenry E. W. (1939) Brit. J. Exp. Pathol. 20:451.

15. Wolbach, S. B. (1937) J. Amer. Med. Assoc. 108:7.

16. Pirani, C. L., Bey C. G., Sutherland K. (1950) Arch. Pathol. 49:710.

17. Robertson, W., Van B. (1950) J. Biol. Chem. 187:673.

18. Wolbach, S. B., Maddoc C. L. (1952) Arch. Pathol. 53:54.

19. Boyle, P. E. (1938) Amer. J. Pathol. 14:843.

20. Boyle, P. E., Bessey O. A., Wolbach S. B. (1937) Proc. Soc. Exp. Biol. Med. 36:733.

21. Boyle, P. E., Bessey O. A., Wolbach S. B. (1937) J. Amer. Dental Assoc. 24:1768.

22. Fullmer, H. H., Lillie R. D. (1958) J. Histochem 6:481.

23. Yale, S. H., Jeffaay H., Mohammed C. L., Wach E. C. (1959) J. Dental Res. 38:396.

24. Halver, J. E., Smith R. R. (1975) Ann. N. Y. Acad. Sci. 258:81.

25. Hojer, J. A. (1924) Acta. Paediat. 3:8.

26. Tinker, D., Rucker R. E. (1985) Physiol. Rev. 65:607.

27. Ginter, E. (1978) Adv. Lipid Res. 16:167.

28. Schwartz, E. R. (1979) Int. J. Vit. Nutr. Res. Suppl. 19:113.

29. Barnes, M. J. (1975) Ann. N. Y. Acad. Sci. 258:264.

30. Stassen, F. L. H., Cardinale G. J., Udenfriend S. (1973) Proc. Nat. Acad. Sci. (USA) 70:1090.

31. Tuderman, L., Myllyla R., Kivirikko K. I. (1977) Eur. J. Biochem. 80:341.

32. Bailey, A. J., Etherington, D. J. (1980) Comp. Biochem. 19:299.

33. Kikuchi, Y., Suzuki, Y., Tamiya, N. (1983) Biochem. J. 213:507.

34. Barnes, M. J. (1975) Ann. N. Y. Acad. Sci. 258:264.

35. Cardinale, G. J., Udenfriend, S. (1974) Adv. Enzymol. 41:245.

36. Critchfield, J. W. Dubick, M., Last, J., Cross, C. E., Rucker, R. B. (1985) J. Nutr. 115:70.

37. Declerck, Y. A., Jones, P. A. (1980) Biochem. J. 186:217.

38. Declerck, Y. A., Jones, P. A. (1980) Cancer Res. 40:3228.

39. Dubick, M. A., Critchfield, J. W., Last, J. A., Cross, C. E., Rucker, R. B. (1983) Toxicology 27:301.

40. Dubick, H. A., Last, J. A., Cross, C. E., Rucker, R. B. (1983) Drug Nutr. Interact 2:105.

41. Dunn, D. M., Franzblau, C. (1981) Biochemistry 21:4195.

42. Hamilton, G. (1971) Prog. Bioorg. Chem. 1:83.

43. Hamilton, S. J., Mehrle, P. M. Mayer, F. I. (1981) Trans. Amer. Fish. Soc. 110:718.

44. Kutnink, M. A., Tolbert, B. M., Richmond, V. L., Baker, E. M. (1969) Proc. Soc. Exp. Biol. Med. 132:440.

45. Murad, S., Grove, D., Lindberg, L. A., Reynolds, G., Sivarajah, A., Pinnell, S. R. (1981) Proc. Nat. Acad. Sci. (USA) 78:2879.

46. Murad, S., Tajima, S., Johnson, G. R., Sivarajah, A., Pinnell, S. R. (1983) J. Invest. Dermatol. 81:158.

47. Myara, I., Charpentier, C., Wolform, C., Gautier, M., Lemonnier, A., Larreque, M., Chamson, A., Frey, J. (1983) J. Inherit. Metab. Dis. 6:27.

48. Peltonen, L., Kvivaniemi, H., Palotie, A., Horn, N., Kaitila, I., Kivirikko K. I. (1983) Biochemistry 22:6156.

49. Peterkofsky, B (1972) Arch. Biochem. Biophys. 152:318.

50. Peterkofsky, B., Kalwinsky, D., Assad, R. (1980) Arch. Biochem. Biophys. 199:3.

51. Ringsdorf, W. M., Cheraskin, E. (1982) Oral Surg. 53:231.

52. Scottburden, T., Davies, P. J., Gevers, W. (1979) Biochem. Biophys. Res. Commun. 91:739.

53. Scottburden, T., Murray, E., Diehl, T., Gevers, W. (1983) Hoppe-Seyler's Z. Physiol. Chem. 364:61.

54. Barrow, M. V., Simpson, C. F., Miller, E. G. (1974) Q. Rev. Biol. 49:101.

55. Mecham, R. P., Lange, G., Madaras, J., Starcher, B. (1981) J. Cell Biol. 90:332.

56. Barnes, M. J., Constable, B. J., Kodicek, E. (1969) Biochem. J 113:387.

57. Barnes, M. J., Constable, B. J., Morton, L. F., Kodicek, E. (1970) Biochem. J. 119:575.

58. Barnes, M. J., Constable, B. J., Morton, L. F., Royce, P. M. (1974) Biochem. J. 139:461.

59. Barnes, M. J., Kodicek, E. (1972) Vit. Horm. 30:1.

60. Urry, D. (1983) Ultrastruct. Pathol. 4:227.

61. Tajima, S., Pinnell, S. R. (1982) Biochem. Biophys. Res. Common. 106:632.

62. Vuust, J., Sobel, M. E., Martin, G. R. (1985) Eur. J. Biochem. 151:449.

63. Spanheimer, R. G., Peterkofsky, B. (1985) J. Biol. Chem. 260:3955.

64. Sodek, J., Feng, J., Yen, E. H., Melcher, A. H. (1982) Calcif. Tissue Int. 34:408.

65. Basu, T. K. (1979) Int. J. Vit. Nutr. Res. Suppl. 19:95.

66. Higuchi, R., Fujinami, T., Nakano, S., Nakayama, K., Hayashi, K., Sakuma, N., Takada, K. (1975) Jpn. J. Atheroscler. 3:303.

67. Nambisan, B., Kurup, P. A. (1974) Atherosclerosis 19:191.

68. Nambisan, B., Kurup, P. A. (1975) Atherosclerosis 22:447.
69. Hatanaka, H., Yamagata, T., Egami, F. (1974) Proc. Jpn. Acad. 50:747.
70. Hornig, D. (1975) Ann. N. Y. Acad. Sci. 258:103.
71. Meier, S., Solursh, M. (1978) J. Ultrastruct. Res. 65:48.
72. Peterkofsky, B., Kalwinsky, D., Assad, R. (1980) Arch. Biochem. Biophys. 199:
73. Naito, M., Sakurai, T., Tezuka, K. (1958) Sinshu. Med. J 7:73.
74. Mueller, P. S., Cardon, P. V. Jr. (1961) J. Lipid Res. 2:83.
75. Mueller, P. S. (1962) J. Lipid Res. 3:92.
76. Banerjee, S., Banerjee, A. (1963) Proc. Soc. Exp. Biol. Med. 112:372.
77. Quastel, J. H., Wheatley, A. H. M. (1934) Biochem. J. 28:1014.
78. Abramson, H. (1949) J. Biol. Chem. 178:179.
79. Rusch, H. P., Kline, B. E. (1941) Cancer Res. 1:465.
80. Banerjee, S. K., Majumder, P. K., Roy, R. K., Chatterjee, G. C. (1972) Indian J. Biochem. Biophys. 9:247.
81. Banerjee, S., Deb, C. (1952) J. Biol. Chem. 194:575.
82. Banerjee, B., Banerjee, S. (1954) J. Biol. Chem. 209:641.
83. Banerjee, S., Singh, H. D. (1957) Amer. J. Physiol. 190:265.
84. Kawishar, W. K., Chakrapani, B., Banerjee, S. (1983) Indian J. Med. Res. 51:488.
85. Rahandraha, T., Ratsimamanga, A. R. (1955) CR. Soc. Biol. 149:1206.
86. Banerjee, S., Banerjee, A. (1965) Amer. J. Physiol. 208:329.
87. Bolker, H. I., Fishman, S., Heard, R. D., O'Donnell, V. J., Webb, J. L., Willis, G. C. (1956) J. Exp. Med. 103:199.
88. Becker, R. R., Burch, H. B., Salomon, L. L., Venkitasubramaniam, T. A., King, C. G. (1953) J. Am. Chem. Soc. 75:2020.
89. Whitehouse, M. W., Staple, E., Gurin, S. (1959) J. Biol. Chem. 234:276.
90. Takeda, Y., Hara, M. (1955) J. Biol. Chem. 214:657.
91. Guchait, R. B., Guha, B. C., Ganguli, N. C. (1963) Biochem. J. 86:193.
92. Ginter, E. (1970) The role of ascorbic acid in cholesterol metabolism Slovak Academy of Sciences, Bratislava.
93. Kirk, J. E. (1973) Monograph on Atherosclerosis, S. Karger, Basel.
94. Nockels, C. F. (1973) Poult. Sci. 52:373.
95. Ginter, E., Nemec, R., Cerven, J., Mikus, L. (1973) Lipids 8:135.
96. Ginter, E., Bobek, P., Ovecka, M. (1968) Int. J. Vit. Nutr. Res. 38:104.
97. Ginter, E., Cerven, J., Mikus, L. (1969) Physiol. Bohemoslov. 18:459.
98. Ginter, E. (1973) Science 179:702.
99. Ginter, E., Cerven, J., Nemec, R., Mikus, L. (1971) Amer. J. Clin. Nutr. 24:1238.
100. Sulimovici, S., Boyd, G. S. (1968) Steroids 12:127.
101. Shimizu, K. (1970) Biochem. Biophys. Acts. 210:333.
102. Kritchevsky, D., Tepper, S. A., Story, J. A. (1973) Lipids 8:482.
103. Wade, F., Hirata, K., Nakao, K., Sakamoto, Y. (1968) J. Biochem. 64:415.
104. Scholan, N. A., Boyd, G. S. (1968) Hoppe-Seyler's Z. Physiol. Chem. 349:1628.
105. Degkwitz, E., Hochli-Kaufmann, L., Luft, D., Staudinger, H. (1972) Hoppe-Seyler's Z. Physiol. Chem. 353:1023.
106. Leber, H. W., Degkwitz, E., Staudinger, H. (1970) Hoppe-Seyler's Z. Physiol. Chem. 351:995.
107. Ginter, E., Nemec, R. (1972) Physiol. Bohemoslov. 21:539.
108. Bjorkhem, I., Kallner, A. (1976) J. Lipid Res. 17:360.
109. Fujinami, T., Okado, K., Senda, K., Nakano, S., Higuchi, R., Nakayama, K., Hayashi, K., Sakuma, N. (1975) Jap. J. Atheroscler. 3:117.
110. Ginter, E., Babala, J., Cerven, J. (1969) J. Atheroscler. Res. 10:341.
111. Hanck, A., Weiser, H. (1977) Int. J. Vit. Nutr. Res. Suppl. 16:67.

112. Ginter, E. (1975) Ann. N. Y. Acad. Sci. 258:410.

113. Hanck, A., Weiser, H. (1979) Int. J. Vit. Nutr. Res. Suppl. 19:83.

114. Glomset, J. A., Wright J. L. (1964) Biochem Biophys Acta 89:266.

115. Bates, C. J., Mandal, A. R., Cole, T. J. (1977) Lancet II:611.

116. Scholz, A. (1973) Klin. Wschr. 51:518.

117. Hall, A. P. (1965) Arthritis Rheum. 8:846.

118. Steim, H. B., Hasan, A., Fox, I. H. (1976) Ann. intern. Med. 84:385.

119. Fujinami, T., Okado, K., Senda, K., Sugimura, M., Kishikawa, M. (1971) Jap. Circulat. J. 35:1559.

120. Ginter, E., Cerna, O., Ondreicka, R., Roch, V., Balaz, V. (1976) Food Chem. 1:23.

121. Sokoloff, B., Hori, M., Sailholf, C., McConnel, B., Imai, T. (1967) J. Nutr. 91:107.

122. Turley, S. D., West, C. E., Horton, B. J. (1976) Atherosclerosis 24:1.

123. Yokota, F., Igarashi, Y., Suzue, R. (1981) Atherosclerosis 38:249.

124. Ginter, E., Adams, M. (1983) Atherosclerosis 46:369.

125. Ginter, E. (1979) Lancet II:958.

126. Holloway, D. E., Peterson, F. S., Prigge, W. F., Gebhard, R. C. (1981) Biochem. Biophys. Res. Commun. 102:1282.

127. Greene, Y. J., Harood, H. J., Stacpoole, P. W. (1985) Biochem. Biophys. Acta. 834:134.

128. Aulinskas, T. H., Vanderwesthoyzen, D. R., Coetzee, G. A. (1983) Atherosclerosis 47:159.

129. Anderson, T. W., Reid, D. B. W., Beaten, G. M. (1972) Lancet II:876.

130. Khan, A. R., Seetharnee, F. A. (1981) Atherosclerosis 39:89.

131. Boxcer, L. A., Watanabe, A. N., Rister, M., Besch, H. R., Allen, J., Baehner, R. L. (1976) New Engl. J. Med. 295:1041.

132. Cameron, E., Pauling, L. (1976) Proc. Nat. Acad. Sci. 73:3685.

133. Cardinale, G. J., Stassen, F. L. H., Cuttan, R., Udenfriend, S. (1975) Ann. N. Y. Acad. Sci. 258:258.

134. Chaokuang, H. (1977) Fed. Proc. 36:177.

135. Ganguli, R., Durieuz, M. F., Waldman, R. H. (1976) Amer. J. Clin. Nutr. 29:762.

136. Goetzl, E. J., Wasserman, S. I., Gigli, I., Austen, K. F. (1974) J Clin. Invest. 52:813.

137. Hahn, G. S., O'Connor, R. (1978) Clin. Res. 26:184.

138. Ross, R., Benditt, E. P. (1962) J. Cell. Biol. 12:533.

139. Schoepflin, G. S., Goetzl, E. J., Austen, K. F. (1977) Fed. Proc. 76:40.

140. Siegel, B. V. (1975) Nature 254:531.

141. Smith, W. B., Shohet, S. M., Zagajeski, E., Lubin, B. H. (1975) Ann. N. Y. Acad. Sci. 258:329.

142. Chatterjee, G. C., Mazumder, P. K., Banerjee, S. K., Roy, R. K., Ray, B., Rudrapal, D. (1975) Ann. N. Y. Acad. Sci. 258:382.

143. Coulehan, J. L., Reisinger, K. S., Rogers, K. D., Bradley, D. W. (1974) New Engl. J. Med. 290:6.

144. Rhead, W. J., Schrauzer, G. N. (1971) Nutr. Rev. 29:262.

145. Soulillou, J. P., Carpenter, C. B., Lundin, A. P., Strom, T. B. (1975) J. Immunol. 115:1566.

146. Delafuente, J. C., Panush, R. S. (1978) J. Allergy Clin. Immunol. 61:132.

147. Panush, R. S., Delafuente, J. C. (1979) Int. J. Vit. Nutr. Res. Suppl. 19:179.

148. Leibovitz, B., Siegel, B. V. (1978) Int. J. Vit. Nutr. Res. 48:159.

149. Siegel, B. V., Morton, J. I. (1977) Experientia. 33:393.

150. Migliozzi, J. A. (1977) Brit. J. Cancer. 35:448.

151. Siegel, B. V. (1974) Infect. Immun. 10:409.

152. Siegel, B. V. (1975) Nature 254:531.

153. Siegel, B. V., Morton, J. I. (1984) Int. J. Vit. Nutr. Res. 54:339.

154. Banic, S. (1975) Nature 258:153.

155. Kuwert, E. K., Marcus, I., Hoher, P. G., Werner, J., Iwand, A., Helm, E. B. (1977) Med. Klinn. 72:797.

156. Banic, S. (1979) Int. J. Vit. Nutr. Res. Suppl. 19:35.

157. Banic, S., Kosac, M. (1979) Int. J. Vit. Nutr. Res. Suppl. 19:41.

158. Ginter, E., Bobck, P., Babala, J., Jakubovsky, J., Zaviacic, M., Lojda, Z. (1979) Int. J. Vit. Nutr. Res. Suppl. 19:55.

159. Heine, H., Norden, C. (1979) Int. J. Vit. Nutr. Res. Suppl. 19:45.

160. Ginter, E., Mikus, L. (1977) Experientia. 33:716.

161. Cameron, E., Campbell, A. (1974) Chem-Biol. Interact. 9:285.

162. Cameron, E., Pauling, L. (1974) Chem-Biol. Interact. 9:273.

163. Basu, T. K., Raven, R. W., Dickerson, J. W. T., Williams, D. C. (1974) Eur. J. Cancer 10:507.

164. Bishun, N., Basu, T. K., Metcalfe, S., Williams, D. C. (1978) Oncology 35:160.

165. Dewys, W., Pories, W. J., Richter, M. C., Strain, W. H. (1970) Proc. Soc. Exp. Biol. 135:7.

166. Schwartz, A. E., Leddicotte, G. W, Fink, R. W., Friedman, E. W. (1974) Surgery 76:32.

167. Rubin, H., Rordi, T. (1973) J. Cell Comp. Physiol. 81:387.

168. Burk, R. R. (1968) Nature 219:1272.

169. Gericke, D., Chandra, P. (1969) Hoppe-Seylers Z. Physiol. Chem. 350:1469.

170. Prasad, K. N., Nobles, E., Sinha, P. K., Ramanuyam, M., Sakamoto, A. (1979) Int. J. Vit. Nutr. Res. Suppl. 19:155.

171. Coulehan, J. L., Reisinger, K. S., Rogers, K. D., Bradley, D. W. (1974) New Engl. J. Med. 290:6.

172. Rhead, W. J., Schrauzer, G. N. (1971) Nutr. Rev. 29:262.

173. Pauling, L. (1970) Vitamin C and the common cold. W. H. Freeman and Co., San Francisco.

174. Hume, R., Weyers, E. (1973) Scot. Med. J. 18:3.

175. Goetzl, E. L., Wasserman, I. G., Austen, K. F. (1974) J. Clin. Invest. 53:813.

176. Yonemoto, R. H. (1979) Int. J. Vit. Nutr. Res. Suppl. 19:143.

177. Richards, R. K., Kueter, K., Klatt, T. I. (1941) Proc. Soc. Exp. Biol. Med. 48:403.

178. Axelrod, J., Udenfriend, S., Brodie, B. B. (1954) J. Pharmacol. Exp. Ther. 111:176.

179. Conney, A. H., Bray, G. A., Evans, C., Burns, J. J. (1961) Ann. N. Y. Acad. Sci. 92:11.

180. Kato, R., Takanaka, A., Oshima, T. (1969) Jpn. J. Pharmacol. 19:25.

181. Degkwitz, E., Kim, K. S. (1973) Hoppe-Seyler's Z. Physiol. Chem. 354:555.

182. Jondorf, W. R., Maiekel, R. P., Brodie, B. B. (1958) Biochem. Pharmacol. 1:352.

183. Sato, P. H., Zannoni, V. G. (1974) Biochem. Pharmacol. 23:3121.

184. Rickans, L. E., Smith, C. R., Zannoni, V. G. (1978) J. Pharmacol. Exp. Ther. 204:702.

185. Zannoni, V. G., Sato, P. H. (1975) Ann. N. Y. Acad. Sci. 258:119.

186. Degkwitz, E., Walsch, S., Dubberstein, M. (1975) Ann. N. Y. Acad. Sci. 258:201.

187. Ginter, E. (1975) Ann. N. Y. Acad. Sci. 258:410.

188. Bjorkham, I., Kallner, A. (1976) J. Lipid Res. 17:360.

189. Holloway, D. E., Rivers, J. M. (1981) J. Nutr. 111:412.

190. Jenkins, S. A. (1980) Br. J. Nutr. 43:95.

191. Zannoni, V. G., Holsztynska, E. J., Lau, S. S. (1982) Adv. Chem. Ser. 200:349.

192. Omaye, S. T., Turnbull, J. D. (1980) Life Science 27:441.

193. Rikans, L. E. (1982) J. Nutr. 112:1796.

194. Holloway, D. E., Peterson, F. J. Rivers, J. M. (1932) Nutr. Rep. Int. 25:941.

195. Sutton, J. L., Basu, T. K., Dickerson, J. W. T. (1982) Biochem. Pharmacol. 31:1591.

196. Peterson, F. J., Holloway, D. E., Duquette, P. H., Rivers, J. M. (1983) Biochem. Pharmacol. 32:91.

197. Peterson, F. J., Babish, J. G., Rivers, J. M. (1982) Nutr. Rep. Int. 26:1037.

198. Kamath, S., Tang, J., Smith, A., Moy, K., Wadhwa-Mehta, S., Bramante, P. (1978) Fed. Proc. 37:589.

199. Hornig, D., Weiser, H. (1976) Experientia. 32:687.

200. Chen, L. H., Chang, H. M. (1979) Int. J. Vit. Nutr. Res. 49:87.

201. Chen, L. H. (1981) Amer. J. Clin. Nutr. 34:1036.

202. Dunlap, C. E., Leshie, F. M., Rado, M., Cox, B. M. (1979) Molec. Pharmacol. 16:105.

203. Brogan, W. C., Miles, P. R., Colley, H. D. (1981) Environ. Health Perspect 38:105.

204. Yau, T. M., Memcl, J. (1981) Int. J. Rad. Biol. 40:47.

205. Heikkila, R. E., Cabbat, F. S., Manzino, L. (1982) J. Neurochem. 38:1000.

206. Ginter, E., Kosinova, A., Hudecova, A., Vejmolova, J. (1982) Biologia. (Bratislava) 37:1195.

207. Ginter, E., Kosinova, A., Hudecova, A., Mlynarcikova, U. (1984) J. Nutr. 114:485.

208. Smith, C. H., Bidlack, W. R. (1980) J. Nutr. 110:1398.

209. Kabrt, J., Oceanaskova, J., Klein, O., Pribyl, T. (1982) Physiol. Bohemoslo. 31:249.

210. Zannoni, V. G., Smith, C. R., Rikans, L. E. (1977) Int. J. Vit. Nutr. Res. Suppl. 16:99.

211. Milne, D. B., Omaye, S. T. (1980) Int. J. Vit. Nutr. Res. 50:301.

212. Arrigoni, O., Dipierro, S., Borraccino, G. (1981) Febs. Lett. 125:242.

213. King, M. M., Lai, E. K., McCay, P. B. (1975) J. Biol. Chem. 250:6496.

214. Chatterjee, G. C., Banerjee, S. K., Rudrapal, D. (1973) Int. J. Vit. Nutr. Res. 43:370.

215. Chatterjee, G. C., Rudrapal, D. (1975) Int. J. Vit. Nutr. Res. 45:284.

216. Rudrapal, D., Chatterjee, J., Chatterjee, G. C. (1975) Int. J. Vit. Nutr. Res. 45:429.

217. Sasmal, N., Kar, N. C., Mukherjee, D., Chatterjee, G. C. (1968) Biochem. J. 106:6.

218. Sasmal, N., Mukherjee, D., Kar, N. C., Chatterjee, G. C. (1968) Indian J. Biochem. Biophys. 5:123.

219. Chatterjee, G. C., Roy, R. K., Sasmal, N., Banerjee, S. K., Majumder, P. K. (1973) J. Nutr. 103:509.

220. Roy, R. K., Banerjee, S. K., Majumder, P. K., Chatterjee, G. C. (1973) Indian J. Biochem. Biophys. 10:202.

221. Wagstaff, D. J., Street, J. C. (1971) Toxicol. Appl. Pharmacol. 19:10.

222. Chatterjee, J., Chatterjee, G. C. (1976) Indian J. Biochem. Biophys. Suppl. 13:42.

223. Chatterjee, K., Chakraborti, D., Mazumder, K., Bhattacharyya, A., Chatterjee, G. C. (1979) Int. J. Vit. Nutr. Res. 49:264.

224. Chatterjee, G. C., Chatterjee, S., Chatterjee, K., Sahu, A., Bhattacharyya, A., Chakraborti, D., Das, P. K. (1979) Toxicol. Appl. Pharmacol. 51:47.

225. Chakraborty, D., Bhattacharyya, A., Majumder, K., Chatterjee, G. C. (1977) Int. J. Vit. Nutr. Res. 47:81.

226. Mukherjee, B., Chakraborty, K., Chatterjee, G. C. (1982) IRCS Med. Sci. 10:379.

227. Bandyopadhyay, S. K., Tiwari, R. K., Bhattacharyya, A., Chatterjee, G. C. (1982) Toxicol. Lett. 11:131.

228. Bandyopadhyay, S. K., Tiwari, R. K., Mitra, A., Mukherjee, B., Banerjee, A., Chatterjee, G. C. (1982) Arch. Toxicol. 50:227.

229. Tiwari, R. K., Bandyopadhyay, S. K., Chatterjee, G. C. (1982) Acta. Vitaminol. Enzymol. 4(3):215.

230. Tiwari, R. K., Bandyopadhyay, S. K., Chatterjee, K., Mitra, A., Banerjee, A., Chatterjee, G. C. (1982) Int. J. Vit. Nutr. Res. 52:448.

231. Chakrabarty, K., Basu, A., Chatterjee, G. C. (1982) IRCS Med. Sci. 10:873.

232. Chatterjee, K., Banerjee, S. K., Tiwari, R. K., Majumder, K., Bhattacharyya, A., Chatterjee, G. C. (1981) Int. J. Vit. Nutr. Res. 51:254.

233. Chakraborty, D., Bhattacharyya, A., Majumder, K., Chatterjee, K., Chatterjee, S., Sen, A., Chatterjee, G. C. (1978) J. Nutr. 108:973.

234. Chakraborty, D., Bhattacharyya, A., Chatterjee, J., Chatterjee, K., Sen, A., Chatterjee, S., Majumder, K., Chatterjee, G. C. (1978) Int. J. Vit. Nutr. Res. 48:231.

235. Attwood, E. C., Robey, E., Kramer, J. J., Ovenden, N., Snape, S., Ross, J., Bradley, F. (1978) Age and Ageing 5:46.

236. Banerjee, A. K., Lane, P. J., Meichen, F. W. (1978) Age and Ageing 7:16.

237. Bowers, E. F., Kubik, M. M. (1965) Brit. J. Clin. Pract. 19:141.

238. Burr, M. L., Elwood, P. C., Hole, D. J., Hurley, R. J., Hughes, R. E. (1974) Amer. J. Clin. Nutr. 27:144.

239. Loh, H. S., Wilson, C. W. M. (1971) Int. J. Vit. Nutr. Res. 41:259.

240. Milne, J. S., Lonergan, M. E., Williamson, J., Moore, F. M. L., McMaster, R., Percy, N. (1971) Brit. Med. J. 4:383.

241. McClean, H. E., Dodds, P. M., Abernethy, M. H., Stewart, A. W., Beaven, D. B. (1976) New Z. med. J. 83:226.

242. Schaus, R. (1957) Amer. J. Clin. Nutr. 5:39.

243. Hughes, R. E., Jones, P. R. (1971) Brit. J. Nutr. 25:77.

244. Siegel, B. V., Leibovitz, B. (1979) Int. J. Vit. Nutr. Res. Suppl. 19:9.

245. Schorah, C. J. (1979) Int. J. Vit. Nutr. Res. Suppl. 19:167.

246. Kinsman, R. A., Hood, J. (1971) Amer. J. Clin. Nutr. 24:455.

247. Sauberlich, H. E. (1975) Ann. N. Y. Acad. Sci. 253:438.

248. Loh, H. S. (1971) Int. J. Vit. Nutr. Res. 42:80.

249. Eddy, T. P. (1979) Int. J. Vit. Nutr. Res. Suppl. 19:103.

250. Eddy, T. P., Taylor, G. F. (1977) Age and Ageing 6:6.

III
PROTEINS, CARBOHYDRATES, AND LIPIDS

10

Dietary Protein and Bone Calcium Metabolism

THOMAS A. EINHORN

Dietary proteins provide the necessary sources of amino acids and nitrogen for the synthesis of body proteins and nitrogen-containing compounds, exclusive of the nitrogen-containing vitamins. Depending on the source of the dietary protein and the physiological state of the individual, the daily requirements for protein may vary widely. Although there are 22 amino acids of biological importance in man, only 16 can actually synthesized. The other eight are so-called "essential" amino acids, and these must be provided by the diet in sufficient quantities to meet the body's structural and metabolic needs. These compounds—lysine, leucine, isoleucine, methionine, phenylalanine, threonine, tryptophan, valine, and, during the early growth and development, histidine—cannot be incorporated into the body from any other source. This chapter will discuss the role of dietary proteins in relation to bone development and calcium metabolism, concentrating on their metabolic functions, effects on the maintainance of mineral homeostasis, and contributions to the development of osteoporosis.

Bone is a complex unit composed of mineral, matrix, and water. By weight, the mineral component accounts for approximately 70 percent of the tissue, water 5–8 percent, and the remainder matrix proteins (1). The mineral exists as imperfect and impure crystals of calcium hydroxyapatite and confers to bone the major portion of its elastic stiffness properties (2). Water provides a medium for nutrient transfer within bone in addition to contributing to the stereodimensional organization of the mineral relative to the collagen framework (1). The predominant component of the matrix is protein, and this exists in the form of collagen, and, to a lesser extent, a variety of noncollagenous proteins, proteoglycans, glycoproteins, phosphoproteins, and lipoproteins (3). Although the proteinaceous matrix is responsible for the bone's plastic stiffness properties, strength is still a function of the mineral phase (2). A major determinant of this strength, however, may be related to the stability of the collagen molecule (4) and the way in which the chemistry and structure of the matrix proteins affect the organization of the mineral phase (2). Dietary protein is important to bone's structural integrity, because it provides the body with the necessary amino acids and nitrogen-containing compounds to synthesize bone matrix. Furthermore, there is evidence that deficiencies in the essential amino acids lysine (5, 6), leucine (7), histidine (8), phenylalanine (9), and tryptophan (10, 11) have negative influences on bone growth and endochondral calcification.

Dietary protein has been shown to have both direct and indirect effects on calcium metabolism. These effects include a dose-dependent inhibition of calcium absorption from the gut (12), a dose-dependent increase in urinary calcium excretion (12, 13), and a resultant alteration in the body's calcium requirements (12). In addition, as will be discussed later in this chapter, protein from the diet may function as a primary source of "acid ash" and, when present in sufficient quantities, may alter the pH of body fluids in such a way as to force the system to turn to the buffering capacity of the basic calcium salts of the skeleton (14).

EFFECTS OF LOW-PROTEIN DIETS

Early studies on the influence of protein-poor diets on bone growth and development did not distinguish between protein and energy deficiencies. In a study by Platt and Stewart (15), histological data from protein- and calorie-deficient young pigs showed reduced proliferation and maturation of cartilage and a reduction in osteoblastic activity. Osteoclastic activity was less severely affected. Measurements of growth revealed retardation, and radiographs demonstrated the characteristic transverse trabecular growth arrest lines in the metaphyses. Both the growth measurements and growth arrest lines were shown to disappear upon repletion with isocaloric amounts of protein (15).

Jha and colleagues (16) examined the bones of rhesus monkeys made protein-deficient by tube feeding with diets containing negligible amounts of protein. They compared the findings to controls fed a 20 percent casein diet. The test monkeys showed histological osteoporosis, decreased endochondral bone formation, and decreased appositional bone growth as assessed by tetracycline labeling. The investigators hypothesized that the osteoblast, a cell with a high protein turnover, is more likely to be affected than the osteoclast, a cell with less protein synthetic activity. Similar findings were made by El-Maraghi et al. (17) when animals were fed protein-poor, normal-calcium diets. Again, there was radiographic osteoporosis as well as a decreased ash content measured in the bones. It was shown that these changes were the result of decreased matrix production and that when dietary protein was repleted, sufficient matrix production occurred to restore normal bone mass and prevent osteoporosis (17).

In more recent times, Shires et al. (18) showed that rats semistarved for 7 weeks lost 28 percent of their body weight and became hypercalcemic and hypophosphatemic, and on histological examination their bones showed reduced bone turnover and osteoporosis without osteomalacia. These changes were attended by reduced levels of insulin, corticosterone, and 1,25-dihydroxyvitamin D_3 but not of parathyroid hormone or 25-hydroxyvitamin D_3 (17).

Studies in human subjects have agreed with the work in animals. Faridi et al. (19) studied 100 children 6 months to 6 years of age suffering from protein–calorie malnutrition. Seventy-five percent showed radiographic osteopenia, 54 percent showed growth arrest lines, and only 5.4 percent had frank rickets. It is therefore apparent, from both animal and human studies, that the major osseous lesions in protein–calorie malnutrition are osteoporosis and growth retardation, with osteomalacia or rickets occurring much less commonly.

To isolate the effects of protein deficiency from energy deficiency, Shenokilar and Rao (20) designed an experiment in which a group of rats was divided into three groups. All three groups were fed diets with normal amounts of calcium, but in Group I the protein content was only 5 percent; Group II, 20 percent (normal dietary protein requirement); and Group III was a weight-control protein group. Groups I and II were pair-fed with respect to calories. Group III was offered the same diet as Group II but in an amount that only allowed the animals to grow at a rate equivalent to Group I. At the end of 5 weeks, all animals were injected with $^{45}CaCl_2$, and calcium balance studies were performed on the bones, urine, and feces. The results showed that there was a slower rate of growth in Group I (low protein) than in either Group II (normal protein) or III (weight-control protein). The rats fed low protein had higher fecal losses of calcium, and these losses were of endogenous rather than dietary origin. The bone accretion rate tended to be greatest in the normal protein group and was greater in the weight-control protein group than in the low-protein group. It was therefore concluded that, between protein and calories, it was protein that was the more important mediator of bone calcium metabolism (20). The findings of this study were confirmed 17 years later when Kuramitsu et al. (21) showed that rats maintained for 45 days on protein-deficient diets showed decreased femoral growth and alkaline phosphatase activity when compared to energy-deficient animals. Serum calcium and bone calcium content were unaffected by either protein or energy deficiency (21).

As mentioned earlier, specific deficiencies in some of the essential amino acids have resulted in diminished growth and an interference with endochondral calcification. Since these effects have never been shown to influence the properties of the organic matrix, apatite particle size, apatite stoichiometry, or carbonate content, it was concluded that specific amino acid deficiencies may simply be related to a failure of matrix production (19). However, since lysine, for example, is a critical amino acid in the formation of collagen intermolecular cross-links (4), it is possible that some or all of these essential amino acid deficiencies may result in specific biochemical defects, which could affect the mechanical integrity of bone tissue.

EFFECTS OF HIGH-PROTEIN DIETS

High-protein diets have been thought to be associated with increased urinary calcium excretion ever since Sherman first made this observation in 1920 (22). In recent times, interest has continued on the effects of excess dietary protein on calcium metabolism, as nearly all studies confirm the findings of persistent negative calcium balance (12). The importance of these findings is that the large excesses of dietary proteins provided by most Western diets may ultimately lead to calcium loss sufficient to induce osteoporosis. Since bone mineral has been suggested as a possible buffer base for the fixed acid load imposed by the ingestion of an "acid ash" diet in man (14), the role of dietary protein in the pathophysiology of bone homeostasis requires serious attention.

Linkswiler et al. (23) studied the effects of low-, medium-, and high-protein intakes on calcium retention in young adult human males when calcium intakes were similarly altered. When consuming low-protein diets (47 g/day), the subjects were consistently in calcium balance, and the amount of calcium retained was unaffected by the calcium intake. When consuming medium-protein diets (95 g/day) no subjects were in calcium balance with low daily calcium intakes of 500 mg, but subjects did achieve calcium balance when the daily calcium intake reached 800 mg. When a high-protein diet (142 g/day) was administered, only three of 15 subjects could maintain calcium balance even with calcium intakes as high as 1400 mg/day (Fig. 10-1). Calcium absorption was not affected by dietary protein when calcium intake was low (500 mg/day), but significantly more calcium was absorbed at medium- or high-protein intakes if calcium intakes were increased from 800 to 1,400 mg/day. Interestingly, the maximal protein effect was reached at the medium protein (95 g/day) intake level (Fig. 10-2).

Urinary calcium was also significantly affected by protein intake. All subjects, regardless of the level of calcium intake, excreted less calcium when given the medium-protein diet, and all but two subjects excreted less calcium when given the medium- than when given the high-protein diet (Fig. 10-3) (23). In a subsequent report from the same laboratory, it was shown that in young adult women the level of dietary protein had no effect on calcium absorption but that urinary calcium excretion was increased, resulting in a negative calcium balance (24). The hypercalciuria was shown to be caused by the tendency of a high-protein diet to reduce fractional tubular reabsorption of calcium and, to a lesser extent, to increase the glomerular filtration rate (24).

The cause and mechanism of dietary protein-induced hypercalciuria in animals and man have been investigated in several laboratories (13, 23–33). In a study of rats fed high-protein diets, it was shown that despite hypercalciuria, intestinal

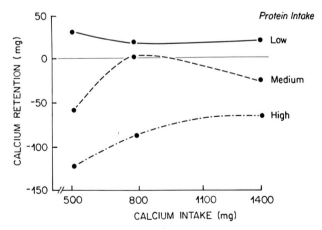

Fig. 10-1 Effects of low-, medium-, and high-protein diets on calcium retention at three levels of calcium intake. [After Linkswiler et al. (23).]

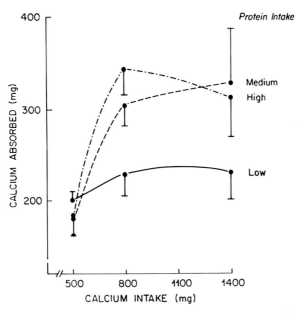

Fig. 10-2 Effects of low-, medium-, and high-protein diets on calcium absorption at three levels of calcium intake. [After Linkswiler et al. (23).]

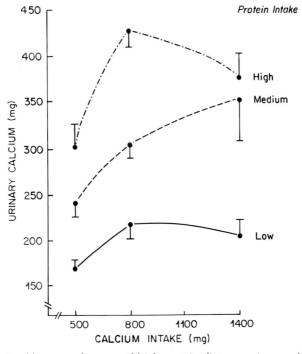

Fig. 10-3 Effects of low-, medium-, and high-protein diets on urinary calcium excretion at three levels of calcium intake. [After Linkswiler et al. (23).]

calcium absorption was not impaired, and intestinal calcium-binding protein activity was unchanged (31). Calvo et al. (33) showed that the hypercalciuria observed in rats fed high-protein diets was not associated with any compositional changes in the femurs or mandibles, thus dismissing bone calcium as the source of the calciuria.

In this study, however, the end products of protein metabolism known to chelate calcium or compete with its renal reabsorption were significantly correlated with urinary calcium. These end products included sulfate, oxalate, and sodium. These findings, in conjunction with those of previous investigators, as well as those cited above, suggested that dietary protein-induced hypercalciuria may not be strictly or even predominantly the result of bone dissolution secondary to hypocalcemia. Instead, other causes such as decreased renal tubular reabsorption (24, 30, 32, 33), an increase in glomerular filtration rate (24, 30, 34), shunting of fecal calcium excretion to the urine (24, 35), and other forms of acid stress such as ammonium chloride loading (12) may be of prime importance.

Dietary proteins have been found to differ in terms of their calciuretic properties, and these differences have been attributed to their sulfated amino acid contents (35). In a report by Schuete et al. (34), it was proposed that the hypercalciuria of high-protein feeding was due to an increase in metabolic acid production from the oxidation of methionine and cystine residues. An example of this phenomenon may exist in the arctic Eskimo. It is true that high-meat diets are rich in sulfated amino acids and that arctic Eskimos, whose diets are very rich in these foods, have a rate of bone loss that is 15–20 percent higher than in U.S. whites (36). One problem with this hypothesis, however, is that the bone loss attributed to a prolonged acidic effect could not be confirmed through measurements of blood pH (36).

In more recent studies, Spencer and co-workers (37, 38) showed that when phosphorus intake in human subjects is allowed to rise with protein (as it normally does in a high meat diet), the hypercalciuric effect of the protein is offset by the hypocalciuric effect of the phosphorus. In both control experiments and those involving high protein/normal calcium (819 mg/day) diets, there were no changes in the amount of calcium excreted in the urine or stool for up to 132 days. As long as meat was the source of the protein, there were no changes in calcium absorption or excretion. These findings were also observed over shorter periods (18–30 days) with large amounts of meat. The authors hypothesized that significant differences may exist between the effects of purified proteins (such as those used in earlier studies) and proteins from meat on calcium metabolism (38). A high phosphorus content such as is found in meat may account for the lack of effect on calcium metabolism when meat is the major source of protein.

The normal Western diet remains high in meat, thereby remaining high in both protein and phosphorus content. Calcium consumption, however, is much more variable from individual to individual and is more frequently than not found to fall below recommended levels (12). The interactions of dietary protein, phosphorus, and calcium, as well as the possible influences of other factors, make the interpretation of even well-designed studies often difficult to evaluate. To make matters worse, information obtained from studies done on rodents are not directly applicable to human bone metabolism (39). In rats, for example, excess dietary protein leads to an increase in urinary calcium excretion but no change in calcium balance. Excess phosphorus leads to a decrease in urinary calcium excretion and a net calcium loss. Furthermore, the stimulus to bone resorption produced by excess dietary phosphorus is unaffected by the level of dietary protein (39). In the absence of a suitable animal model, continued clinical experiments remain the best means of studying human bone metabolism.

TREATMENT AND PREVENTION OF BONE LOSS IN RELATION TO DIETARY PROTEIN

A dietary means of treating or preventing progressive bone loss and osteoporosis could have a major impact on public health. To address this issue, several investigators (once again using the rat model) have studied the interactions of dietary elements in relation to acidity, calcium absorption, and hypercalciuria. In a well-controlled study by Petito and Evans (40), the question of the relative contributions of increased dietary protein and acid phosphate mixture to the diet acid load was addressed. These two dietary components were compared to the effects of ingestion of ammonium chloride, an acid known to cause bone loss in rats (41–44). It was shown that acid phosphate, ammonium chloride, and protein all potentially influenced blood pH and hence calcium loss in the urine and feces, with a resultant lowered bone density. However, when less acidic phosphate sources were used, bone loss was either reduced or prevented (40). The significance of this study appears to be that diet acidity may be the final common denominator of the effects of certain dietary components on bone calcium loss. Although performed in rats, this study may be of importance to the current-day management of patients at risk for developing osteoporosis, since calcium supplements can be more or less acidic as a result of their composition. Calcium carbonate, for example, is a basic molecule, whereas calcium lactate is potentially acid (40).

As was discussed in the previous section, a sustained increase in urinary calcium has been shown to occur when dietary protein is increased and calcium is held constant (23, 26–28, 30, 34). Regardless of the actual level of calcium and phosphorus in the diet, a 100 percent increase in protein intake causes a 50 percent rise in urinary calcium excretion, and a 200 percent protein increase causes a 100 percent increase in urinary calcium loss (23). The actual level of dietary calcium and phosphorus, however, has been shown to modify the effects of protein on calcium balance (23, 45). This suggests that dietary calcium requirements are increased by high levels of dietary protein. Because increases in protein and phosphorus intakes have opposite effects on calcium metabolism (45), a simultaneous increase in both may have a less dramatic effect than an increase in one or the other. Since calcium absorption is enhanced by increases in protein intake when calcium intake is moderate to high, but not when it is low (23), the effect of dietary protein on calcium retention is likely to be influenced by phosphorus as well as by calcium.

Foods that are rich in protein, such as meat, are high in phosphorus but low in calcium. Milk products, however, are high in both calcium and phosphorus. Diets that contain both meat and milk are therefore high in protein but also high in calcium and phosphorus. Based on these facts, Schuette and Linkswiler (46) examined the effects of adding meat, meat plus milk, or purified proteins plus calcium and phosphorus to a low-protein diet in adult men. They showed that on the low-protein diet, calcium was not lost but phosphorus was. When meat was added (increased dietary protein), phosphorus retention increased but calcium retention decreased. When meat plus milk was consumed (also a high protein diet), the subjects retained substantial amounts of both calcium and phosphorus. With the simulated purified protein and calcium and phosphorus-supplemented diet, however, calcium was retained but phosphorus was lost (46). This study suggests that in Western diets high in meat, an adequate consumption of dairy products may be a means of preventing bone loss.

In the United States, 75 percent of dietary calcium comes from dairy products (47). This is a potential problem for certain individuals, since lactose deficiency is common (48). Although there are certain means available to counter this problem, such as the addition of enzyme preparations to milk products thereby predigesting the lactose, severe lactose deficiency often renders the individual afraid or simply averse to the consumption of dairy products. To provide an alternate dietary method for the prevention diet acid load-induced bone loss, Lutz (49) examined the use of oral sodium bicarbonate as a buffer. The study succeeded in demonstrating that ingestion of sodium bicarbonate alkalinized the urine and reversed the increase in urinary calcium associated with high-protein intake (Fig. 10-4). The results further suggested that in women with protein-induced hypercalciuria, the ingestion of small amounts of sodium bicarbonate may be an effective way to increase calcium retention and possibly prevent osteoporosis (49).

EFFECTS OF DIETARY PROTEIN ON BOTH FORMATION AND REPAIR

Although several of the above reports have shown that high-protein diets are associated with hypercalciuria and an increased risk of osteoporosis, the effects of dietary protein on bone formation and repair have received far less attention. To answer this question, two types of studies have been performed. The first type employed the demineralized bone matrix-induced model of endochondral bone formation to study the effects of diet on discrete stages of bone development (50). The second type employed a clinically applied model of fracture healing (51).

Implantation of demineralized bone matrix into an extraskeletal site in a laboratory animal results in a sequence of synchronous phases of endochondral bone development (52). On day 3 after implantation, there is histological evidence of mesenchymal cell proliferation. On day 7, cartilage differentiation occurs. This is followed by calcification of the cartilage by day 10, and from days 14 to 21, the tissue undergoes ossification with the development of an hematapoetic marrow space (52). By assessing the ^{3}H-thymidine incorporation and ornithine decarboxylase activity in 28-day-old rats, Weiss et al. (50) showed that mesenchymal cell proliferation was unchanged on high-protein, normal calcium (80 percent casein, $Ca/P = 1.5$) diets. Assessement of ^{45}Ca incorporation showed that osteogenesis was reduced by 75 percent, and there was increased matrix turnover with de-

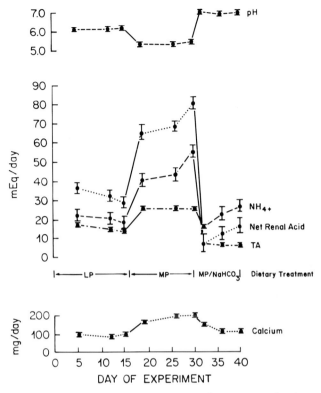

Fig. 10-4 Effects of three dietary treatments on renal excretion of calcium and acid in women. LP = low (44 g) protein; MP = moderate (102 g) protein; MP/NaHCO₃ = 102 g protein plus 5.85 g (70 mEq) sodium bicarbonate. Urinary calcium and acid indices were determined on 3 days of each dietary period. Protein intake was increased on day 17. Sodium bicarbonate was added to the moderate protein diet on day 31. TA = titratable acid; NH_4 = ammonium ion concentration. [After Lutz (49).]

creased remodeling. Moreover, there was no evidence of marrow formation (Figs. 10-5, 10-6) (50). These findings suggest a strong negative influence of a high-protein/normal-calcium diet on all but the very early stages of endochondral bone formation. When a high-protein/low-calcium diet was tested, these early stages were also affected, showing a 62 percent reduction in cell proliferation and chondrogenesis and a 98 percent reduction in bone formation (Fig. 10-7) (50). Although it is difficult to extrapolate from the rat to the human, these results suggest that Western diets high in protein and normal with respect to calcium could lead to osteoporosis due to a failure of osteoid formation and mineralization but not to cell proliferation nor chondrogenesis. Diets high in protein and low in calcium, however, may depress cell proliferation and chondrogenesis. This could lead to inadequate repair of trabecular microfractures and ultimately result in osteoporotic fractures involving the vertebrae, proximal femur, and distal radius.

To examine the role of dietary protein in relation to bone repair, Einhorn et al. (51) created closed femoral fractures in rats, placed the rats on high-protein/normal-calcium, protein-free/normal-calcium, and regular diets, and subjected the

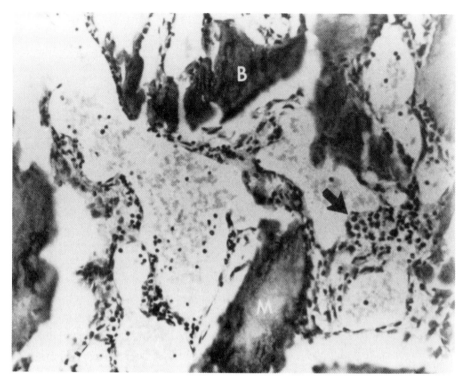

Fig. 10-5   Day-14-implanted matrix of rat fed normal-protein/normal-calcium diet. M, implanted matrix; B, bone; arrow, bone marrow. 120×. [Reprinted with permission from Weiss et al. (50).]

5-week calluses to mechanical testing. It was shown that protein deprivation resulted in a significant reduction in strength-related parameters of bone; however, the stiffness properties were unchanged. Through a set of calculations relating the cross-sectional geometry of the bones to the mechanical properties, it was determined that the reduction in callus strength was a function of the smaller radii of the calluses rather than an effect on the material composition. When the calluses of animals fed high-protein/normal-calcium diets were tested and compared to those of the animals fed regular diets, no differences were found (51). These findings may reflect the need for adequate dietary protein intake during early fracture healing. However, since calcium is mobilized from other skeletal sites in response to a skeletal injury (53, 54), the calciuretic effects of a high-protein diet may be rendered insignificant in relation to the accumulation of calcium in the callus.

SUMMARY

The proper dose of dietary protein is important to bone homeostasis in terms of supplying adequate substrates for anabolic processes and controlling calcium balance. Low dietary protein results in decreased osteoblastic activity, osteoporosis,

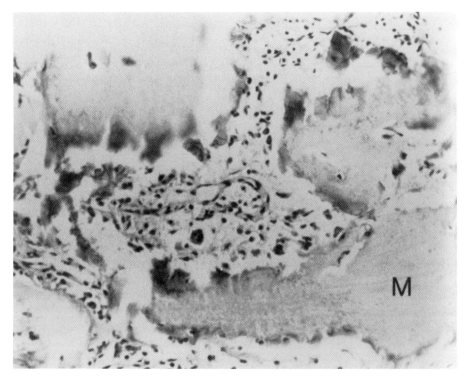

Fig. 10-6   Day-14-implanted matrix of rat fed high-protein/normal-calcium diet. Note the absence of marrow. M, matrix. 120×. [Reprinted with permission from Weiss et al. (50).]

and growth retardation. Although protein deficiency is most commonly associated with a caloric deficit as well, studies have shown that the deleterious effects on skeletal tissues are predominantly the result of insufficient protein intake. In addition, certain essential amino acids from the diet may be required for normal processes of endochondral ossification to take place.

High dietary protein results in hypercalciuria and decreased calcium retention. These effects are subject to partial protection by increased dietary calcium. The effects may be caused by reduced fractional renal tubular reabsorption of calcium, increased glomerular filtration of calcium, or the use of skeletal calcium as a base to buffer a fixed acid load imposed by a protein-rich "acid ash" diet. Although increased calcium intake only partially offsets the calcium loss associated with a high-protein diet, the combinations of dietary phosphorous with calcium may offer greater protection. Meat, though high in protein, is also high in phosphorus, thereby offering partial protection against hypercalciuria. Introducing more calcium into the diet may be even more effective. Since certain foods such as milk are high in both phosphorus and calcium, it is suggested that in Western diets high in meat, an adequate consumption of dairy may be a means of preventing bone loss. The ingestion of an alkalizing agent such as sodium bicarbonate may offer an alternate means of offsetting the acidic effects of a high-protein diet.

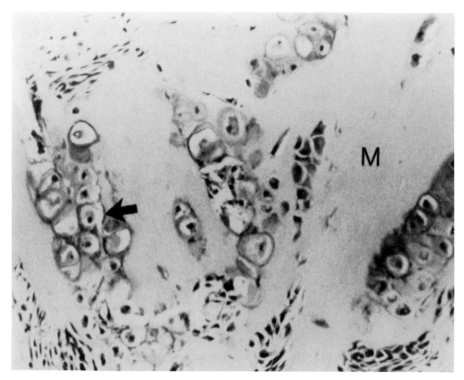

Fig. 10-7 Day-14-implanted matrix of rat fed high-protein/low-calcium diet. Note the absence of bone formation. Only chondrocytes (arrow) are present. M, matrix. 120×. [Reprinted with permission from Weiss et al. (50).]

Studies on bone formation models suggest that high dietary protein inhibits osteoid formation and mineralization as opposed to cell proliferation and chondrogenesis. Fracture healing, another form of bone formation, appers to be unaffected by protein-enriched diets but does require adequate dietary protein for fracture callus to achieve normal strength.

REFERENCES

1. Lane, J. M. (1978) In: AAOS-Monterey Seminar, p. 141.

2. Burstein, A. H., Zilka, J. M., Heiple, K. G., Klein L. (1975) J. Bone Joint Surg. 57A:956.

3. Boskey, A. L. (1981) Clin. Orthop. 157:225.

4. Triffit, J. T. (1980) In: Urist, M. R. (ed) *Fundamental and Clinical Bone Physiology*. Philadelphia: J. B. Lippincott, p. 50.

5. Gillespie, M., Neuberger, A., Webster, T. A. (1945) J. Biochem. 39:203.

6. Likins, R. C., Bavetta, L. A., Posner, A. S. (1957) Arch. Biochem. Biophys. 70:401.

7. Maun, M. E., Cahill, W. M., Davis, R. M. (1945) AMA Arch. Pathol. 40:173.

8. Maun, M. E., Cahill, W. M., Davis, R. M. (1946) AMAM Arch. Pathol. 41:25.
9. Maun, M. E., Cahill, W. M., Davis, R. M. (1945) AMA Arch. Pathol. 39:294.
10. Bavetta, L. A., Bernick, S. (1956) Oral Surg. Oral Med. Oral Pathol. 9:308.
11. Bavetta, L. A., Bernick, S. (1956) Oral Surg. Oral Med. Oral Pathol. 9:906.
12. Review (1981) Nutr. Rev. 39:11.
13. Widhe, T. (1982) Clin. Orthop. 162:304.
14. Wachman, A., Bernstein, D. S. (1968) Lancet 1:958.
15. Platt, B. S., Steward, R. J. C. (1962) Br. J. Nutr. 16:483.
16. Jha, G., Deo, M. G., Ramalingasiwami, V. (1968) Am. J. Pathol. 53:1111.
17. El-Maraghi, N., Platt, B. S., Stewart, R. J. C. (1965) Br. J. Nutr. 191:491.
18. Shires, R., Avioli, L. V., Bergfeld, M. A., Fallon, M. D., Slatopolsky, E., Teitelbaum, S. L. (1980) Endocrinology 107:1530.
19. Faridi, M. M. A., Ansari, Z., Bhargava, S. K. (1984) J. Trop. Pediat. 30:150.
20. Shenokilar, I. S., Rao, B. S. N. (1968) Indian J. Med. Res. 56:1412.
21. Kuramitsu, N., Matsui, T., Yano, H., Kawashima, R. (1985) J. Nutr. Sci. Vitaminol. 31:189.
22. Sherman, H. C. (1920) J. Biol. Chem. 44:21.
23. Linkswiler, H. M., Joyce, C. L., Anand, C. R. (1974) Trans. NY Acad. Sci. 36:333.
24. Hegsted, M., Linkswiler, H. M. (1980) Fed. Proc. 39:901.
25. Hawks, J. E., Bray, M. M., Wilde, M. O., Dye, M. (1942) J. Nutr. 243:283.
26. Johnson, N. E., Alcantara, E. N., Linkswiler, H. (1970) J. Nutr. 100:1425.
27. Walker, R. M., Linkswiler, H. M. (1972) J. Nutr. 102:1297.
28. Margen, S., Chu, J.-Y., Kaufman, N. A., Calloway, D. H. (1974) J. Clin. Nutr. 27:584.
29. Spencer, H., Kramer, L., Osis, D., Norris, C. (1978) Am. J. Clin. Nutr. 31:2167.
30. Allen, L. H., Bartlett, R. S., Block, G. D. (1979) In: Barzel, U. S. (ed) Osteoporosis II New York: Grune & Stratton, p. 245.
31. Allen, L. H., Hall, T. E. (1978) J. Nutr. 108:967.
32. Chu, J.-Y., Margen, S., Costa, F. M. (1975) Am. J. Clin. Nutr. 28:1028.
33. Calvo, M. S., Bell, R. R., Forbes, R. M. (1985) J. Nutr. 112:1401.
34. Schuette, S. A., Zemel, M. B., Linkswiler, H. M. (1980) J. Nutr. 110:305.
35. Whiting, S. J., Draper, H. H. (1980) J. Nutr. 110:212.
36. Mazess, R. B., Mather, W. (1974) Am. J. Clin. Nutr. 27:916.
37. Spencer, H., Kramer, L., Osis, D., Norris, C. (1978) Am. J. Clin. Nutr. 33:2128.
38. Spencer, H., Kramer, L., DeBartolo, M., Norris, C., Osis, D. (1983) Am. J. Clin. Nutr. 37:924.
39. Bell, R. R., Engelmann, D. T., Sie, T.-Y., Draper, H. H. (1975) J. Nutr. 105:475.
40. Petito, S. L., Evans, J. L. (1984) J. Nutr. 114:1049.
41. Barzel, U. S. (1969) Calcif. Tissue Res. 4:94.
42. Barzel, U. S. (1975) Endocrinology 96:1304.
43. Barzel, U. S., Jowsey, J. (1969) Clin. Sci. 36:517.
44. Lemann, J., Litzow, J. R., Lennon, E. J. (1966) J. Clin. Invest. 45:1608.
45. Hegsted, M., Schuette, S. A., Zemel, M. B., Linkswiler, H. M. (1981) J. Nutr. 111:553.
46. Schuette, S. A., Linkswiler, H. M. (1982) J. Nutr. 112:338.
47. Martson, R., Friend, B. (1976) Nutritional Review, Natl. Food Supply 158:25.
48. Newcomer, A. D., Hodgson, S. F., McGill, D. B. (1978) Ann. Intern. Med. 89:218.
49. Lutz, J. (1984) Am. J. Clin. Nutr. 39:281.
50. Weiss, R. E., Gorn, A., Dux, S., Nimmi, M. E. (1981) J. Nutr. 111:804.

51. Einhorn, T. A., Bonnarens, F., Burstein, A. H. (1986) J. Bone Joint Surg. 68A:1389.

52. Reddi, A. H., Huggins, C. B. (1975) Proc. Natl. Acad. Sci. USA 69:1601.

53. Lane, J. M., Betts, F., Posner, A. S., Yue, D. W. (1984) J. Bone Joint Surg. 66A:1289.

54. Singh, L. M., Rocco, J. D. R., Dunphy, J. E. (1968) Surg. Gynecol. Obstet. 126:243.

11

Stimulation of Intestinal Calcium and Phosphorus Absorption by Carbohydrates

H. J. ARMBRECHT

That certain sugars can enhance calcium absorption has been known for many years (1, 2). The effect of the milk sugar lactose on calcium absorption has been studied in the most detail. This interaction is important nutritionally because of the high concentrations of both calcium and lactose in milk (3). Recent studies have also suggested that lactose may enhance phosphorus absorption and balance. Therefore, this review will concentrate on the stimulation of calcium and phosphorus absorption by lactose. Lactose tends to supplement the action of vitamin D in enhancing calcium absorption. Lactose is also effective throughout the lifespan. Thus, lactose may be important nutritionally in older individuals with decreased capacity to absorb calcium and decreased serum levels of vitamin D metabolites.

STIMULATION OF CALCIUM ABSORPTION BY LACTOSE

In Vivo Studies of Lactose and Calcium Absorption

Several studies have examined the effect of lactose on calcium absorption and balance in infants (4), children (5), young adults (6–8), and older adults (9). These studies have shown that calcium absorption (7, 8) and calcium balance (6, 9) are improved by lactose in lactose-tolerant individuals. This improvement is seen whether the lactose is administered in water or milk. On the other hand, most (6–8), but not all (10), studies have found that lactose does not improve calcium absorption and balance in lactose-intolerant individuals. This may be due to the osmotic effects of the unabsorbed lactose. These effects include a reduction in the intraluminal calcium concentration (11) and an acceleration in the small intestine transit time (12).

The effect of lactose on calcium absorption and balance has also been studied in rats. Dietary lactose (12–15%) significantly improves calcium retention and balance (13, 14). The effect of lactose is more pronounced in rats fed a low-calcium diet than in rats fed a high-calcium diet. Interestingly, feeding lactose and a moderate diet of calcium mimics the effects of a high-calcium diet (15). Absorption of calcium from *in situ* duodenal loops is depressed, and the amount of intestinal calcium-binding protein is decreased.

In Vitro Studies of Lactose and Calcium Absorption

The *in vitro* effects of lactose on calcium absorption have been explored in the rat. The presence of lactose in a ligated intestinal segment increases the absorption of radioactive calcium from that segment (16, 17). These studies showed that lactose acts within 30 min and that lactose has to be present in the same intestinal segment as calcium to exert its effect. In these studies, lactose caused the greatest enhancement of calcium absorption in the ileum, although an appreciable response was also seen in the duodenum and jejunum. It was also found that lactose increases calcium absorption in vitamin D-deficient rats. This is in agreement with a more recent study, which found that the effect of lactose is independent of the vitamin D status of the animal (18). Using a different *in vitro* system, perfusion with a low concentration of lactose (10 mM) did not affect calcium absorption by intestinal segments (19).

Everted intestinal sacs have also been used to study calcium uptake in the presence and absence of lactose (20). These studies have shown that lactose does not need to be physically present with the calcium to enhance calcium uptake. This suggests that lactose interacts with the tissue to alter its permeability rather than interacting with the calcium ion itself. The effect of lactose is not inhibited by metabolic inhibitors that block calcium transport. This suggests that lactose alters the passive pathways of calcium uptake. It was also found that lactose enhances calcium uptake to a similar degree over a wide range of calcium concentrations. This again suggests that lactose alters the passive permeability to calcium.

Recently, the effect of lactose on calcium absorption has been studied using ileal segments mounted in Ussing chambers (21). Net intestinal calcium absorption was determined by measuring unidirectional steady-state calcium fluxes *in vitro* under short-circuit conditions. Iso-osmotic replacement of sodium chloride by lactose produced an increased net calcium absorption. This net calcium absorption resulted from an increased absorptive flux from mucosa to serosa and a reduced secretory flux from serosa to mucosa. The effect of lactose was additive to that of 1,25-dihydroxyvitamin D administration. These results show that replacement of sodium by lactose increases calcium absorption in the absence of transepithelial gradients. However, this study could not differentiate between the effects of lactose and the effects of sodium removal, since sodium removal alone mimicked the efffects of lactose.

The question of whether there are age changes in the ability of lactose to stimulate calcium absorption in mammals has been examined using everted sacs (18). This may be of some importance nutritionally, since calcium absorption and serum 1,25-dihydroxyvitamin D levels decline with age in both rats (22, 23) and man (24). Using everted intestinal sacs (20), the effect of lactose on intestinal calcium uptake was determined in young, adult, and old rats (Table 11-1). In the absence of lactose, calcium uptake significantly decreased with age in the duodenum ($p < .001$, one-way ANOVA) but did not change with age in the ileum. Lactose significantly increased calcium uptake in the duodenum in all age groups ($p < .001$, two-way ANOVA). The effect of lactose in the duodenum did not change significantly with age ($p < .231$). In the ileum, lactose also significantly increased calcium uptake in all age groups ($p < .001$, two-way ANOVA), and the effect of lactose did not change with age ($p < .336$).

Mechanism of Lactose Action

The mechanism by which lactose stimulates active and/or passive calcium absorption is not yet known, but several have been proposed. Lactose may interact directly with the calcium ion to enhance its absorption (25), it may remove an energy-dependent epithelial cell barrier to calcium movement (26), or it may modify the transmural or transcellular potential of the intestine (21, 27).

The concept that lactose interacts directly with calcium to facilitate absorption is based on early studies showing that lactose may form an uncharged complex with calcium (25) and that lactose may cocrystallize with calcium (28). However, more recent *in vitro* experiments have shown that preincubation with lactose alone is enough to increase subsequent calcium uptake (20). In the same experiments, the lactose effect was independent of the ratio of lactose to calcium, and no evidence was found for the coabsorption of lactose and calcium as a complex. These results suggest that lactose interacts with the tissue to enhance calcium permeability rather than with calcium itself to facilitate calcium absorption.

The fact that lactose depresses oxygen consumption by the intestinal tissue has led to the hypothesis that lactose enhances permeability by removing an energy-dependent epithelial barrier (26). However, *in vitro* experiments have shown that lactose enhances calcium uptake even in the absence of metabolic energy (20). This suggests that calcium modifies the passive component of calcium absorption.

It has also been suggested that lactose modifies the potential across the intes-

Table 11-1   Effect of Age and Lactose on Intestinal Uptake of Calcium

Age	Segment	Calcium uptake ($pmoles/mg$)	
		Control	Lactose
Young	Duodenum	289 ± 26	348 ± 20
Adult	Duodenum	192 ± 17	296 ± 15
Old	Duodenum	143 ± 7	186 ± 17
Young	Ileum	170 ± 16	276 ± 15
Adult	Ileum	210 ± 17	307 ± 32
Old	Ileum	154 ± 11	218 ± 23

Everted intestinal sacs from young (2–3 months), adult (12–14 months), or old (22–24 months) rats were used to measure calcium uptake. Sacs were preincubated for 45 min in the presence or absence of buffer containing 150 mM NaCl (control) or 70 mM NaCl plus 160 mM lactose (lactose). Sacs were then transferred into buffer containing 0.25 mM radiolabeled calcium for the measurement of calcium uptake. Table entries are the mean and standard error of six sacs [Data tabulated from Armbrecht (41)]. Lactose significantly enhanced calcium uptake in the duodenum and ileum in all age groups ($p < .001$, two-way ANOVA).

tinal tissue or the potential across the brush border membrane. That lactose stimulates calcium absorption even with the tissue potential short-circuited (reduced to zero) demonstrates that lactose does not work solely by altering tissue potential (21). Since lactose replaced sodium chloride iso-osmotically in these experiments, the authors have proposed that lactose works by hyperpolarization of the brush border membrane (21). This theory needs experimental verification, perhaps by using isolated intestinal brush border membranes.

Finally, there is conflicting evidence as to whether lactose affects the active component of calcium absorption, the passive component, or both. That lactose exerts its effect in the absence of metabolic energy (20), in the absence of vitamin D (16), in the ileum (16, 20), and in older animals (Table 11-1) again suggests that it affects primarily the passive component. Direct measurement of calcium fluxes in the ileum has been made in the presence and absence of lactose (21). Iso-osmotic replacement of sodium chloride by lactose increases the mucosal to serosal flux and decreases the serosal to mucosal flux (presumably passive). Further studies are needed to determine the exact site of lactose action.

STIMULATION OF PHOSPHORUS ABSORPTION BY LACTOSE

The effect of lactose on phosphorus absorption has been less studied than the effect of lactose on calcium absorption. However, there is evidence that lactose enhances both phosphorus absorption and phosphorus balance. In humans the phosphorus balance as well as calcium balance is improved by the feeding of lactose (6). In rats, feeding lactose enhances phosphorus balance and net intestinal absorption of phosphorus (14). This effect of lactose is seen in rats fed both high- and low-phosphorus diets.

Recently, the effect of lactose on phosphorus transport has been studied using everted intestinal sacs (18, 41). Phosphorus transport was studied in both duodenal and ileal sacs from young, adult, and old rats (Table 11-2). In the absence of lactose, phosphorus uptake declined significantly with age in the duodenum ($p <$

Table 11-2 Effect of Age and Lactose on Intestinal Uptake of Phosphorus

Age	Segment	Phosphorus uptake ($p$moles/mg)	
		Control	Lactose
Young	Duodenum	736 ± 73	1,187 ± 169
Adult	Duodenum	492 ± 51	641 ± 34
Old	Duodenum	300 ± 42	532 ± 59
Young	Ileum	288 ± 27	453 ± 13
Adult	Ileum	395 ± 23	512 ± 40
Old	Ileum	294 ± 20	350 ± 36

Phosphorus uptake was measured in the same experiment as in Table 11-1. After preincubation in the presence or absence of lactose, everted sacs were transferred into buffer containing 1.0 mM phosphorus for the measurement of phosphorus uptake. Table entries are the mean and standard error of six sacs. [Data tabulated from Armbrecht (41)]. Lactose significantly enhanced phosphorus uptake in the duodenum and ileum of all age groups ($p < .001$, two-way ANOVA).

.001, one-way ANOVA) but did not change with age in the ileum. In the duodenum, lactose significantly increased phosphorus uptake in all age groups ($p <$ .001, two-way ANOVA), and the effect of lactose did not change significantly with age ($p < .201$). Lactose also significantly increased phosphorus uptake in the ileum of all age groups ($p < .001$, two-way ANOVA), and the effects of lactose were not significantly different in each age group ($p < .169$). These experiments demonstrate that lactose enhances the uptake of phosphorus into the intestine *in vitro* as it does calcium uptake (Table 11-1). In addition, the effect of lactose on phosphorus uptake is similar in all age groups.

The mechanism by which lactose stimulates phosphorus absorption is still under investigation. However, some experiments suggest that lactose may work differently to enhance phosphorus uptake from how it does to enhance calcium uptake. Under anaerobic conditions, the effect of lactose on phosphorus uptake is inhibited, but the effect of lactose on calcium uptake is not inhibited (18). This suggests that lactose stimulates the *active* component of phosphorus absorption. A recent report suggests that lactose works by increasing the intestinal brush border permeability to phosphorus (29). Incubation of brush border membrane vesicles with lactose causes an enhancement of phosphorus uptake. Lactose specifically enhances the diffusional component of phosphorus uptake in this system. Interestingly, it has been reported that sugars stimulate the activity of purified intestinal alkaline phosphatase (30). However, the role of alkaline phosphatase in the intestinal absorption of phosphorus and/or calcium is still not known.

STIMULATION OF CALCIUM ABSORPTION BY OTHER SUGARS

There is evidence that other complex sugars in addition to lactose enhance calcium absorption. Sucrose and cellobiose enhance calcium uptake *in vitro* (20), and glucose polymers enhance the appearance of radioactive calcium in bone after oral administration to rats (31). The reported effects of glucose and galactose, the monosaccharide components of lactose, on calcium absorption are more variable. Glucose and galactose do not enhance calcium uptake by intestinal sacs at the same concentrations that lactose enhances uptake (20). However, glucose has been reported to enhance calcium absorption in the intact animal (32). Glucose and galactose mimic the effect of lactose in Ussing chamber experiments (21), but these effects may be due to the substitution of the sugars for sodium. When given by gavage, lactose enhances calcium absorption in the rat, but glucose and sucrose do not enhance absorption in this experimental system (33).

EFFECT OF LACTOSE ON SKELETAL MINERALIZATION

There is experimental evidence that the stimulation of calcium and phosphorus absorption by lactose results in enhanced bone mineralization. In rats, lactose enhances the deposition of radioactive calcium from the intestine into the skeleton (16, 31, 32, 34, 42). Feeding diets containing 12–15 percent lactose to young rats for a period of weeks significantly increases bone calcification (13, 14). It has been suggested that lactose has a direct effect on bone calcification (32, 38). However, it is difficult to separate out the effects of lactose on bone calcification from its effects on absorption. Human studies have shown that lactose or milk improves calcium balance (6–9) and bone mineralization (9) in lactose-tolerant individuals. On the other hand, lactose intolerance is associated with bone loss (35) and osteoporosis (36, 37).

CONCLUSIONS

In summary, there is evidence from both animal and human studies that dietary lactose influences calcium and skeletal metabolism. Lactose stimulates intestinal absorption of calcium and phosphorus, improves calcium and phosphorus balance, increases deposition of calcium into bone, and increases long-term bone mineralization. These effects of lactose may be nutritionally important, since they are independent of vitamin D status and tend to supplement the action of vitamin D. Lactose enhances calcium absorption in the ileum, which shows decreased responsiveness to 1,25-dihydroxyvitamin D compared to the duodenum. The effect of lactose in the ileum may be nutritionally important, since large amounts of lactose are found in the ileum after lactose administration (39). Lactose also works to stimulate intestinal absorption of calcium in all age groups. This may be important in older mammals, which have decreased capacity to absorb calcium (22, 24). In older individuals the role of vitamin D in enhancing intestinal absorption of calcium may be diminished. Animal studies have shown that the capacity to synthesize and respond to 1,25-dihydroxyvitamin D decreases with age (23, 40). Further research is needed to understand and utilize the beneficial effects of lactose on intestinal absorption of the minerals found in bone. Studies of ways to improve calcium absorption in lactose-intolerant individuals of all ages are also needed.

Acknowledgments: The author acknowledges the excellent technical assistance of Susan Porter. This work was supported by the Veterans Administration and by the National Dairy Board in cooperation with the National Dairy Council.

REFERENCES

1. Bergeim, O. (1926) J. Biol. Chem. 70:35.
2. Kline, O. L., Keenan, J. A., Elvehjem, C. A., Hart, E. B. (1932) J. Biol. Chem. 98:121.
3. Dittmer, D. S. (1961) Blood and other body fluids. Fed. Am. Soc. Exptl. Biol., Washington, D.C., p. 459.
4. Ziegler, E. E., Fomon, S. J. (1983) J. Pediatr. Gastroenterol. Nutr. 2:288.
5. Mills, R., Breiter, H., Kampster, E., McKey, B., Pickens, M., Outhouse, J. (1940) J. Nutr. 20:467.
6. Condon, J. R., Nassim, J. R., Millard, F. J. C., Hilbe, A., Stainthorpe, E. M. (1970) Lancet I 7655:1027.

7. Kocian, J., Skala, I., Bakos, K. (1973) Digestion 9:319.

8. Cochet, B., Jung, A., Griessen, M., Bartholdi, P., Schaller, P., Donath, A. (1983) Gastroenterology 84:935.

9. Recker, R. R., Heaney, R. P. (1985) Am. J. Clin. Nutr. 41:254.

10. Pansu, D., Chapuy, M. C. (1970) Calcif. Tiss. Res. 4(suppl.):155.

11. Debongnie, J. C., Newcomer, A. D., McGill, D. B., Phillips, S. F. (1979) Dig. Dis. Sci. 24:225.

12. Pirk, F., Skala, I. (1972) Digestion 5:89.

13. Evans, J. L., Ali, R. (1967) J. Nutr. 92:417.

14. Schaafsma, G., Visser, R. (1980) J. Nutr. 110:1101.

15. Pansu, D., Bellaton, C., Bronner, F. (1979) J. Nutr. 109:508.

16. Lengemann, F. W., Wasserman, R. H., Comar, C. L. (1959) J. Nutr. 68:443.

17. Lengemann, F. W. (1959) J. Nutr. 69:23.

18. Armbrecht, H. J. (1986) Fed. Proc. 45:709.

19. Urban, E., Pena, M. (1977) Digestion 15:18.

20. Armbrecht, H. J., Wasserman, R. H. (1976) J. Nutr. 106:1265.

21. Favus, M. J., Angeid-Backman, E. (1984) Am. J. Physiol. 246:G281.

22. Armbrecht, H. J., Zenser, T. V., Gross, C. J., Davis, B. B. (1980) Am. J. Physiol. 239:E322.

23. Armbrecht, H. J., Forte, L. R., Halloran, B. P. (1984) Am. J. Physiol. 246:E266.

24. Gallagher, J. C., Riggs, B. L., Eisman, J., Hamstra, A., Arnaud, S. B., DeLuca, H. F. (1979) J. Clin. Invest. 64:729.

25. Charley, P., Saltman, P. (1963) Science 139:1205.

26. Wasserman, R. H. (1964) Nature 201:997.

27. Martin, D. L., DeLuca, H. F. (1969) Am. J. Physiol. 216:1351.

28. Bugg, C. E. (1973) J. Amer. Chem. Soc. 95:908.

29. Debiec, H., Lorenc, R. (1985) J. Nutr. 115:1168.

30. Dupuis, Y. Digaud, A., Fontaine, N. (1977) Calcif. Tiss. Res. 22(suppl.):556.

31. Zheng, J., Wood, R. J., Rosenberg, I. H. (1985) Am. J. Clin. Nutr. 41:243.

32. Lengemann, F. W., Comar, C. L. (1961) Am. J. Physiol. 200:1051.

33. Ghishan, F. K., Stroop, S., Meneely, R. (1982) Pediatr. Res. 16:566.

34. Sato, R., Noguchi, T., Naito, H. (1983) J. Nutr. Sci. Vitaminol. 29:365.

35. Kocian, J., Vulterinova, M. Bejblova, O., Skala, I. (1973) Digestion 8:324.

36. Birge, S. J., Keutmann, H. T., Cuatrecases, P., Whedon, G. D. (1967) New Engl. J. Med. 274:445.

37. Pacifici, R., Drake, D., Avioli, L. V. (1985) Calcif. Tiss. Int. 37:101.

38. Finlayson, B. (1970) Investigative Urology 7:433.

39. Dahlquist, A., Thomson, D. L. (1964) Acta. Physiol. Scand. 61:20.

40. Armbrecht, H. J., Zenser, T. V., Davis, B. B. (1980) Endocrinology 106:469.

41. Armbrecht, H. J. (1987) Nutr. Res. 7:1167.

42. Miller, S. C., MIller, M. A., Omura, T. H. (1988) J. Nutr. 118:72.

12

Dietary Lipids and
the Calcifying Tissues

H. GILDER AND A. L. BOSKEY

METABOLISM OF LIPIDS

The need for dietary lipid has been known for centuries, long before the discovery of fat-soluble vitamins and the essential fatty acids. Out of taste and habit, affluent societies have come to glut themselves with an excess of fatty foods and calories, whereas in underdeveloped countries, where the chief sources of food are grains, people may be as well nourished while consuming very little fat. The body is capable of adapting to a large variety of foods and different relative amounts of the three major foodstuffs—protein, carbohydrate, and fat.

Recent nutritional studies have emphasized the unfavorable health consequences of dietary overindulgence. But little is known about optimal diets for human beings, although it is clear that at different stages of the life-span the optimal intake varies in health and disease (1).

The nonprotein portion of the diet, which comprises as much as 70 percent of the total caloric intake, may be composed of any proportion of fat (lipid) and carbohydrate, provided the fat-soluble vitamins and essential fatty acids are supplied. Fat supplies flavor and variety as well as assuring the required essential fatty acids. The average intake of fat in the United States and other affluent societies is 42 percent of the total calories, a figure physicians and nutritionists believe should be reduced to 30 percent (2). The consequences of some nutritional regimens that deviate markedly from the normal intakes suggests that it is foolhardy to use diets that are drastically different from the norm.

Roles of Lipids in the Body

Dietary lipids provide a major source of energy. Although all three nutrient classes supply energy for the body economy, fats have the advantage of being concentrated, containing per gram more than twice the caloric value of carbohydrate or protein.

Lipids, chiefly the phospholipids and cholesterol, are the principal components of cell membranes. These membranes have been likened to a sea of lipid in which proteins are intercalated. The phospholipids, which comprise the structural basis for biomembranes, are synthesized *de novo* in the smooth endoplasmic reticulum from dietary lipid. Membranes of subcellular organelles with different biological roles vary in lipid composition.

The principal role of lipids within the membrane is structural. The rigidity of the membrane core is largely determined by the nature of the fatty acid side chains. Usually the carbon 1 of the glycerol moiety of the phospholipid is occupied by a saturated fatty acid while the 2 position has an unsaturated fatty acid. At most of the double bonds the fatty acid chains are kinked in the *cis* configuration, causing loose packing, facilitating insertion of cholesterol in the spaces, and resulting in more fluidity of the membrane. In the phosphatidylcholine molecule, there seems to be preferential pairing of saturated and unsaturated fatty acids. For example arachidonic acid (20:4) prefers to pair with palmitic acid (16:0), and docosahexanoic acid (22:6) with stearic acid (18:0) (3).

The "essential" fatty acids (EFA), those that the body cannot synthesize *de novo*, have a number of vital roles (4). They are constituents of the phospholipids and cholesterol esters in all membranes, they are precursors for the prostaglandins, and they are utilized in cholesterol metabolism.

Most cells are capable of synthesizing *de novo* from simple precursors all of the lipid classes—phospholipids, cholesterol, glycerides, glycolipids, etc., and their constituent fatty acids. However, Burr (5) demonstrated in 1929 that rats fed fat-free diets developed a syndrome of poor growth, dermatitis, degenerative changes in certain organs, and sterility. The condition could be reversed by the addition of unsaturated fatty acids, especially linoleic acid, to the diet. In 1971, Prout showed that an EFA deficiency caused abnormalities in dentin and enamel development in growing rats (6). By analogy with dentin one might assume comparable effects on osteogenesis. For years, essential fatty acid deficiency was not observed in humans except in infants on low-fat intakes or with intestinal disease. It was not until the late 1950s that the deficiency was shown to occur in adults when long-term total parenteral nutrition became a form of therapy for patients who were unable to take oral nourishment (7). This was well before the advent of safe intravenous fat emulsions.

The biochemical defect in essential fatty acid deficiency is the inability of mammalian tissues to introduce double bonds into long-chain fatty acids nearer than 9 carbons from the methyl group. The significant dietary EFA are linoleic acid [18:2ω6(9,12)] and linolenic acid [18:3ω3(9,12,15)] (Table 12-1). These can be replaced by some of the polyunsaturated fatty acids (PUFA) occurring naturally in vegetable oils having carbon lengths of 18, 20, and 22 atoms, and having two to six double bonds all in the *cis* configuration. Nevertheless, from the practical point of view, it is recommended that 1–3 percent of the total caloric intake consist of linoleic acid (7, 8). The ingested unsaturated fatty acids in the diet are variously modified by elongation, shortening, and desaturation within the cells to form the polyunsaturated fatty acids (PUFA) before they become part of the membrane structures.

The requirement for linolenic acid is about one-tenth that of linoleic acid. The two produce separate and different PUFAs, and there is no crossover between them. Linolenic acid is found in large amounts in the central nervous system

Table 12-1 Families of Unsaturated Fatty Acids and Their Derivatives

Family[a]	Fatty acid[b]	Structure[c]	Major metabolites[d]	PGs[e]	Source
ω9	18:1ω9(9) oleic acid	C(C)₇C=C(C)₇COOH	20:3ω9 eicosatrienoic acid		Animal and vegetable oils
ω6	18:2ω6(6,9) linoleic acid	H₃C(C)₄C=CCC= C(C)₇COOH	20:3ω6 eicosatrienoic acid	PGE₁	Vegetable oils
			20:4ω3 arachidonic acid	PGE₂	
ω3	18:3ω3(9,12,15) linolenic acid	H₃CCC=CCC=CCC= C(C)₇COOH	20:5ω3 eicosapentaenoic acid	PGI₃	Vegetable oils
			22:6ω3 docasahexaenoic acid		Marine oils

[a]Omega number, *viz.* ω3, refers to the carbon number counting from the methyl terminus at which the first double bond is situated.

[b]Number after the colon is the number of double bonds. Numbers in parentheses show the position of the double bonds.

[c]Hydrogens have been omitted to simplify the drawing.

[d]These are only a few of the many metabolites derived from these fatty acids.

[e]Prostaglandins.

lipids. Signs of EFA deficiency occur not only owing to dietary deficiency but also to dietary imbalance of the two EFAs or their metabolic products (8).

Dietary considerations of lipids during pregnancy are important for human fetal development (9). Infants or malnourished mothers are susceptible to EFA deficiency (10). The placenta is impermeable to most lipids, but the EFAs are transported directly from the maternal diet. The placenta synthesizes the other fatty acids, and they are actively transported to the fetus (11). In a recent study of moderately malnourished mothers, the postpartum placental weights were reduced, but their lipid constituents comprised relatively high concentrations of high-carbon PUFA (12). This was apparently due to the failure of the transfer of the unsaturated fatty acids to the fetus. Retained in the placenta, these became further elongated. The failure of transfer was presumed to be due to the EFA deficiency.

In the newborn, 40–50 percent of the dietary energy is provided as fat from well-nourished lactating mothers (13). Human milk contains four times more EFA and less protein and calcium than cow's milk. This may reflect the greater lipid requirements of the highly developed central nervous system of the human but a slower body growth in comparison to those of the calf. Thus it is not surprising that premature infants and infants on low-fat formulas are particularly susceptible to EFA deficiency (8).

The plasma and tissue lipids of EFA-deficient subjects are characterized by an abnormal elevation of the triene, eicosatrienoic acid (20:3ω9) (5, 8, 11), a product of oleic acid, relative to the tetraenes which include arachidonic acid (Table 12-1). An assay for EFA deficiency has been developed that is based on the increase of the ratio of trienes to tetraenes in the plasma (14). The rapidity with which an EFA deficiency can develop in man is exemplified in studies of McCarthy on surgical patients on fat-free parenteral nutrition in which after 1 week, the ratio of triene to tetraene in plasma decreased strikingly (15).

The prostaglandins, leukotrienes, and thromboxanes are a class of cyclic 20-carbon fatty acids that are synthesized in plasma membranes from the 18-carbon fatty acids (16). They act as short-range hormones and affect cell membrane function by serving as second messengers. The prostaglandins modulate the activities of a number of hormones. There is experimental evidence that the prostaglandins take part in bone development (17). Abnormal patterns of prostaglandins result from a deficiency of EFA.

PUFAs that are synthesized from the EFA are also required in the esterification of cholesterol and in the excretion of sterols.

Lipids serve as vehicle for transporting the fat-soluble vitamins in the blood. They are the principal form in which energy is stored in the body. The adipocyte, a specialized connective tissue cell, is capable of storing enormous quantities of triglycerides for future needs. These depots of fat also serve as thermal insulation and as mechanical buffers to protect organs from physical damage from the outside. Finally, dietary lipids make food palatable; they slow gastrointestinal motility and they have high satiety value.

Metabolism of Dietary Fats

Most of the dietary fats consumed by humans are triglycerides. Phospholipids, cholesterol, and other lipid classes comprise only about one-tenth of total fat intake in the normal diet. Digestion of fats commences in the duodenum with the action of intestinal and pancreatic enzymes and the bile acids. The resulting monoglycerides, long-chain fatty acids (containing more than 12 carbon atoms) released from the triglycerides, and cholesterol, pass through the mucosal cell membranes and are resynthesized into triglycerides and cholesterol esters in the endoplasmic reticulum. Phospholipids and specific proteins are added to form lipid globules (100–1,000 μm in diameter), known as chylomicrons, which are released from the cells by exocytosis and pass into the lymph channels and the thoracic duct. The fatty acids of medium chain length (6–10 carbon atoms) pass through the cells into the portal blood to reach the liver directly.

Combinations of phospholipids, cholesterols, cholesterol esters, triglycerides, and fatty acids are assembled with specific proteins to form lipoproteins. The lipoprotein particles vary in size from 7 to 25 μm in diameter and are designated as high-, low-, and very low-density lipoproteins (HDL, LDL, and VLDL), respectively, according to their densities, which in turn depend on their relative content of lipid and protein. The lipoproteins are involved in transport of lipids, especially cholesterol. Free fatty acids are also transported in the bloodstream bound to plasma albumin.

A fatty acid-binding protein (FABP) has been identified in the intermyocyte spaces of the heart muscle. FABP is believed to control the passage of lipid into myocytes and thus also to control energy release (18). Since fatty acid is the preferred substrate for heart muscle metabolism and since FABP increases with the lipid content of the diet, this is conjectured to be a new mechanism for regulating energy in this tissue.

When lipoproteins and chylomicrons reach the peripheral tissues, they are adsorbed on the surface of capillary endothelial cells and then hydrolyzed to glycerol and fatty acids by specific lipoprotein lipases. Cleavage of triglycerides is 30 times more active than that of phospholipids. The fatty acids and monoglycerides released are absorbed directly into the cells and are used as membrane components and for energy. Other lipids are recognized by specific receptors on the cell surfaces and are endocytosed. The spent chylomicrons and lipoproteins return to the liver for reloading.

Fatty acids not only originate in the diet but also are synthesized endogenously from the metabolic breakdown product of sugars, some amino acids, and other fatty acids.

Effect of Dietary Fat Intake on Body Fats

Lipids are synthesized by most tissues in the body. Nevertheless dietary lipids may govern the lipid composition of some tissues. The fatty acid composition of the triglycerides in storage fats is in a state of continuous flux, varying in response to changes in the dietary fat. The intermolecular rearrangement of fatty acids in triglyceride occurs relatively slowly and comes about by hydrolysis and reesterification of the more recently synthesized depot triglycerides (3, 19). When a diet high in saturated fatty acid is consumed, the proportion of these fatty acids in the adipose tissue triglycerides may increase to the extent of changing the physical properties such as the fluidity of the adipose tissue (19).

In breeding studies, free-living animals (bovids and pigs) were shown to have less body fat but seven times more unsaturated fatty acids and fewer saturated and monounsaturated fatty acids in adipose tissue than did genetically similar domesticated animals (20). This was due to the fact that muscles of meat-producing animals that have been force-fed for profit have more infiltrated fat, which is high in saturated fats. Also domesticated animals are genetically selected for fast growing, they are fed high-energy foods, and their exercise is restricted.

To prevent an essential fatty acid deficiency, a balanced intake of saturated and unsaturated fatty acids in the diet is as important as the actual amount present. Crawford showed that an existing EFA deficiency can be exacerbated by loading animals with dietary fat containing excessive amounts of saturated fatty acids, since these fatty acids compete for enzyme systems that metabolize the essential fatty acids of similar length (20).

The phospholipids and, particularly, phosphatidylcholine of different tissues of the same animal vary considerably in composition, positional distribution, and species of fatty acid (3). The variability reflects the different functions of these tissues. The fatty acid composition of membrane lipids, chiefly cholesterol esters and phospholipids, changes less in response to dietary changes than does that of the triglycerides. In studies of brain lipids in different species of animals, the fatty acid distribution of cholesterol esters and phospholipids was remarkably similar even among the species, and it remained the same under a variety of food intakes (9).

Kramer studied the experimental myocardial necrosis induced in rats on high-fat intakes (21). He tested diets consisting of oils with different proportions of saturated and unsaturated fatty acids. As with the studies of muscle described above, the lesions were due not to any specific fat in excess but to an imbalance of the fatty acids. For example, if the intake of linolenic acid (ω3) was increased to more than 5 percent of the total ingested fat, cardiac necrosis developed. The linolenic acid apparently inhibited the desaturation and elongation of arachidonic acid and thus deprived the cells of the fatty acids needed for membrane phosphatidylcholine and phosphatidylethanolamine formation. The heart lesions were abolished by increasing the intake of saturated fatty acids, thus supplying a more balanced mixture of fatty acids for phospholipid synthesis.

The type of fat ingested may influence not only the fatty acid composition of membrane lipids but also the spectrum and quantity of prostaglandins produced (22). For example, feeding arachidonic acid to humans increased the PGE_2 levels in plasma, which resulted in an increase in the reactivity of the platelets. On the other hand, the Eskimo diet containing large amounts of fish, which are rich in ω3 fatty acids, alters the array of prostaglandins produced. Relatively less of the prostaglandins that cause platelet aggregation and more of the prostaglandins that disaggregate them are synthesized with the resulting bleeding tendencies in Eskimos (23, 24).

Hydrogenated vegetable oils have become a major fat source in modern food manufacture. In view of the trend toward higher consumption of vegetable oils, many have investigated the nutritional effects of these products (22, 25). When vegetable oils are hardened by partial hydrogenation, 5–8 percent of the fatty acids may be converted from the biologically more common *cis* double bonds to those in the *trans* configuration. Many of the double bonds are moved to abnormal positions on the chain. Since the metabolism of fatty acids and their incorporation into membranes depends on their geometry and double bond position, using abnormal isomers could produce unusual membrane structure.

Rats fed hydrogenated oil showed large increases of abnormal fatty acids in tissue and in plasma lipoprotein (26). Furthermore when the intake of linoleic acid was already low, an essential fatty acid deficiency was accentuated. Adding linoleic acid to the diet did not significantly diminish the amount of retention of the isomeric acids in the tissues. *Trans* fatty acids in culinary fats have been shown experimentally to influence the rate of oxidation of heart muscle mitochondria, the synthesis of the prostaglandins, and the fluidity of the membranes (27, 28).

Studies with humans cannot be so well controlled. In a retrospective postmortem study of 20- to 60-year-old subjects who throughout their lives had consumed a common mixed diet containing an estimated 6–8 percent of commercially modified fatty acid, Ohlrogge observed that the lipids of several tissues reflected this intake in varying degrees (29). The *trans* fatty acids were present in highest levels in the triglycerides of plasma, liver, and heart. Significant amounts also accumulated in the cholesterol esters and phospholipids. There was a trend toward the accumulation of fatty acids with double bonds farthest from the carbonyl group. Emken fed deuterium-labeled octadecanoic acid isomers to humans (28). Traced to the tissue, some of the resulting unsaturated isomers were concentrated, and others were excluded from the lipids in various tissues.

The observation of abnormal fatty acids in human tissues was not thought to be a matter of concern by the group of scientists studying hydrogenated fats (25). They contend that there is always some variation in the fatty acid content of lipids of most tissues. At current levels of consumption, persons on normal balanced diets are able to utilize unusual isomers at rates sufficient to prevent any undue accumulation in the tissue lipids. The hydrogenated fats serve well as a source of fuel, and no reasonable diet is apt to contain sufficient nonnatural fatty acids to change the lipid class composition or to interfere with the function of the membranes.

These generalizations are probably valid for the population as a whole. Nevertheless, physicians with patients with nutritive disorders, as well as the diet- and health-conscious public, should be alerted to the possibility of biological defects after long term utilization in excess of certain man-made lipids that have been shown in animals to cause abnormalities in membranes and lipoprotein composition. That hydrogenated fatty acids do not interfere with the metabolism of the EFA may be comforting, but on the other hand these abnormal fatty acids have atherogenic effects comparable to those of their natural saturated counterparts (30, 31), so they are not nutritionally desirable except as a source of energy.

LIPIDS IN BONE DEVELOPMENT

Presence of Lipids in Bone and Teeth

The metabolism of lipid in bone is under the same controls as in other tissues. However, analysis of lipids in calcifying tissues is made difficult because of the presence of mineral. Relatively recent studies have revealed that in addition to the roles they play in the nonmineralizing tissues, lipids have special functions in the calcification process in most mineralizing tissues.

Histochemical Demonstration of Lipids in Bone

The presence of lipid in bone and other calcified tissue was demonstrated by Von Bibra as far back as 1884 (32). In the 1960s, using histochemical techniques with Sudan black and other fat-soluble dyes, Irving and, soon after, Enlow, observed the presence of lipid in both cells and matrix at the calcifying front in the epiphyseal plate and spread throughout the extracellular matrix of long bones (33, 34). In bones of young animals, lipid dyes tended to be localized in pericellular regions, while in mature bones, the dyes were scattered more diffusely (35). Later, electron microscopic studies showed that lipid droplets were situated within cartilage cells at the zone of calcification and also in the cytoplasm of some bone cells. The ultrastructure of the lipid within these cells is visibly distinguishable from that in the vascular channels. Lipids are generally found concentrated at the boundary between calcifying and noncalcified tissue (36).

Extraction of Lipids

The total lipid content of mineralizing tissues ranges from 1.7 percent of the dry weight of calcified cartilage to 0.2 percent of bone and dentin (36–38). Table 12-2 is derived from analysis of the lipids of bovine bone by Shapiro as recalculated by Dirkson (37–39). Data from human bone are incomplete and inaccurate (37, 38). Of the total lipid about 65 percent may be extracted from ground bone with-

Table 12-2 Lipid Composition of Bovine Bone

	mg/100 g Calcified Tissue		
Lipid class	Predemineralization	Postdemineralization	Acid extraction
Tri-, di-, monoglycerols	702	67	19
Cholesterols and cholesterol esters	17	159	60
Fatty acids	8	64	20
Phospholipids	13	5	1
Fraction of total lipids	65%	26%	9%

Source: Dirksen (37).

out demineralization. Most of the lipid readily extracted from bone is derived from vascular channels or bone marrow. Its composition is comparable to that of lipids normally extractable from soft tissue. Another 26 percent of the total lipids is extracted with neutral solvents from the tissue after demineralization with EDTA. It contains relatively less triglyceride and a larger proportion of cholesterols and phospholipids. Acidic solvent extraction is required to release the remaining lipids, which comprises 9 percent of the total lipid. Table 12-3 indicates the distribution of phospholipid species in these extracts (37–39). The relative amounts of the acidic phospholipids, phosphatidylserine (PS), phosphatidylinositol (PI), and phosphatidic acid (PA) are increased in lipid extracts of bone after demineralization.

Lipids at the Site of New Mineralization

Lipid is found both in the cells and in the matrix of developing bone and dentin. The consistent histological detection of lipid at the site of active calcification led Irving and Wuthier to investigate the lipids of epiphyseal cartilage and bone during the process of endochondral ossification (40–42). Wuthier dissected out the epi-

Table 12-3 Distribution of Phospholipids in Bovine Bone

	mg PL/100 g Calcified Tissue		
Phospholipid (PL)	Predemineralization	Postdemineralization	Acid extraction
Sphingomyelin	5.49	1.82	0.08
Phosphatidylcholine	4.75	1.07	0.19
Phosphatidylethanolamine	2.56	1.12	—
Phosphatidylserine	—	0.85	0.13
Phosphatidylinositol	—	0.27	0.13
Phosphatidic acid	—	0.27	0.06
Cardiolipin	0.58	0	0
Total phospholipid	13.38	5.40	0.59

Sources: Dirksen (37), Shapiro (38, 39).

physeal apparatus of long bones from full-term bovine fetuses and analyzed six maturational zones of the epiphyseal plate and bone: resting, proliferating, hypertrophic and calcifying cartilage, and cancellous and compact bone. Since the epiphyseal growth plate is extremely uneven and its dissection is difficult, the data should be interpreted as showing trends rather than the absolute values in a given zone. The lipid fraction extracted only after demineralization of the six zones rose from 1 percent of the demineralized weight of resting cartilage to a peak of 8.5 percent of the hypertrophic cartilage. Lipid content decreased to near 1 percent in the two bone fractions. Phospholipid represented between 20 and 36 percent of total lipid in all of the samples. The total phospholipid content increased from 180 mg% of demineralized dry weight in resting cartilage to 295 mg% of demineralized dry weight in calcified cartilage. The phospholipid content dropped to a low figure in cancellous and compact bone.

Characteristic of Phospholipid Associated with Calcified Tissue

Wuthier examined the species of phospholipids extracted from the cartilage and bone fraction (42). Similar phospholipid species were found in the total lipid extracted from the epiphyseal plate at various stages of maturation. The ethanolamine phospholipids were present in higher proportions in proliferating cartilage. Bone phospholipids were similar to those of cartilage but contained somewhat more sphingomyelin, phosphatidylserine, and phosphatidylinositols and less of the phosphatidylethanolamines. Before demineralization, the serine and inositol phospholipid fractions were decreasingly extractable in proportion to the degree of calcification of the cartilage and bone. This reduced extractability indicated a possible interaction between the acidic phospholipids and the newly formed mineral and matrix protein and is the basis for the current theory that the strong affinity for calcium of the acidic phospholipids is associated with the calcification mechanism (38, 43).

Roles of Lipid in Bone Metabolism

Membrane Composition

Lipids play multiple roles in bone structure, function, and development. To begin with, they are essential components of all membranes including those of the cellular elements of both cartilage and bone. The integrity and function of membranes depend on the optimal distribution of saturated and unsaturated phospholipids in their structure.

Matrix Vesicles

The extracellular matrix of the epiphyseal cartilage as well as of several other calcified tissues contains membrane-bound, lipid-rich vesicles that are believed to be the site of initial mineral deposition (Fig. 12-1) (36, 43–45). Extracellular matrix vesicles range in diameter from 30 nm to 1 μm (average 0.1 μm). When examined at the electron microscopic level, the vesicles are observed to be surrounded by a trilamellar membrane 8–9 nm thick (47). By morphological and biochemical evidence the vesicles have been shown to be derived by budding from the chondrocyte plasma membrane (36, 44–49). Whether this occurs at specific

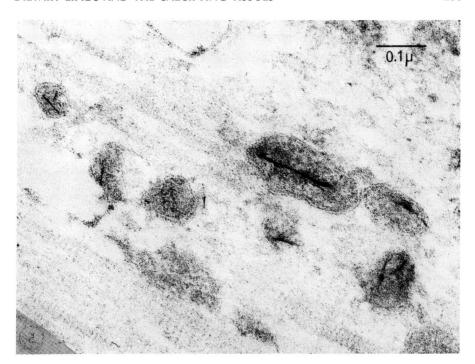

Fig. 12-1 Electron micrograph of matrix vesicles containing clumps of apatite crystals in osseous matrix of a 7-day-old chick femur. Stained with lead acetate and uranyl acetate (152,000×). [Photomicrograph kindly provided by Dr. H. C. Anderson (61).]

regions on the membrane or is a random process is yet to be determined. Concurrent with matrix calcification in the growth plate, a progression may be observed from mineral-free organelles to vesicles covered or filled with masses of mineral clumps (50, 51). Similar vesicles have been observed in some types of bone, in mantle dentine, and in other types of physiological and pathological calcifications (45, 46). However, vesicles have not been found to be associated with mineral deposition in all calcifying tissues.

Matrix vesicle membranes have alkaline phosphatase activity and contain a variety of other phosphatase-related enzyme activities. In cartilage they are distinguished from chondrocyte membranes in their enrichment in phospholipids and, in particular, cardiolipin, phosphatidic acid, sphingomyelin, and phosphatidylserine (Table 12-4) (48, 52, 53). The acidic phospholipids are concentrated in the inner membrane of the vesicle. It is believed that the affinity of these acidic phospholipids for calcium serves to concentrate calcium within the vesicle, where, in an environment of increased calcium and phosphate-producing enzymes, initiation of calcification occurs with the formation of the first calcium phosphate crystals (50, 54, 55). Some of the calcium that accumulates within the matrix vesicles may be derived from the mitochondria of the chondrocytes (38, 49).

In spite of their active participation in mineralization, certain findings argue that the vesicles once free in the matrix are degenerative products of the cell. First, their appearance suggests that they are degradative. They contain amorphous

Table 12-4 Phospholipid Content of Cells, Chondrocyte Membranes, and Vesicles of Chick Epiphyseal Plate

		μg/g Tissue	
Lipid	Cells[a]	Membranes	Vesicles
Sphingomyelin	16	4	7
PC and lyso-PC[b]	172	40	21
PE and lyso-PE	70	14	12
PS and lyso-PS	9	2	9
PI and lyso-PI	13	4	3
PA, PG, and CDL	6	2	4
Total phospholipid	288	68	58
Total lipid	800	310	360

Source: Wuthier (52).

[a]Cells from proliferating cartilage.

[b]Abbreviations: PC, phosphatidylcholine; PE, phosphatidylethanolamine; PS, phosphatidylserine; PI, phosphatidylinositol; PA, phosphatidic acid; PG, phosphatidylglycerol; CDL, cardiolipin.

material, vacuoles, and remnants of other organelles. Unlike the chondrocytes, which are known to synthesize fatty acids *de novo* from ^{14}C-labeled acetate and actively incorporate serine and acetate into phosphatidylserine and lysophosphatidylserine, the vesicles lack these synthetic capacities (55, 56). In the end stages of epiphyseal differentiation, the phospholipid content of the matrix vesicles and the level of their metabolism typify a degradative state in that phospholipases are more active, and the lyso- forms of the phospholipids increase at the expense of the diacyl forms, implying the loss of synthetic enzymes. Furthermore, the fatty acids in the remaining phospholipids reflect the activity of the specific phospholipases present. The dominant proportion of the phosphatidylserines in vesicles (Table 12-4) may be explained by the fact that these are more slowly degraded than other phospholipids (53).

Calcium–Acidic Phospholipid Phosphate (CaPLP) Complexes

Associated closely with mineralizing tissues are complexes of calcium, acidic phospholipids, and phosphate (53, 57, 58). They have been isolated from chondrocyte membranes, from the matrix vesicles, and from a variety of other mineralizing tissues, but they are absent from nonmineralized tissues (38). Their presence signals nucleation and apatite formation, and they appear when the microenvironment is suitable for the formation of hydroxyapatite. The evidence for their involvement is based on the sites where they are found and on their ability to cause *in vitro* hydroxyapatite deposition (59). That the complexes are absolutely required for calcification to occur is yet to be proved.

The mean molar ratio of components of the CaPLP complexes is variable and depends on the availability of the phospholipids in the tissue from which it is isolated as well as the method of isolation and the amount of final rinsing of the particles. Generally the calcium:phospholipid ratio varies between 2:1 and 5:4 (38, 53, 58).

The CaPLP complexes can be produced *in vitro* from a metastable calcium phosphate solution when phosphatidylserine or phosphatidylinositol is introduced into the medium (60). The optimal conditions for their formation *in vitro* are a high pH and concentrations of calcium and phosphate comparable to those present in osteoid tissue. Phosphate must be bound to the phospholipid before calcium. This was shown by the finding that calcium salts of phospholipids are not able to cause hydroxyapatite formation (38, 50, 60, 61). Once phosphate and calcium bind to the phospholipids, the lipid-soluble particles that are formed can promote hydroxyapatite growth.

Although vitamin D, which is a cholesterol derivative, will be dealt with elsewhere in this book, it is important to note that $1,25(OH)_2$ vitamin D is involved in the regulation of phospholipid metabolism in kidney, intestine and bone. Boskey studied vitamin D-deficient, phosphate-depleted immature rachitic rats to test the hypothesis that CaPLP complexes, as components of vesicles and cell membranes, played a role in initiating mineralization *in vivo* (62). The content of CaPLP complex in the nonmineralizing epiphyseal cartilage was the same in controls as in rachitic rats. On the other hand the rapidly remodeling metaphyseal bone of the rachitic rats contained fewer complexes than did that of the control rats suggesting some kind of role of the complexes in mineralization. Further evidence for the contribution to calcification of the D vitamins in the formation of lipid complexes were experiments in rachitic rats which showed that several vitamin D metabolites, but most actively 1,25 dihydroxyvitamin D, fed to rachitic rats, caused significant increases of complexed acidic phospholipids in bones as well as normalizing the histomorphic and mineral parameters (63).

Proteolipids

Proteolipids are a special class of proteins that are fat-soluble because of their lipid components and their high content of hydrophobic amino acids. They are present in most cells but in large quantities only in the nervous system tissues. A proteolipid has been isolated from calcifying tissue that appears to be associated with calcification. Ennever fractionated crude acetone-precipitated phospholipid extracts of lyophilyzed cartilage on hydroxypropylated dextran gel (64, 65). The proteolipid eluted in the void volume contained 80 percent of lipid and 20 percent of protein. It represented one-half of the total phospholipid by weight extracted from cartilage. The proteolipid induced apatite formation at low pH (7.2) *in vitro*, whereas the phospholipid eluted from the gel in later fractions did not, implying that the protein was essential for the activity at this pH.

Proteolipids that supported *in vitro* calcification were present in resting as well as in calcifying cartilage and thus they are components of chondrocyte plasma membranes before matrix vesicles are formed (65). The calcified zone of fetal calf epiphyseal cartilage contained tenfold the proteolipid of the reserve cell zone (66). The ratio of proteolipid to phospholipid is increased in calcifying areas and this ratio is reduced in rachitic animals. Furthermore proteolipid from rachitic animals fails to cause calcification *in vitro*. These findings suggest a role of the proteolipids in matrix vesicles formation. The proteolipids and the CaPLP complexes can be coisolated from calcifying tissue. However the precise relationship of the proteolipids to the complexes is unclear. One hypothesis is that the complexes are synthesized on the proteolipid surfaces and that this facilitates calcification.

Prostaglandins

There is increasing evidence that prostaglandins exert control over bone cell function and bone remodeling. The PGE_2 series plays a role in bone formation and resorption, and the PGI_2 series is active in regulating blood flow (69). Prostaglandins are synthesized and secreted locally in calcifying tissue (17). Using a matrix-induced endochondral bone formation system, Weintroub showed that various prostaglandin metabolites peaked at discrete stages in bone development, suggesting that specific cell types are associated with a unique assortment of prostaglandins (68). Studies of cultured fetal and young rat bones (70, 71) and adult human femur trabecular bone (72) have shown that PGE_2 causes resorption of calcium. PGE_2 was also shown to stimulate bone formation along the periosteum (71). The action of the prostaglandin is similar to that of parathormone and 1,2-dihydroxy vitamin D and appears to be mediated by an increase in the activity of the existing osteoclasts (70). At high concentrations the prostaglandins inhibit bone resorption.

The PGE_2 also stimulate the synthesis of collagen in embryonic chick bone cultures (69). Experiments were carried out in the presence of cortical hormones in order to inhibit the endogenous prostaglandins. Raisz postulated that the PGE_2s are involved in all aspects of bone remodeling including enhancing replication of the periosteal osteoblasts (69).

Evidence from *in vivo* studies corroborates the *in vitro* experiments. When high doses of PGE_2 were administered to weanling rats for 3 weeks, major bone changes were observed, including a narrowing of the growth plate, depression of longitudinal and radial bone growth rates, and increased metaphyseal hard tissue mass (71). This was associated with an increase in the calcified cartilage core and in the number of osteoclasts. In adult rats, similar doses of PGE_2 increased cortical endosteal bone formation of the tibial shaft. In view of the large doses required to produce them, the significance of these effects of the prostaglandins is difficult to assess.

Role of Inositol Phospholipids

Inositol was once believed to be a vitamin, but subsequently it was shown that its metabolic role involves the phospholipids of which it is a component (74). These are phosphatidylinositol (PI) and the polyphosphoinositols, namely phosphatidylinositol-4 phosphate and phosphatidylinositol-4,5-diphosphate, which contain a second and third phosphate at the 4 and 5 positions of the inositol molecule. Michel (75) showed that the phosphatidylinositides were associated with calcium mobilization by a mechanism that is initiated when a cell receptor is occupied, setting off the action of a phospholipase C functioning as a second messenger, which catalyzes the breakdown of the phosphatidylinositide. The products of the hydrolysis then cause the transport of calcium, which may move either into or out of the cell organelles (76). This appears to be an important mechanism for calcium transport but not the only one. The phosphatidylinositides are present in minute amounts in most cells. Even in the nervous system and adrenal medulla, where they occur in largest quantities, they account for only 6 percent of the total lipid phosphorus (74). The precise role of the inositol phospholipids in bone metabolism remains to be determined.

Role of Phosphatidylserine

The possibility that PS has a role similar to that of PI as second messenger in bone calcification has not been explored. There is some evidence, however, that PS acting as an ionophore mediates the translocation of calcium across the lipid barrier (76, 77). Tyson (78) showed *in vitro* that cardiolipin and phosphatidic acid were by far the most active ionophores in translocating calcium through a membrane. Lysophosphatidylethanolamine was next. Of the remaining phospholipids, phosphatidylserine was twice as active as phosphatidylethanolamine or phosphatidylinositol.

Glycolipid

Attention has been given to the glycolipids in calcifying tissues because of their relatively high content in cartilage. The glycolipids are important constituents of most cell membranes. Kensett showed that increasing the fat content of diets of dwarf and nondwarf chicks resulted in increased glycolipid concentrations in the epiphyseal cartilage with no significant changes in neutral lipids or phospholipids (79). To our knowledge, no other studies have investigated the effects of glycolipids on hard tissue mineralization.

Dietary Deficiencies and the Effects on Bone Development

Bone development is vulnerable to dietary deficiencies, as is the maturation of other organs and tissues. The important role of lipid in cell membranes suggests that more attention should be given to the dietary lipid and its influence on the function of all organs and tissues. The consequences of deficiencies of the fat-soluble vitamins on bone and tooth development are understood. In view of the known changes that occur in other tissues when fat intake is manipulated experimentally, it is possible that bone and tooth function may also be altered by modifying dietary fat.

Effects of Essential Fatty Acid Deficiency on Teeth and Bones

The major function of the EFA is to maintain normal membrane structure. A deficiency in the diet leads to alteration in the composition of membrane phospholipids, resulting in changes of their properties. This was observed by Prout in studies of the effects of an EFA deficiency on enamel and dentine in rats (6). He compared a stock rat diet to a high-sugar, fat-free diet with or without 1.5 percent of corn oil supplements. When corn oil was added to the deficient diet, the morphological and biochemical properties of the teeth were comparable to those of rats on the stock diet. In rats on the deficient diet, the teeth loosened, the gingival color was poor, and abnormal calculus was deposited. Histologically, the fiber bundle patterns were irregular and abnormally oriented, and there appeared to be a defective union between cementum and dentine. The alveolar bone of control rats showed osteoblastic activity and no osteoclasts, whereas in the deficient rats there were resorptive changes, increased vascularity, and signs of active remodeling.

Prout and co-workers also compared the organic matrix of the teeth of EFA-deficient rats with that of normal animals (6, 80). The total lipid, representing 0.35 percent of the dentine and 0.56 percent of the enamel, and the fraction of each lipid species, were the same in both diet groups. The fatty acid composition of individual lipids, however, representing about 50 percent of total lipids, was altered in the EFA-deficient animals. In general, the amounts of palmitic and linoleic acids in the phospholipids were lower, and those of stearic and oleic acids were higher. A unique fatty acid with gas liquid chromatography characteristics of docasahexanoic acid (22:6) represented 10–20 percent of the total fatty acids (80). A group of phospholipids isolated together, which included phosphatidylethanolamine, phosphatidic acid, and cardiolipin, was found to be abnormally low in the EFA-deficient rats.

The importance of linoleic acid in dentine development was further confirmed by radioactive studies showing the rapid uptake of this fatty acid into the phospholipids and particularly into the acidic phospholipids of dentine (81).

Dietary Modification of Membranes

Although studies comparable to those above on tooth structure have not been done on bone, the magnitude of the changes and the similarity of the two types of tissue suggest that EFA deficiency may have comparable effects.

The lipid composition of various membranes is not fixed but differs with their function and their required physical characteristics (80). Dietary manipulations are capable of altering several characteristics of membranes. Membranes become unstable if the average length of the fatty acid chains of phospholipids is reduced or the proportion of unsaturated fatty acids is increased. Changes due to diet are often compensated for, however, by secondary action of enzymes. For example, Neudorffer compared the muscle membrane lipids in turkeys fed beef fat with those fed anchovy oil (83). The animals on the oil diet had a large decrease in the oleic acid content of their membrane lipids and an increase in the PUFA. At the same time, the 1:1 ratio between unsaturated and saturated fatty acids remained the same in the two groups, presumably because of a secondary adaptation by tissue enzymes to protect the membranes from nonphysiological changes due to diet. The protective device may be brought about by the specificity of action of the phospholipid-synthesizing enzymes or by changes in the phospholipases.

Nutritionally induced changes in membranes may result from a number of factors yet to be investigated (84). Some of these are the changes in polar head groups of the phospholipids, the changes of the ratio of cholesterol to phospholipid in the membranes, hormonal changes, lipid–enzyme interactions, and the interrelationship of any of these factors. Since calcium is an activator, or essential cofactor for many of the enzymes involved in lipid metabolism such as the transacylase, the base-exchange enzyme, and several of the phospholipases, there could also be a relationship between tissue lipid content and the hormones involved in calcium homeostasis. The studies done to date have shown only that diet will effect a few measurable aspects of membranes, making the picture appear to be less complicated than it actually is.

In spite of the significant changes in membrane constituents in several tissues that the above studies describe, to date no deleterious effects on function or structure have been observed (82). Comparable studies have not been carried out on cell membranes in bone. In view of the importance of phospholipid in mineralization, such dietary manipulations might alter the function of chondrocytes, osteoblasts, and the osteocytes.

Potential Risks to Bone Development of Certain Diets

Although data are not available on the affects of bone development of changes in lipid consumption, the danger to bone function in deviating too far from normal nutritional intake is presumably the same as the danger to the function of other cells. Examples of nutritional intake that deviate sufficiently to affect tissue composition are given below.

Low-Fat and Fat-Free Intakes

A low fat intake is often recommended for body weight reduction and for gallbladder disease. If the fat intake is reduced to below 25 percent of the total calories, there is a risk of EFA deficiency. It is recommended that the subject receive at least 3 percent of total calories in the form of linoleic acid. Supplements of the fat-soluble vitamins must of course be taken.

The biological effects of eliminating fat from the diet, except for the amount required to supply the fat-soluble vitamins and the EFA, are not well defined. Substantial changes have been observed in tissues of experimental animals fed solely carbohydrate and protein as sources of energy. If adequate calories are provided, the body will convert the excess carbohydrate and some amino acid side chains to fat, and fat will continue to be the primary source of energy. But under these conditions the fat that the body is capable of synthesizing tends to contain predominantly saturated fatty acids, such as palmitic acid, and monosaturated fatty acids, such as palmitoleic and oleic acids, compared to the spectrum of fats present in tissues of animals on normal diets (85). Consequently the tissue must modify the endogenous fatty acids secondarily to produce the PUFA for the phospholipid and cholesterol esters of the new membrane (85). This strains the cells' synthetic capacity and limits the range of fatty acids that can be synthesized. When a low-fat diet is fed, care should be taken to supply enough EFA to assure a normal ratio of PUFA to saturated fatty acid (86). A low-fat diet may also alter the variety and amount of prostaglandins produced by the cells (22).

Intravenous Nutrition

The situation above, that is, the omission of fat from the diet, often occurs in patients on total parenteral nutrition (TPN). The intravenous route is frequently used in the surgical patient for all nutrients if the patient is unable to take oral feeding in the postoperative period for 5 or more days (8, 87, 88). The formula for surgical patients consists in solutions of glucose and amino acids, to satisfy energy and nitrogen requirements, and essential vitamins and minerals. In the past, the use of intravenous fat was often avoided, because the period of time on nullus per os was too short to introduce the danger of EFA deficiency, and because the administration of intravenous lipid was an extra hazard, an extra bother, and an added expense. With the recent advent of safe and easy-to-administer lipid emulsions that are free of side affects (87), intravenous lipids are now given more frequently, but probably still not often enough. Malnourished surgical patients seem to respond well to intravenous infusions that contain fat to satisfy 35–50 percent of the total nonprotein energy (88, 89, 90).

Lipid supplied to postoperative patients on TPN has a number of advantages (11, 88, 90, 91). It has a high caloric density, thus reducing the volume of fluid required. The infusion is isotonic, permitting it to be safely infused into peripheral veins. Finally, it prevents the excessive stimulus to secrete insulin that occurs when glucose is infused. Insulin promotes an anabolic mode in the peripheral tissues which is contraindicated when free glucose and amino acids are needed for tissue repair. Lipid and carbohydrate are equally efficient for energy, and both spare amino acid (88). It is possible, but has not yet been investigated, that an important advantage of lipid supplementation for post operative patients is the one pointed out above (85), and that is that it supplies a rich assortment of fatty acids for the manufacture of membranes. In surgical convalescence, where tissue repair is taking place, it may be prudent to supply an adequate mixture of lipids rather than rely on endogenous lipids for membrane repair.

Nonsurgical patients with a variety of gastrointestinal abnormalities have been maintained for long periods of time on TPN (89, 92). The most successful preparation of lipid used is Intralipid, a 10 or 20 percent soybean oil triglycerides emulsion containing small quantities of purified egg phospholipid as emulsifier and glycerol to make the solution isotonic (93). Soybean oil triglycerides contain 54 percent of linoleic acid, 26 percent of oleic acid, 8 percent of linolenic acid, 9 percent of palmitic acid, and 3 percent of stearic acid (94).

The solution containing amino acids, glucose, vitamins, and minerals, without the lipid, is regularly administered over an extended period of time during the day, whereas the lipid is given in a bolus, two or three times a week (95). Recent reports now indicate that it is safe to mix all of the nutrients in advance and administer them from a single container (96). Besides simplifying the feeding routine, there is evidence that lipid given continuously throughout the day with the rest of the ingredients in the parenteral feeding is preferable because it provides a sustained lipid source for the tissues (97). It might also be argued that efficient membrane synthesis can occur only if an optimal concentration of the lipid components is available during the manufacturing process, in analogy with the requirement of all of the amino acids for protein synthesis.

Long-term TPN must be carefully monitored. If the ingredients are chemically pure, there is a danger that some unknown nutrient that is normally present in trace amounts in food is absent. Some minerals and biochemical factors for which requirement has not been proved are added to the feedings in an attempt to avoid this type of deficiency (87, 89). Nevertheless, some studies have discovered possible dietary deficiencies in patients on long-term TPN. They have been found to require more EFA than subjects on oral intake (91, 98). Even when 2–3 percent of the total calories are in the form of linoleic acid in the Intralipid, and no clinical signs of a deficiency are apparent, patients still show low levels of linoleic acid in plasma and red cell membranes. A possible explanation for this finding is an imbalance or deficiency of fatty acid varieties in a diet in which there is only one lipid source.

Metabolic bone disease has been observed in long-term TPN (76, 98). The condition is characterized by abnormal calcium absorption, decreased bone mineralization, hypercalcuria without hypercalcemia, and an elevated plasma alkaline phosphatase level. Skeletal pain is a clinical feature. The levels of phosphate, parathyroid hormone, and 25-OH vitamin D remain within normal limits. The etiology is still in question. Some speculate that the high level of sulfur-containing amino acids in the nutrient solution induces calcium loss (99) or that vitamin D metabolites are altered (98, 100). The condition can be reversed by withholding vitamin D (99).

Diets Rich in Polyunsaturated Fatty Acids

Eskimos and other inhabitants of arctic countries live on diets of fish that are rich in PUFA (23, 24). These people are relatively free of many of the degenerative diseases that afflict citizens of warmer climates, for example, arteriosclerotic heart disease, cancer, and diabetes. Their plasma cholesterol is low. However, their plasma arachidonic acid level is lower than that of inhabitants of temperate climates. A low level of the ω6 series of fatty acids leads to a reduced level of prostaglandins 1 and 2. Although the level of the ω3 series of fatty acids is high, the fatty acid precursor, 20:5ω3, converts slowly to the product prostaglandin 3 series, with a resulting defect in the balance of prostaglandins and the well-known bleeding tendency of Eskimos (23, 24). It is of interest to note that Eskimos have an increased incidence of osteoporosis (101). Whether this is directly associated with their diet is not known.

Linoleic acid is toxic if taken in excessive quantities (7). Subjects receiving very high fat diets (i.e., 35% of the total calories or more) should see that not more than 10 percent of the total calories are in the form of EFA.

SUMMARY

The requirement for dietary lipids was first realized with the discovery of the fat-soluble vitamins and more recently with the recognition of the essential fatty acids. These cannot be synthesized *in vivo,* yet they and their derivatives are necessary components of cell membranes as well as precursors of the prostaglandins. A deficiency of the essential fatty acids in the diet results in a syndrome that affects most of the body tissues and organs. Not only are these fatty acids required to supply optimal components for the construction of the various classes of lipids, but they are also needed to assure a proper balance of the prostaglandins. The amounts and types of lipids in the diet have effects, sometimes subtle, sometimes major, on the composition and function of many of the organs and tissues.

Lipids are involved in several aspects of bone development. Phospholipids and cholesterol are essential components of bone and cartilage cell membranes. The matrix vesicles derived from the chondrocytes contain a high content of acidic phospholipids, which facilitate the trapping of calcium and aid in producing the ambience for mineralization. Specific proteolipids that appear to stimulate nucleation have been isolated from cartilage and bone matrix and from a number of other calcifying tissues. The prostaglandins in osteoid cells have been shown to modulate bone formation.

Incontrovertible evidence is mounting that lipids have a vital role in bone and tooth growth. Tooth development is compromised in animals on essential fatty acid-deficient diets. Prostaglandins, given to laboratory animals, cause changes in bone architecture. Patients on long-term total parenteral nutrition may develop osteomalacia which may in part be due to unbalanced intravenous fat intake.

Although few studies have shown effects of dietary manipulation on the lipids involved in bone and tooth growth, it is certain that dietary changes affect cell membranes in other tissues. Diets deficient in essential fatty acids, for example, modify the immune capacity of the white blood cells and change the physical characteristics of their membranes. In practice, and to assure normal bone and tooth development during illness, dietary fat should be considered in planning an intake for any ill infant, for any patient with gastrointestinal disease, and for patients who must be subjected to any artificial diet for extended periods of time.

REFERENCES

1. *Nutrition Education in US Medical Schools* (1985) Washington DC: National Academy Press.
2. *Recommended Dietary Allowances,* Ninth Edition (1980) Washington DC: NCR National Academy of Sciences.
3. Kuksis, A. (1970) Progr. in the Chem. of Fats and other Lipids 12:1.
4. Holman, R. T. (ed) (1986) Prog. Lipid Res. Vol. 25.
5. Burr, G. O., Burr, M. M. (1929) J. Biol. Chem. 82:345.
6. Prout, R. E. S., Tring, F. C. (1971) J. Periodont. Res. 6:182.
7. Krause, M. V., Mahan, L. K. (1984) *Food Nutrition and Diet Therapy,* 7th Edition. Philadelphia: WB Saunders.
8. Yamanaka, W. K., Clemans, G. W., Hutchinson, M. L. (1982) Progr. in Lipid Res. 19:187.
9. Crawford, M. A., Hassam, A. G., Stevens, P. A. (1982) Progr. in Lipid Res. 20:31.
10. Galli, C., Socini, A. (1983) In: Perkins, E. G. and Visek, W. J. (eds) *Dietary Fats in Health.* Champaign, Ill: Amer. Oil Chemists Soc., p. 278.
11. Kuhn, D. C., Crawford, M. (1986) Progr. in Lipid Res. 25:345.
12. Araya, J., Aguilera, A. M., Soto, C., Molina, R. (1985) Nutrition Res. 5:1065.
13. Walker, W. A., Watkins, J. B. (1985) *Nutrition in Pediatrics.* Boston: Little Brown.
14. Horrobin, D. F., Cunnane, S. C. (1982) Progr. in Lipid Res. 20:831.
15. McCarthy, M. C., Cottam, G. L., Turner, W. W. (1981) Amer. J. Surg. 142:747.
16. Bailey, J. M. (ed) (1984) *Prostaglandins, Leukotrienes and Lipoxins.* New York: Plenum.
17. Raisz, L. G., Martin, T. G. (1984) In: Peck, W. A. (ed) *Bone and Mineral Research,* Annual 2. Amsterdam: Elsevier, p. 286.
18. Fournier, N. C., Rahim, M. (1985) Biochemistry 24:2387.

19. Privett, O. S., Blank, M. L., Verdino, B. (1965) J. Nutr. 85:187.

20. Crawford, M. A., Stevens, P., Williams, G., Turner, R. W. D. (1982) Progr. in Lipid Res. 20:589.

21. Kramer, J. K. G., Farnworth, E. K., Thompson, B. K., Corner, A. H. (1982) Progr. in Lipid Res. 20:491.

22. Emken, E. A. (1984) Annual Rev. Nutr. 4:339.

23. Sinclair, H. M. (1982) Progr. in Lipid Res. 20:897.

24. Vahouny, G. V., Chen, I. S., Satchithanandam, S., Cassidy, M. M., Sheppard, A. J. (1984) In: Bailey, J. M. (ed) op cit, p. 393.

25. Perkins, E. G., Visek, W. J. (eds) (1983) *Dietary Fats in Health*. Champaign, Ill: Amer. Oil Chemists Soc.

26. Holman, R. T., Mahfouz, M. M., Lawson, L. D., Hill, E. G. (1983) In: Perkins, E. G., Visek, W. J. (eds) op cit, p. 320.

27. Kummerow, F. A. (1983) In: Perkins, E. G., Visek, W. J. (eds) op cit, p. 391.

28. Emken, E. A. (1983) In: Perkins, E. G., Visek, W. J. (eds) op cit, p. 302.

29. Ohlrogge, J. B., Gulley, R. M., Emken, E. A. (1982) Lipids 17:551.

30. Gottenbos, J. J. (1983) In: Perkins, E. G., Visek, W. J. (eds) op cit, p. 375.

31. Kummerow, F. A. (1982) Progr. in Lipid Res. 20:743.

32. Bibra, E. von (1884) Schweinfurt, Germany 1:114.

33. Irving, J. T. (1963) Arch. Oral Biol. 8:735.

34. Enlow, D. H., Conklin, J. L., Bang, S. (1964) Anat. Rec. 148:279.

35. Mankin, H. J. (1984) In: Cruess, R. L., Rennie, W. R. J. (eds) *Adult Orthopedics*, Vol. 1, New York: Churchill Livingstone, p. 163.

36. Wuthier, R. E. (1982) In: Anghileri, L. J., Tuffet-Anghileri, A. M. (eds) *The Role of Calcium in Biological Systems,* Vol. 1. Boca Raton: CRC Press, p. 41.

37. Dirksen, T. R. (1977) In: Snyder, F. (ed) *Lipid Metabolism in Mammals,* Vol. 2. New York: Plenum, p. 237.

38. Shapiro, I. M. (1971) Arch. Oral Biol. 16:411.

39. Shapiro, I. M. (1970) Calcif. Tiss. Res. 5:21.

40. Irving, J. T., Wuthier, R. E. (1968) Clin. Orthop. 56:237.

41. Irving, J. T. (1973) Clin. Orthop. 97:225.

42. Wuthier, R. E. (1968) J. Lipid Res. 9:68.

43. Boskey, A. L. (1981) In: Veis, A. (ed) *The Chemistry and Biology of Mineralized Connective Tissue,* Elsevier/N. Holland, p. 531.

44. Bonucci, E. (1969) J. Ultrastruct. Res. 20:33.

45. Anderson, H. C. (1969) J. Cell Biol. 41:59.

46. Anderson, H. C. (1986) Bone and Mineral Res. 3:109.

47. Glimcher, M. J. (1976) In: *Handbook of Physiology,* Endocrinology Section VII, Baltimore: Wilkins and Williams, p. 25.

48. Peress, N. S., Anderson, C., Sajdera, S. W. (1974) Calcif. Tiss. Res. 14:275.

49. Wuthier, R. E. (1982) Clin. Orthop. 169:219.

50. Ali, S. Y., Wisby, A., Evans, L., Craig-Gray, J. (1977) Calcif. Tiss. Res. 22S:490.

51. Anderson, H. C., Cecil, R., Sajdera, S. W. (1975) Amer. J. Path. 79:237.

52. Wuthier, R. E. (1975) Biochim. Biophys. Acta 409:128.

53. Wuthier, R. E., Gore, S. T. (1977) Calc. Tiss. Res. 24:163.

54. Wuthier, R. E. (1984) In: Sigel, H. (ed) *Metal Ions in Biological Systems,* Vol. 17, Calcium and its Roles in Biology, New York: M. Dekker, p. 412.

55. Majesta, R. J., Holwerda, D. L., Wuthier, R. E. (1979) Calcif. Tiss. Res. 27:41.

56. Wuthier, R. E., Wians, F. H., Jr., Giancola, M. S., Dragic, S. S. (1978) Biochemistry 17:1431.

57. Boskey, A. L., Posner, A. S. (1976) Calcif. Tiss. Res. 19:273.

58. Boskey, A. L., Goldberg, M. R., Posner, A. S. (1978) Proc. Soc. Exp. Biol. Med. 157:59.

59. Boskey, A. L. (1978) Metab. Bone Dis. 1:137.

60. Boskey, A. L., Posner, A. S. (1982) Calcif. Tiss. Int. 34:S1.

61. Anderson, H. C., Reynolds, J. J. (1973) Develop. Biol. 34:211.

62. Boskey, A. L., Timshak, P. L. (1983) Metab. Bone Dis. 5:81.

63. Boskey, A. L., DiCarlo, E. F., Gilder, H., Donnelly, R., Weintroub, B. (1988) Bone 9:309.

64. Ennever, J., Boyen-Salyers, B., Riggan, L. J. (1977) J. Dent. Res. 56:967.

65. Boyan-Salyers, B. D., Vogel, J., Riggan, L. J., Summer, F., Howell, R. (1978) Metabol. Bone Dis. 1:143.

66. Boyan, B. D., Ritter, N. M. (1984) Calc. Tiss. Res. 36:332.

67. Boyan-Salyers, B. D. (1981) In: Veis, A. (ed) op cit, p. 539.

68. Weintroub, S., Wahl, L. M., Feuerstein, N., Winter, C. C., Reddi, A. H. (1983) Biochem. Biophys. Res. Com. 117:746.

69. Raisz, L. G. (1984) Hormone Res. 20:22.

70. Holtrop, M. E., Raisz, L. G. (1979) Calc. Tiss. Res. 29:201.

71. Nefussi, J. R., Baron, R. (1984) Anat. Rec. 211:9.

72. Schartl, A., Keck, E., Kruskemper, H. L. (1985) In: Schror, K. (ed) *Prostaglandins and other Eicosanoids in the Cardiovascular System*. Basel: Karger, p. 548.

73. Ueno, K., Haba, T., Woodbury, D., Price, P., Anderson, R., Jee, W. S. S. (1985) Bone 6:79.

74. Hawthorne, J. N. (1985) Proc. Nutr. Soc. 44:167.

75. Michel, R. H. (1975) Biochim. Biophys. Acta 415:81.

76. Weiser, M. M. (1984) In: Solomons, N. W., Rosenberg, I. H. (eds) *Current Topics in Nutrition and Disease*. Vol. 12. Absorption and Malabsorption of Mineral Nutrients, New York: AK Liss, p. 15.

77. Yaari, A. M., Shapiro, I. M., Brown, C. E. (1982) Biochem. Biophys. Res. Comm. 105:778.

78. Tyson, C. A., Zande, H. V., Green, D. E. (1976) J. Biol. Chem. 251:1326.

79. Kensett, B. C., Ho, S. K., Touchburn, S. P. (1978) Internat. J. Vit. Nutr. Res. 48:84.

80. Odutuga, A. A., Prout, R. E. S. (1974) Arch. Oral Biol. 19:911.

81. Prout, R. E. S., Odutuga, A. A. (1974) Arch. Oral Biol. 19:1167.

82. Lee, A. G. (1985) Proc. Nutr. Soc. 44:147.

83. Neudoerffer, T. S., Lea, C. H. (1967) Brit. J. Nutr. 21:691.

84. Gurr, M. I. (1985) Proc. Nutr. Soc. 44:231.

85. Mattson, F. H. (1981) In: Perkins, E. G., Visek, W. J. (eds) op cit, p. 241.

86. Judd, J. T. (1982) Progr. Lipid Res. 20:571.

87. Wretland, A. (1981) Nutr. Rev. 39:257.

88. Jeejeebhoy, K. N. (1985) In: Deitel, M. (ed) *Nutrition in Clinical Surgery*, 2nd Edition, Baltimore: Williams and Wilkins, p. 121.

89. Silberman, H., Eisenberg, D. (1982) *Parenteral and Enteral Nutrition for the Hospitalized Patient*, Norwalk: Appleton–Century–Croft, Chap. 7, p. 182.

90. Gilder, H. (1986) J. Parent. Enter. Nutr. 10:88.

91. Howard, L., Michalek, A. V. (1984) Ann. Rev. Nutr. 4:69.

92. Jeejeebhoy, K. N., Anderson, G. H., Nakhooda, A. F., Greenberg, G. R., Sanderson, I., Marliss, E. B. (1976) J. Clin. Invest. 57:125.

93. Wretland, A. (1976) In: Meng, H. C., Wilmore, D. W. (eds) *Fat Emulsions in Parenteral Nutrition*. Chicago: AMA, p. 109.

94. Dowling, R. J., Alexander, M. A. J., Mullen, J. L. (1985) In: Deitel, M. (ed) op cit, p. 139.

95. Dudrick, S. J. (1983) In: Dudrick, S. J., Baue, A. E., Eiseman, B., Maclean, L. D., Rowe, M. I. (eds) *Manual of Preoperative and Postoperative Care*, Am. Coll. Surg. p. 86.

96. Jacobson, S., Christenson, I., Kager, L., Kallner, A., Ljungdahl, I. (1981) Amer. J. Clin. Nutr. 34:1402.

97. Abbott, W. C., Grakauskas, A. M., Bistrian, B. R., Rose, R., Blackburn, G. L. (1984) Arch. Surg. 119:1367.

98. Shike, M., Harrison, J. E., Sturtridge, W. C., Tam, C. S., Bobechko, P. E., Jones, G., Murray, T. M., Jeejeebhoy, K. N. (1980) Ann. Intern. Med. 92:343.

99. Klein, G. L., Ament, M. E., Bluestone, R., Norman, A. W., Targoff, C. M., Sherrard, D. J., Young, J. H., Coburn, J. W. (1980) Lancet II:1041.

100. Cole, D. E. L., Slotkin, S. H. (1983) Amer. J. Clin. Nutr. 37:108.

101. Thompson, D. D., Posner, A. S., Laughlin, W. S., Blumenthal, N. C. (1983) Calc. Tiss. Res. 35:392.

IV
TRACE ELEMENTS AND METABOLIC BONE DISEASE

13

Aluminum Metabolism and the Uremic Patient

WILLIAM G. GOODMAN

Knowledge about the metabolism and toxicity of aluminum has expanded considerably during the past 10 years. Before the mid-1970s, analytical methods for measurement of aluminum in biological samples were inadequate to detect microgram quantities of the metal, and the potential for interactions between aluminum and biological systems was unknown (1). This technical limitation precluded accurate studies of the tissue distribution and metabolism of aluminum in humans and experimental animals (1, 2).

With the development of more precise methods for quantitative aluminum determinations, several clinical and pathological conditions in man were described in which the content of aluminum in specific tissues was elevated. High levels of aluminum were detected in brain in hemodialysis patients dying from a clinically distinctive and rapidly progressive encephalopathy, and evidence of substantial aluminum deposition in bone was noted in dialysis patients with severe osteomalacia that was refractory to treatment with active vitamin D sterols (3–9). Subsequent investigations into the toxicity and metabolism of aluminum have provided considerable amounts of new information about the response of different tissues to aluminum deposition. These studies constitute a rapidly expanding literature on the biological effects of aluminum.

PHYSICAL AND CHEMICAL PROPERTIES OF ALUMINUM

Aluminum is the third most abundant element in the outer layer of the earth's crust (10). It accounts for approximately 8 percent of the weight of the crust, and it is the most common metal in this geological layer (10, 11). Aluminum is predominantly found in mineral form as silicates of aluminum, and these are a major component of many rocks and soils. Surface water generally contains low levels of aluminum, but the aluminum content of water samples from different geographic areas varies widely (10, 11).

The solubility of aluminum in aqueous solutions is strongly influenced by pH and by the respective concentrations of other ionic constituents, such as phos-

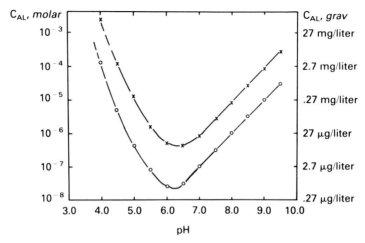

Fig. 13-1   Equilibrium solubility of microcrystalline Al (OH)$_3$ at 25°C. and 1 atm pressure (upper curve). Ionic strength = 0.0; total concentration of dissolved F = 10^{-8} molar. [Reprinted with permission from Hem (10).]

phorus, in solution (10, 11). In highly acid or highly alkaline conditions, aluminum is soluble in aqueous solutions (Fig. 13-1) (10). However, microcrystalline aluminum hydroxide, Al(OH)$_3$, precipitates from solution at pH levels within the physiologic range to form insoluble cationic polymers (10, 11). This property of aluminum presents methodologic difficulties for investigators using experimental procedures in which aluminum is added to aqueous solutions for administration to test subjects or for *in vitro* studies. The low solubility of aluminum in aqueous solutions must be appreciated and confirmation that experimental conditions actually conform to theoretical projections with regard to the concentration of aluminum in solutions should be obtained using precise analytical methods whenever possible (123).

METABOLISM OF ALUMINUM

Tissue Distribution

Although aluminum is present in large amounts in the immediate environment, the aluminum content of most tissues in normal man is quite low (1, 12, 13). The plasma concentration of aluminum is normally less than 10 μg/L, and a large percentage of aluminum is bound to plasma proteins, including albumin (1, 12, 14, 15). After single intravenous injections in dogs, plasma aluminum values are markedly elevated, and the initial volume of distribution of aluminum is approximately twice the blood volume, or 5 percent of total body weight (16). The subsequent clearance of aluminum from plasma is rapid, with a half-life of 276 ± 52 min, but renal excretion accounts for less than 50 percent of the total plasma clearance (16). This finding indicates that aluminum is readily transferred from plasma into other tissues (16).

The extent of aluminum binding by plasma proteins has not been established precisely. Estimates of the protein-bound fraction of plasma aluminum range from 80 percent to 95 percent (1, 16–21). Thus, only a small fraction of aluminum in plasma is in the non-protein-bound, diffusible state (21). Aluminum can bind specifically to high-affinity iron-binding sites on transferrin (22). Since most iron-binding loci on the transferrin molecule are normally unoccupied, transferrin represents a potential reservoir for aluminum in plasma (11). High-affinity metal-binding sites are also present on albumin, and these may further contribute to the protein binding of aluminum in plasma (11, 15). Although albumin contains a large number of metal-binding sites, the affinity of aluminum for the metal-binding sites on transferrin is considerably greater than that for albumin (124). Aluminum also has a higher affinity for transferrin than for citrate, the main organic substrate in plasma that forms soluble complexes with aluminum (123). Consequently, most aluminum in plasma ultimately becomes bound to transferrin (123). Internalization of transferrin-bound aluminum via the pathway normally utilized for the cellular uptake of iron through the transferrin receptor complex may be an important mechanism by which aluminum gains access to the intracellular compartment (125).

The aluminum content of most other tissues is 4 mg/kg dry weight or less (1, 12, 13). In the lung, higher values are found, and these increase with age (2). The inhalation of dust particles from the atmosphere that contain aluminum may account for this observation. Brain is the only other tissue in which an increase in aluminum content has been noted with age (23). Overall, the total body burden of aluminum in normal man is approximately 30–35 mg (1, 14).

In contrast to these findings in normal subjects, the aluminum content of several tissues is commonly elevated in patients with chronic renal failure (Fig. 13-2) (13). Bone, liver, and spleen exhibit the highest concentrations of aluminum, but increases in aluminum content also occur in brain, parathyroid gland, and possibly red cell (2, 3, 13, 24, 25). Studies of the distribution of aluminum in experimental animals given repeated injections of aluminum demonstrate a similar pattern of aluminum deposition in tissues. Although bone and liver represent the major sites of aluminum accumulation when renal function is either normal or reduced, the uremic state may affect the specific organ distribution of aluminum (26–28). Thus, aluminum levels are higher in bone but lower in liver in aluminum-treated uremic rats than in rats with normal renal function given equal amounts of aluminum by repeated parenteral injections (28, 29).

Available evidence indicates that aluminum loading in patients with chronic renal failure occurs by two predominant mechanisms: the gastrointestinal absorption of aluminum from aluminum-containing, phosphate-binding antacids that are given therapeutically in large quantities for the control of secondary hyperparathyroidism, and parenteral exposure to dialysis solutions that contain aluminum (see later) (1, 2, 14). In addition to exposure to aluminum from these sources, reductions in renal function contribute greatly to the tissue retention of aluminum in patients with chronic renal failure (1, 2, 14). The tissue levels of aluminum are generally higher in patients with chronic renal failure who are undergoing maintenance dialysis than in nondialyzed uremics (2, 13, 14). Such differences may reflect the severity and duration of uremia, the cumulative dose

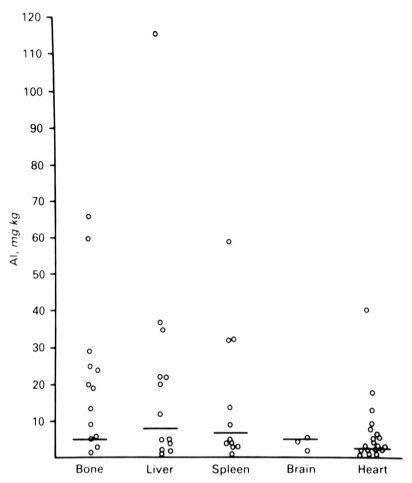

Fig. 13-2 Aluminum concentration in various tissues obtained from nondialyzed adult uremic patients. Horizontal lines represent the upper limits of normal for values determined in tissues obtained from nonuremic subjects. [Reprinted with permission from Alfrey (1).]

of orally ingested aluminum, or exposure to dialysate that contains aluminum (6, 36). The most substantial elevations in tissue aluminum content are found in the subgroup of patients with chronic renal failure in whom the highest prevalence of aluminum-related disease has been documented (3, 9, 14, 30–35).

The tissue content of aluminum is increased by several orders of magnitude in patients with clinical disorders associated with aluminum toxicity (3, 13, 32, 33, 35, 36). Bone aluminum levels often exceed 100 mg/kg dry weight of tissue (normal <5–7 mg/kg) in dialysis patients with histopathological evidence of aluminum-related bone disease (31–33). In patients with aluminum-related encephalopathy or dialysis dementia, the aluminum content of brain gray matter is 10–20 times greater than values determined in nonuremic subjects (3, 13, 35). Marked elevations in bone aluminum content are also found in patients with aluminum-related encephalopathy, which indicates that the high levels of aluminum in brain are part of a more generalized state of aluminum loading in such patients (4). Thus, aluminum-related bone disease and encephalopathy may be seen concurrently in individual patients (3, 6, 7). The total body aluminum content in dialyzed subjects with aluminum-related diseases is approximately 2–3 g (1, 2).

Intestinal Absorption

The gastrointestinal tract is a substantial but incomplete barrier to the absorption of aluminum from ingested foods and medications (1, 2, 42). Despite the general abundance of aluminum in the environment, the amount ingested daily is quite small. Reported values for dietary aluminum intake range from 3–5 mg/day to 30–35 mg/day (37–39).

Some balance studies have suggested that normal subjects absorb as much as several hundred milligrams of aluminum from an oral load of 1–3 g. Such doses are similar to those commonly used in patients with chronic renal failure (38, 40, 41). These results are inconsistent, however, with data that indicate that the total body burden of aluminum is only 2–3 g in uremic patients with aluminum-related disease who have ingested large amounts of aluminum-containing antacids for many years (1, 2, 13). Other studies, in subjects with normal renal function, indicate that aluminum balance remains close to zero when the daily oral intake of aluminum is several hundred milligrams (39). The precision of measurement of the aluminum content of biological samples is probably insufficient to accurately determine its fractional absorption by the gut using balance techniques, and no stable isotopes of aluminum are currently available for radioisotope tracer studies of aluminum transport by the gastrointestinal tract. Thus, the capacity of the gut to absorb aluminum remains to be established.

Approximately 15–55 µg of aluminum is excreted in the urine each day in subjects with normal renal function ingesting normal amounts of aluminum in the diet, and the biliary excretion of aluminum is negligible even following large parenteral aluminum loads (1, 20, 38–40). Because the aluminum content of most tissues does not increase with age, the total body balance of aluminum probably remains close to zero during life in normal man (2). Since renal clearance is the primary route of aluminum elimination from the body, the low daily rate of aluminum excretion in the urine suggests that the amount of aluminum entering the body each day is small (16–18, 40–42). On the basis of these observations, it is likely that the fractional absorption of ingested aluminum by the gut is less than 1 percent (1, 42). In normal subjects the urinary excretion of aluminum appears to be a reasonable indicator of the total amount of aluminum absorbed by the gastrointestinal tract (1, 39, 42).

The absorption of even small fractions of ingested aluminum may have very important physiologic consequences for subjects with impaired renal function (1, 2, 14). This mode of aluminum entry is particularly relevant because such patients ingest large doses of aluminum-containing medications (43, 44). Consider, first, that the serum levels of aluminum and the urinary excretion of aluminum both increase after large oral aluminum loads (37–41). Second, serum aluminum levels have been correlated with oral aluminum intake in several studies of uremic patients undergoing chronic dialysis (45–47). These findings indicate that ingested aluminum can enter the plasma and that this source represents a potential route of aluminum uptake into tissues in patients with persistently high levels of oral aluminum intake.

The mechanism of aluminum transport by the intestine is not well understood. The solubility of aluminum in aqueous solutions, the pH of luminal fluid in various segments of the intestine, and the interaction of aluminum with other constituents in gut luminal fluid such as fluoride, citrate, or carbonate are physical–chemical factors that may modify the intestinal absorption of aluminum (1, 48). Theoretically, the pH conditions in the stomach and duodenum would favor aluminum transport in these two segments, (48). Recent preliminary data suggest that alterations in gastric pH may affect intestinal aluminum absorption in man (126), and citrate has been documented to markedly enhance intestinal aluminum transport (127, 128). Thus, the ingestion of aluminum-containing compounds in conjunction with citrate can markedly enhance aluminum absorption by the gut, and this can contribute to marked increases in aluminum retention in tissues in patients with renal insufficiency (129). Intestinal aluminum absorption may also be enhanced by uremia (130).

In short-term studies in man, the urinary excretion of aluminum increases as a function of increasing amounts of orally ingested aluminum (38–41). These limited data are consistent with a diffusional, load-dependent mechanism for intestinal aluminum transport. However, in studies of vitamin D-deficient and vitamin D-replete rats, both a saturable and a nonsaturable component of duodenal aluminum transport have been described using the everted gut sac technique (49, 50). The presence of aluminum in luminal perfusate decreased the saturable component of calcium absorption in these studies (50). It has been suggested, therefore, that aluminum may compete with calcium for vitamin D-dependent transport in the intestine.

In separate studies, it has been noted that aluminum makes vitamin-D a less effective stimulator of intestinal calcium transport. The intestinal absorption of calcium was blunted during the administration of 1,25-dihydroxvitamin D in vitamin D-deficient chicks that had been pretreated with aluminum for 5 days (51). The increment in intestinal calcium-binding protein during treatment with vitamin D analogs was also reduced in aluminum-loaded animals (51). These observations suggest that aluminum impairs the function of vitamin D-dependent transport mechanisms in the intestine. Such changes could not only modify the transport of aluminum and calcium but they may also affect the intestinal absorption of other ions.

Iron transport mechanisms in the gut may be involved in the transepithelial movement of aluminum, and the absorption of ingested aluminum appears to increase under clinical conditions of iron deficiency (48, 52). Theoretically, age-related differences in the intestinal transport of aluminum could contribute to the development of aluminum-associated bone disease in pediatric patients with renal failure (48); other metals, such as lead, are absorbed by the intestine to a greater extent in children than in adults. However, differences in intestinal aluminum transport with age have not been documented (53). It is more likely that the development of aluminum-related bone disease in children undergoing chronic dialysis reflects the higher doses of aluminum-containing antacids per unit body weight in such patients (43, 46).

Renal Excretion

The urinary excretion of aluminum is approximately 15–55 μg/day in normal man (1, 38, 39). As noted previously, available evidence indicates that excretion by the kidneys is the major route for the elimination of aluminum from the body (1, 2, 42). In studies of dogs with normal renal function given aluminum parenterally during hemodialysis with aluminum-containing dialysate, 48 percent of the administered load of aluminum was excreted in the urine within 8 h, and virtually no biliary excretion of aluminum was documented (20). In contrast, there are data from studies in humans which indicate that some aluminum is excreted in the bile (131). Kaehney et al. reported that the renal clearance of aluminum was 5.5 ml/min during oral aluminum loading in normal human subjects, and most reported values for the renal clearance of aluminum are 10 percent or less of the glomerular filtration rate (16, 18, 54, 55).

The renal clearance of aluminum is usually insufficient to remove the daily load of aluminum during ongoing parenteral aluminum administration (1, 2, 16, 42). Aluminum balance remained positive in dogs with normal renal function given daily intravenous injections of aluminum for several weeks, and the renal contribution to the clearance of aluminum from plasma was less than 50 percent (16). Similar findings have been reported in patients with normal renal function who inadvertently received total parenteral nutrition with solutions contaminated with aluminum (18, 56). In these studies, less than one-half of the daily load of 2.0–3.5 mg of aluminum was excreted in the urine, and the renal clearance of aluminum was approximately 10 ml/min (56). Such clinical and experimental findings regarding the plasma and renal clearances of aluminum are primarily attributable to the high degree of protein and tissue binding of aluminum and to the small fraction of ultrafiltrable aluminum in plasma available for glomerular filtration. The renal tubule may also reabsorb a portion of the filtered load of aluminum (57). Thus, normal renal excretory function does not preclude aluminum accumulation in tissues during the administration of aluminum, and net aluminum balance remains positive in patients and in experimental animals with normal renal function during periods of sustained aluminum loading.

Experimental studies indicate that the amount of aluminum retained in tissues is higher in rats with impaired renal function than in animals with normal renal function given equal amounts of aluminum parenterally (28, 29). These data further support the contention that the rate of renal aluminum excretion is an important determinant of aluminum accumulation in tissues.

In the absence of ongoing aluminum loading, aluminum excretion in the urine continues at increased rates in patients with adequate renal function who have previously accumulated aluminum in tissues. Urinary aluminum levels increase following renal transplantation in patients who have been treated in the past by maintenance dialysis, and these values remain elevated for months thereafter (59). Also, after the removal of aluminum from total parenteral nutrition solutions, high levels of urinary aluminum excretion were documented in patients with aluminum-related bone disease, and several years were required for bone aluminum levels to fall substantially (18, 58). Such observations indicate that aluminum is mobilized from tissues at relatively low rates even when renal function is well maintained, and they suggest that the total capacity of the kidney to excrete aluminum is rather limited (1, 14, 42).

Hormonal Factors

The results of several investigations suggest that calcium-regulating hormones are involved in the metabolism of aluminum. Serum aluminum levels have been reported to increase during treatment with active vitamin D sterols in rats fed diets supplemented with aluminum (60). It is unclear, however, whether this finding is due to vitamin D-mediated increases in the intestinal absorption of aluminum or to alterations in the tissue distribution of aluminum.

Mayor et al. reported that exogenously administered parathyroid hormone (PTH) enhanced the intestinal transport and total body retention of aluminum in rats (26). The importance of this observation has been questioned on the basis of results that fail to document a positive relationship between the serum levels of immunoreactive PTH (iPTH) and the bone aluminum content in chronic dialysis patients (61). Current evidence indicates that serum iPTH values are actually lower in hemodialysis patients with evidence of aluminum deposition in bone than in others undergoing maintenance dialysis, and increases in the rate of accumulation of aluminum in bone have been demonstrated after parathyroidectomy in patients undergoing long-term hemodialysis (31, 32, 62–64, 132).

Although the results of several clinical studies suggest that low rather than high levels of PTH in serum contribute to the pathogenesis of aluminum-related disease, it is possible that high rates of PTH secretion enhance the uptake of aluminum into bone during periods of active bone formation and turnover (65). Skeletal turnover is increased in secondary hyperparathyroidism, and this disorder commonly develops during the course of progressive renal insufficiency (66). Additional investigations are required, therefore, to fully evaluate the respective roles of PTH and of PTH-induced changes in the metabolism of vitamin D as potential modifiers of both the intestinal absorption and the tissue toxicity of aluminum.

SOURCES OF ALUMINUM IN UREMIC PATIENTS

The documentation of aluminum retention in tissues and the description of the clinical manifestations of aluminum-related disease were initially reported in studies of patients undergoing maintenance hemodialysis (3–8). Case clusters, or "epidemics," of dialysis encephalopathy and of osteomalacia resistant to treatment with analogs of vitamin D were related to parenteral aluminum loading via contaminated dialysate in certain dialysis units and within specific geographical areas where the concentration of aluminum in water supplies was high (4–8).

It is common practice to add alum, or aluminum sulfate, to municipal water supplies for the purpose of removing particulate matter, and the concentration of aluminum in water may reach several hundred micrograms per liter as a result of this process (67, 68). Although the ingestion of water containing high aluminum levels is of little consequence in man owing to the low rate of intestinal absorption of aluminum, dialysis patients are routinely exposed to 90–180 L or more of water as dialysate during conventional hemodialysis treatments. The use of water containing high concentrations of aluminum in the preparation of dialysis solutions can, therefore, result in the administration of large parenteral loads of aluminum (4–8, 69, 70). Before the widespread availability of reverse osmosis for water purification and adequate removal of aluminum in the manufacture of hemodialysis solutions, this mode of aluminum loading was not uncommon (4–8). The absence of adequate renal excretory function in dialysis patients assures that virtually all aluminum that enters the plasma from dialysate will be retained.

Because of the extensive protein binding of aluminum in plasma, dialysate aluminum levels that exceed 10 μg/L result in positive aluminum balances during individual hemodialysis treatments, and dialysate aluminum levels greater than 50 μg/L have been associated with a high incidence of aluminum-related bone disease (1, 14, 70). Conversely, the net removal of aluminum during routine hemodialysis sessions is quite limited because of the small fraction of non-protein-bound, ultrafilterable aluminum in plasma water available for transfer across dialysis membranes (19, 21, 67). Even under optimal treatment conditions in which the aluminum concentration in dialysate is low (i.e., less than 10 μg/L), the amount of aluminum removed during conventional hemodialysis procedures does not exceed 1–2 mg (71). Available data indicate that net aluminum removal during dialysis is largely dependent on the concentration of aluminum in plasma (19, 21, 71, 138). Thus, hemodialysis alone is not an effective therapeutic approach to remove aluminum in patients with evidence of extensive tissue aluminum accumulations.

Peritoneal dialysis fluid can also serve as a source of aluminum loading in patients undergoing chronic dialysis. High levels of aluminum in serum were documented in patients using dialysis solutions that contained 23–54 μmol/L of aluminum for continuous ambulatory peritoneal dialysis (CAPD); serum aluminum levels fell rapidly after aluminum was removed from the solutions (72). Aluminum levels in most commercially available peritoneal dialysis solutions are generally low however, and this source does not currently represent a major route of aluminum loading in patients undergoing CAPD (14).

The transport of aluminum across the peritoneal membrane is influenced by the same factors that limit the net removal of aluminum during hemodialysis, although the presence of small amounts of protein in peritoneal dialysis effluent may slightly enhance aluminum removal (73). Current evidence indicates that the total amount of aluminum removed over a 24-h period during CAPD is similar to or slightly greater than that observed during a single hemodialysis procedure (73, 139).

Aluminum-containing, phosphate-binding antacids currently represent the major source of aluminum exposure in the dialysis population. Prevention of hyperphosphatemia is a major therapeutic objective in the management of secondary hyperparathyroidism (75), and phosphate-binding agents are used extensively for the control of serum phosphorus levels in patients with renal insufficiency both during the period of progressive renal failure prior to the initiation of dialysis and after the institution of maintenance dialysis (43–45, 74).

Aluminum-related bone disease can develop in patients undergoing long-term dialysis despite the regular use of high quality dialysate containing aluminum levels that are not associated with positive aluminum balances (9, 30–32). The aluminum content of bone and other tissues is substantially increased in such patients (9, 30–33). Aluminum absorption from antacid preparations represents the probable source of aluminum loading under these clinical conditions, and the results of several studies indicate that the serum levels of aluminum correspond to the dose of orally ingested aluminum (45–47). Because of the introduction of adequate procedures for the removal of aluminum from water used to prepare dialysis solutions, aluminum loading via the gastrointestinal tract currently accounts for the majority of cases of aluminum-related bone disease in patients undergoing this treatment. Available data indicate that the prevalence of aluminum-related bone disease in the general dialysis population is approximately 25–30 percent (30, 76).

BONE DISEASE AND ALUMINUM

Aluminum accumulation in tissues has been implicated in the pathogenesis of encephalopathy, microcytic anemia, and certain histologic lesions of renal osteodystrophy in patients undergoing long-term dialysis (4, 9, 25, 30–35). High levels of aluminum in bone have also been associated with the development of metabolic bone disease in adults with normal renal function inadvertently given solutions containing aluminum during total parenteral nutrition (18, 58). This last observation indicates that aluminum may have specific adverse effects on the metabolism of bone even in nonuremic patients who have sequestered aluminum in tissues.

The present discussion addresses the relationship between aluminum deposition in bone and the pathogenesis of several histologic subtypes of renal osteodystrophy. A substantial body of evidence indicates that aluminum can alter the formation and mineralization of bone both in man and in experimental animals (9, 29–32, 77–79, 81–83). Whether the accumulation of aluminum in bone is the proximate cause of certain skeletal lesions in patients with chronic renal failure and high levels of aluminum in bone remains the subject of considerable controversy (14, 80, 84).

Classification of Renal Osteodystrophy

Renal osteodystrophy occurs in most patients with chronic renal failure, but several quite different histopathological lesions of bone are seen (66, 85). The five major subtypes of renal osteodystrophy and the bone biopsy features of each are presented in Table 13-1 (66, 133). Based on available data, two pathogenic processes account for the development and progression of renal osteodystrophy in

Table 13-1 Histopathologic Classification of Renal Osteodystrophy

	Osteitis fibrosa	Mild lesion	Osteomalacia	Adynamic lesion (aplastic bone)	Mixed renal osteodystrophy
Osteoid volume	Normal or moderately increased	Normal	Increased	Normal or decreased	Increased
Osteoid seam width	Normal	Normal	Increased	Normal or decreased	Increased
Osteoid surface	Normal or moderately increased	Normal or moderately increased	Increased	Normal or decreased	Increased
Resorption surface	Increased, often extensive	Moderately increased	Normal or decreased	Normal or decreased	Increased
Fibrosis	Present, often extensive	Absent or minimal	Absent	Absent	Present, often extensive
Bone formation rate	Markedly increased	Increased	Decreased, may be unmeasurable	Decreased, may be unmeasurable	Decreased
Serum iPTH	Markedly increased	Moderately elevated	Low, normal, or moderately increased	Low, normal, or moderately increased	Increased
Bone aluminum content (mg/kg)	Often normal[a], may be high	Often normal[a], may be high	High	High	Normal[a] or high
Histochemical stain for aluminum (% of trabecular bone surface)	<30%	<30%	>50%	>30%	Variable

[a]For uremic patients, normal values are higher than for nonuremic subjects.

most patients with renal failure. These are secondary hyperparathyroidssm and aluminum accumulation in bone (30, 66).

Hyperparathyroid Bone Disease and High Turnover States

Osteitis fibrosa is the most common skeletal lesion in patients with chronic renal failure (30, 66, 85, 133). In this disorder, there is histologic evidence of active bone resorption and tissue fibrosis, and the severity of the histological findings on bone biopsy generally corresponds to the serum level of iPTH (66). Bone formation is increased when measured using the technique of double tetracycline labeling (30, 85). Both the volume of osteoid and the width of osteoid seams are usually normal; thus, there is no histologic evidence of defective mineralization. Moderate increases in the volume of osteoid may be seen in osteitis fibrosa, but this finding is predominantly due to increases in the extent of trabecular bone surface covered by osteoid. Such changes are commonly observed when bone formation and turnover are increased (66).

The mild lesion of renal osteodystrophy represents the initial skeletal response to secondary hyperparathyroidism in uremic subjects, and it can progress to overt osteitis fibrosa if serum PTH levels increase further (66, 85). It most often occurs early in the clinical course of patients with end-stage renal disease, but the disorder is also seen in dialysis patients in whom secondary hyperparathyroidism has been moderately well controlled. The predominant histologic features in bone are moderate increases in resorption surface and in the percentage of trabecular bone surface covered with osteoid (30, 66). Fibrotic changes are minimal or absent. Bone formation may be normal, but values are frequently moderately elevated (30, 66). The volume of osteoid and the width of osteoid seams are within the normal range.

In dialysis patients with osteitis fibrosa and the mild lesion of renal osteodystrophy, evidence of marked aluminum accumulation in bone is uncommon (Fig. 13-3) (9, 14, 30, 66). When deposits of aluminum are present as judged by histochemical methods, they are generally less extensive in these two disorders than in either osteomalacia or the aplastic lesion of renal osteodystrophy (14, 30, 66, 133).

Aluminum-Related Bone Disease and Low Turnover States

In contrast to the findings in hyperparathyroid bone disease, the aluminum content of bone is usually substantially elevated in dialysis patients with osteomalacia and the aplastic lesion of renal osteodystrophy (Fig. 13-3) (9, 30, 66, 133).

In osteomalacia, the volume of unmineralized bone matrix is increased, and osteoid seams are widened; both histologic changes may be quite extensive (9, 30, 66). Bone formation is markedly reduced, and it is frequently unmeasurable (9, 16, 30, 66, 133). The mineralization lag time is prolonged in renal osteomalacia, which indicates that the calcification of newly formed osteoid is delayed. There is little histologic evidence of either active bone resorption or active bone formation, and both the number of osteoblasts and the number of osteoclasts are diminished. Fibrotic changes in bone are distinctly absent (30, 66, 85).

The histologic appearance of bone in the aplastic, or adynamic, lesion of renal osteodystrophy differs substantially from that of renal osteomalacia in several re-

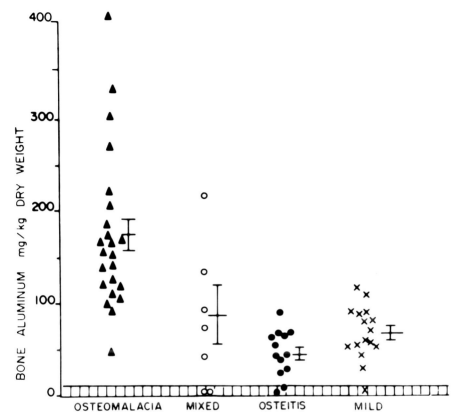

Fig. 13-3 Bone aluminum content for individual dialysis patients classified according to histologic subtype of renal osteodystrophy. Brackets indicate mean values ± SE for patients with each histologic lesion. Normal values for bone aluminum content are indicated by the area depicted by the vertical lines. [Reprinted with permission from Hodsman et al. (31).]

spects (30, 66, 86). Measurements of osteoid volume and osteoid seam width are often within the normal range, but both values may actually be reduced (66, 86). These features contrast with the marked increases in osteoid volume and osteoid seam width that characterize osteomalacia. However, similar to the findings in osteomalacia, bone formation is diminished in patients with the aplastic lesion of renal osteodystrophy, and there is a paucity of osteoblasts and osteoclasts in bone (30, 66, 86). The hypocellular changes in aplastic bone parallel those noted in renal osteomalacia.

Other than reductions in the numbers of cells, the aplastic lesion of bone cannot easily be distinguished by light microscopy from mild renal osteodystrophy using conventional histomophometric criteria. Bone formation is reduced, however, in the aplastic lesion, whereas it is normal or increased in the mild lesion of renal osteodystrophy (14, 66). Measurements of bone formation using double tetracycline labeling are important, therefore, for the histopathological diagnosis of aplastic bone, and they serve to differentiate this disorder from the mild lesion of renal osteodystrophy (14, 66, 133).

Mixed Lesion of Renal Osteodystrophy

In the mixed lesion of renal osteodystrophy, there is histologic evidence of both excess parathyroid hormone secretion and defective mineralization (66, 85). Bone resorption surfaces are increased, and the degree of tissue fibrosis can equal that observed in overt osteitis fibrosa. Such changes are consistent with the high serum levels of PTH reported in this disorder (85). However, bone formation is frequently diminished in the mixed lesion, and this feature differs substantially from the findings in patients with osteitis fibrosa (66, 85). Increases in the volume of osteoid and in the width of osteoid seams are also prominent. Thus, in addition to skeletal changes attributable to high serum levels of PTH, there is histological evidence of impaired mineralization (66, 85).

Aluminum levels in bone vary widely in patients with the mixed lesion of renal osteodystrophy (Fig. 13-3). Some patients have extensive skeletal aluminum accumulation, whereas others have minimal evidence of aluminum deposition in bone (9, 66).

Pathological Significance of Aluminum Deposition in Bone in Renal Osteodystrophy

The results of epidemiologic and histologic studies of bone disease in chronic dialysis patients and the data from evaluations of the response to treatment using active vitamin D sterols in patients with renal osteodystrophy initially suggested that aluminum was pathogenic for certain histologic subtypes of renal osteodystrophy (4–9, 30, 87–90). A severe form of fracturing osteomalacia was reported in dialyzed patients from localized geographic areas, particularly in England, where the prevalence of dialysis encephalopathy was also high (4–8, 87, 88). Subsequent investigations documented that tissue aluminum levels were markedly elevated in specimens of brain and bone from such patients, and aluminum-contaminated dialysate was identified as the source of aluminum loading (4–8). Adequate water treatment and effective aluminum removal from dialysate solutions reduced the incidence of both dialysis encephalopathy and the osteomalacic form of renal osteodystrophy in several dialysis centers (134).

In addition, osteomalacia in patients undergoing long-term dialysis was frequently noted to be unresponsive to treatment with various vitamin D sterols, including 1 α-hydroxyvitamin D and 1,25-dihydroxyvitamin D (9, 89, 90). The etiology of the mineralization defect in such patients was unknown, and several possibilities were considered but later rejected; these included phosphorus depletion, fluoride intoxication, and defective renal production of 24,25-dihydroxyvitamin D (91–93). However, systematic evaluations of patients with renal osteodystrophy who did not exhibit clinical and bone biopsy improvement during calcitriol therapy revealed that many such patients had evidence of aluminum deposition in bone (9). Importantly, the predominant histologic lesion in such "treatment failures" was osteomalacia (9).

Cross-sectional studies of large groups of dialysis patients with renal osteodystrophy have confirmed that the aluminum content of bone is higher in patients with osteomalacia and aplastic bone than in other forms of renal osteodystrophy

(9, 30–33, 135). Measurements of the bone aluminum content by flameless atomic absorption spectroscopy frequently exceed 100 mg/kg of dry tissue, and histochemical staining of biopsy specimens demonstrates extensive deposits of aluminum along the surface of bone (9, 33, 136). These are most prominent at the junction between mineralized bone and osteoid seams. Deposits of aluminum may also be seen within cement lines and long neutral or inactive bone surfaces (9, 30, 33).

Several observations suggest that aluminum is pathogenic for both osteomalacia and aplastic bone. Bone formation is markedly reduced in both lesions, and the degree of impairment in bone formation corresponds to the extent of aluminum deposition in bone (9, 30–32, 66). Some patients with the aplastic lesion of bone will progress and develop overt histologic osteomalacia as documented by bone biopsy (14, 66). Thus, aplastic bone may represent an early histologic phase of aluminum-related bone disease that can evolve into osteomalacia (14, 77, 78).

In contrast to these findings, the aluminum content of bone is only moderately elevated in most dialysis patients with osteitis fibrosa and mild renal osteodystrophy (9, 30–33, 66, 133). Aluminum levels in bone often reach 30–50 μg/kg dry weight of tissue, but higher values for bone aluminum content are less frequently encountered (14, 33). When histochemical methods are used to determine the aluminum content of bone, both the extent and intensity of histochemical staining for aluminum at the surface of bone are minimal to moderate (9, 33, 66). The proportion of trabecular bone surfaces that stain positive for aluminum is usually less than 30 percent (133).

Some patients with the mixed lesion of renal osteodystrophy also exhibit deposits of aluminum in bone, and the presence of aluminum at bone-forming surfaces may contribute to defective mineralization in certain cases (66). In other patients, hypocalcemia and/or hypophosphatemia are present (66, 85). Hypocalcemia may result in further increases in serum PTH levels, and low serum levels of both calcium and phosphorus can contribute to defects in the mineralization of newly formed bone.

The mixed lesion of renal osteodystrophy can represent a state of transition from secondary hyperparathyroidism to aluminum-related bone disease or vice versa in some patients with renal osteodystrophy (14, 66). Occasional patients with bone biopsy evidence of osteitis fibrosa subsequently develop histologic changes of osteomalacia with concurrent evidence of increasing aluminum deposition in bone (14, 66). Tissue fibrosis may persist in such cases, but it is less extensive and qualitatively less well organized than in overt osteitis fibrosa. Bone formation is often reduced in such cases, and measurements of bone formation decrease substantially in the interval between bone biopsy evaluations. Conversely, patients with osteomalacia or the aplastic lesion of renal osteodystrophy may develop tissue fibrosis during the course of treatment for aluminum-related bone disease with the chelating agent deferoxamine (14, 66). Increases in bone formation and in the serum levels of iPTH accompany these histologic changes (94, 95, 136). Moreover, the extent of aluminum deposition at the surface of bone decreases after treatment with deferoxamine, although the total aluminum content of bone as measured by chemical methods may not change substantially (14, 93, 136). These observations suggest that the deposition of aluminum along the surface of bone is an important determinant of the skeletal response to aluminum accumulation (137).

Although the observations from clinical studies strongly suggest that aluminum contributes to the development of certain histologic lesions of renal osteodystrophy, the data fail to establish a pathogenic role for aluminum in the evolution of bone disease. Subsequent *in vivo* and *in vitro* investigations have addressed two major issues with regard to the actions of aluminum on bone: the effects of aluminum on the mineralization process, and the role of aluminum deposition in bone as a modifier of collagen production and bone formation.

ALUMINUM AND THE MINERALIZATION OF BONE

The mechanism by which osteomalacia develops in conjunction with evidence of aluminum deposition in bone remains uncertain. When evaluated using histochemical methods, deposits of aluminum are prominent at the junction between osteoid seams and mineralized bone in dialysis patients with biopsy-proven osteomalacia but not in those with osteitis fibrosis (9, 30–33). This localized accumulation of aluminum within the mineralization front has been confirmed using electron microprobe techniques (96). Moreover, the extent of aluminum deposition at the surface of bone correlates with the severity of osteoid accumulation not only in dialysis patients with histologic osteomalacia but also in experimental animals given repeated parenteral injections of aluminum (31, 93). These observations suggest that aluminum deposited within the mineralization front of bone may act as a physical–chemical inhibitor of skeletal calcification.

Observations regarding the uptake of tetracycline into bone are also consistent with an adverse effect of aluminum on the mineralization of osteoid. The tetracyclines are deposited in bone at sites of active mineralization along developing osteoid seams (97, 98). In several conditions characterized by impaired mineralization, such as vitamin D-deficient osteomalacia, the uptake of tetracycline into bone is diminished (98, 99). This disturbance may be attributable to low serum levels of calcium and/or phosphorus in vitamin D deficiency, but reductions in tetracycline deposition in bone are viewed by most workers as a qualitative marker of defective calcification (98–101). Reductions in the uptake of tetracycline are a consistent finding in dialysis patients with osteomalacia and evidence of aluminum deposition in bone (9, 30–33, 102). These observations are of particular interest, however, because the serum levels of calcium and phosphorus are usually normal or increased in aluminum-related osteomalacia (14, 62). Similar reductions in tetracycline uptake have been noted in studies of experimental animals given aluminum parenterally (28, 29, 81–83).

The pattern of tetracycline uptake along osteoid seams is often discontinuous in specimens of bone in which there is substantial aluminum deposition (33, 102). At osteoid surfaces where aluminum has accumulated, there is frequently no evidence of tetracycline uptake (33, 102). In contrast, tetracycline labels are identified along bone-forming surfaces that exhibit no histochemical evidence of aluminum deposition (33, 102). Thus, aluminum may disrupt the process of mineralization within the developing osteoid seam, and this impairment in mineralization may contribute to the accumulation of osteoid and to the development of histologic changes of osteomalacia.

Despite substantial indirect evidence, confirmation that aluminum was actually responsible for a defect in the mineralization of bone could not be obtained from studies of clinical bone biopsy material. Subsequent studies in rats and dogs demonstrated that the administration of aluminum by repeated parenteral injections over several weeks induced skeletal lesions of osteomalacia in animals with previously normal bone (28, 29, 81–83). The presence of renal insufficiency enhanced the adverse effect of aluminum on skeletal mineralization in several experiments, and this difference was attributed to more extensive aluminum retention in bone during aluminum loading in animals with impaired renal function (29, 82). The histologic severity of osteoid accumulation in aluminum-loaded dogs was also correlated with the bone aluminum content, and these findings are similar to those noted in patients with aluminum-related osteomalacia. (9, 16, 31). Moreover, in rats given repeated daily injections of aluminum for up to 15 weeks, Ellis et al. reported that bone formed during the administration of aluminum was inadequately mineralized as judged by qualitative histologic criteria (81); the localized defect in skeletal mineralization persisted after the injections of aluminum were stopped (81).

High concentrations of aluminum in tissue culture media reduce the incorporation of radioactive calcium into embryonic chick bone *in vitro* (103, 104). The specific role of alterations in the function of bone cells under these experimental conditions has yet to be established. Thus, the inhibition of mineralization in the presence of aluminum may be due either to direct physical–chemical effects on the mineralization process or to alterations in the function of osteoblasts. However, aluminum impairs the formation and growth of hydroxyapatite crystals in a concentration-dependent manner in cell-free systems *in vitro* (105, 121), and complexes of citrate and aluminum diminish the rate of growth of calcium phosphate crystals in solution *in vitro* (106, 107, 122) (Figs. 13-4, 13-5). These findings demonstrate that aluminum can act as a physical–chemical inhibitor of mineralization under certain experimental conditions. Changes in the local microenvironment within the mineralization front induced by aluminum may therefore account for alterations in the calcification of osteoid in aluminum-related osteomalacia.

Some investigators have disputed the putative role of aluminum in the pathogenesis of osteomalacia (80, 84). In vitamin D-deficient dogs with osteomalacia, aluminum is deposited at the mineralization front following parenteral aluminum loading in a manner similar to that described in dialysis patients with aluminum-related bone disease (84). However, the subsequent administration of active vitamin D sterols resolved the histologic changes of osteomalacia in these animals (84). Similar observations were reported by Hodsman et al. in the rat, and the results are consistent with the view that aluminum may accumulate passively within unmineralized osteoid (108). Thus, the observed relationship between aluminum accumulation in bone and the severity of histologic osteomalacia reported in clinical studies could represent a coincidental finding. Moreover, increases in bone aluminum content achieved by various experimental procedures *in vivo* have not

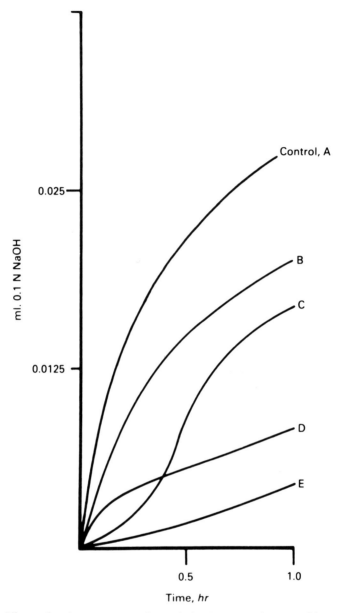

Fig. 13-4 Effects of various concentrations of aluminum on the rate of formation of hydroxyapatite crystals in solution. Concentration of aluminum (mM): A, 0; B, .021; C, .042; D, .063; E, .125. [Reprinted with permission from Posner et al. (121).]

induced an entirely consistent lesion of bone as judged by quantitative histologic methods (80). On the basis of these findings, the role of aluminum as a specific modifier of skeletal mineralization has been challenged (80, 84).

Despite such observations, the development of osteomalacia in previously normal bone following aluminum loading in experimental animals indicates that alu-

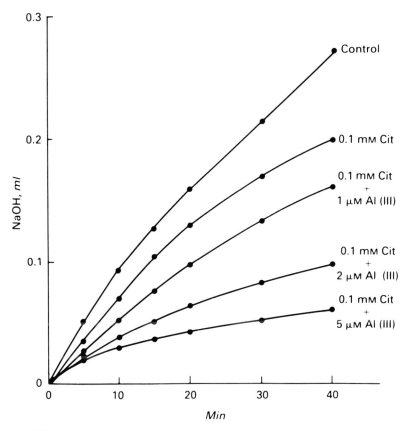

Fig. 13-5 Effect of citrate and aluminum citrate complexes on the rate of crystal growth of calcium phosphate. The volume of 0.1 M NaOH required to maintain pH constant at 7.4 during the precipitation of calcium phosphate from solution is plotted as a function of time. [Reprinted with permission from Meyer et al. (122).]

minum contributes to an alteration in skeletal mineralization (28, 29, 81–83). A considerable body of experimental data suggests that the effect of aluminum on bone is mediated locally at the tissue level. Thus, histologic changes of osteomalacia were noted in trabecular bone but not in cortical bone in rats given repeated injections of aluminum intraperitoneally for 4 weeks (79). Extensive deposits on aluminum were confined to trabecular bone surfaces in this experiment, whereas aluminum deposition was minimal or absent at the surfaces of cortical bone (79). It is possible that hormonal and metabolic factors may be important modulators of the differing skeletal responses to aluminum loading, and this issue requires further investigation. One such factor is parathyroid hormone, and there are preliminary data to suggest that reductions in the serum levels of PTH may substantially alter the tissue response to aluminum deposition (63, 84, 109, 110, 113, 114).

Furthermore, the studies of vitamin D-deficient dogs treated with aluminum do not directly address the issue of aluminum-mediated changes in the calcification of bone (84). The defect in skeletal mineralization in vitamin D deficiency differs substantially from that observed in aluminum-related bone disease. Serum calcium and phosphorus levels are reduced and serum PTH values are increased in vitamin D deficiency (99, 100). In contrast, the levels of PTH in serum are frequently normal or low in patients with aluminum-related bone disease, and the defect in skeletal mineralization in this disorder occurs in the presence of normal or increased levels of calcium and phosphorus in serum (14, 16, 62, 77–79, 81–83). Thus, it is unlikely that disturbances in the mineralization of bone in aluminum-related osteomalacia and vitamin D-deficient osteomalacia share a common mechanism. Indeed, vitamin D-deficient osteomalacia is reversible when serum calcium concentrations are restored to normal either with or without vitamin D repletion, whereas aluminum-associated osteomalacia does not respond to the administration of active vitamin D sterols (9, 31, 32, 99–101, 118). The failure of aluminum to block vitamin D-mediated calcification does not, therefore, exclude the existence of other pathways by which aluminum can alter the mineralization of osteoid.

ALUMINUM AND THE FUNCTION OF OSTEOBLASTS

In addition to evidence of defective mineralization, bone formation is diminished in patients and in experimental animals with aluminum-associated osteomalacia (9, 30–33, 38, 77, 78, 81–83). The synthesis of collagen and, therefore, the production of osteoid, is a function of the osteoblast, and adverse effects of aluminum on bone cell metabolism represent another potential mechanism for skeletal aluminum toxicity (77, 78, 82, 83). Despite marked differences from osteomalacia in the histologic appearance of bone, the aplastic lesion of renal osteodystrophy is characterized by reductions in the number of osteoblasts and by low rates of bone formation, and these changes are quantitatively similar to those observed in aluminum-related osteomalacia (66, 86, 133). Thus, a disturbance in the synthesis of collagen by the osteoblast may be common to both the osteomalacic and adynamic lesions of aluminum-related bone disease (77, 78, 81–83).

Several studies of bone formation and mineralization using quantitative histologic techniques in experimental animals have established that mineralized bone formation decreases during aluminum administration (77, 78, 81–83). The magnitude of the reduction in bone formation corresponds to the extent of aluminum deposition in bone (29, 77, 78, 82). However, isolated reductions in the mineralization of newly formed osteoid do not fully account the low rate of mineralized bone formation. Both bone and matrix formation fall in parallel as early manifestations of the skeletal toxicity of aluminum in the rat, and these changes result in the aplastic lesion of bone (77, 78, 109). Mineralized bone formation is impaired during experimental aluminum loading whether or not there is concurrent histologic evidence of a defect in the mineralization of osteoid. Such findings suggest that changes in the synthesis of bone collagen during aluminum loading contribute substantially to impaired bone formation in aluminum-related bone disease.

Robertson et al. reported that the number of osteoblasts was diminished in rats that developed osteomalacia after 9 weeks of parenteral aluminum loading (82).

These observations are consistent with changes noted in clinical bone biopsy material from patients with aluminum-related bone disease (66, 82, 102). Similar histologic findings have been reported in trabecular bone from young growing pigs that were given intravenous injections of aluminum for 8 weeks (115). In addition to histologic evidence of osteomalacia, bone formation was markedly reduced in these animals, and changes in the rate of bone formation were due primarily to reductions in the number of sites of active bone formation as assessed by the presence of double tetracycline labels (115). However, at sites within bone where the uptake of tetracycline was maintained, the width of separation of bands of tetracycline fluorescence was normal (115). The finding of widened osteoid seams was confined to bone surfaces that did not label with tetracycline, whereas the width of osteoid seams was normal at bone-forming surfaces where cellular indices of active bone formation were maintained (115).

These data in the pig correspond to the observations of Evans et al. in dialysis patients with renal osteodystrophy and evidence of aluminum deposition in bone, and they are also similar to reports of patchy osteomalacia in patients undergoing total parenteral nutrition who developed aluminum-related bone disease (58, 102). The results of these studies suggest that the total number of osteoblasts is reduced in association with the deposition of aluminum in bone; however, the function of remaining osteoblasts is normal with regard to osteoid production and mineralization.

Whether alterations in the number of cells or in the function of individual cells can be ascribed to a direct adverse effect of aluminum on the skeleton remains controversial (14, 80). Localized deposits of aluminum along bone-forming surfaces may interfere with the calcification of osteoid directly, or such deposits may have toxic effects on the osteoblast (33, 79, 102). PTH is an important modulator of bone formation, and reductions in the secretion of PTH induced by aluminum could also account for diminished numbers of osteoblasts and for low rates of bone formation in the lesions of osteomalacia and adynamic bone (31, 116). Serum PTH levels are often, but not invariably, low in patients with aluminum-related bone disease (14, 32, 62, 66, 132). Such findings are distinctly unusual for individuals with advanced renal failure, and they suggest that the function of the parathyroid glands is impaired in aluminum-related bone disease. The secretion of PTH in response to hypocalcemic stimuli is reduced in hemodialysis patients with aluminum-associated osteomalacia (111, 112), and aluminum has been shown to directly inhibit the release of PTH from dispersed bovine parathyroid cells *in vitro* (117).

Despite these findings, persistent elevations in serum calcium concentrations are a common biochemical finding in patients with aluminum-related bone disease. This disturbance may suppress the secretion of PTH *in vivo* and contribute to the lower serum levels of PTH in patients with evidence of aluminum deposition in bone (119).

Several studies indicate that PTH and aluminum interact to modify the histology of bone and the dynamics of bone formation and turnover. Preliminary data suggest that high levels of aluminum in bone reduce the histologic severity of secondary hyperparathyroidism in pediatric patients undergoing chronic dialysis (120). Conversely, some patients with osteitis fibrosa do not develop histologic osteomalacia even in the presence of high levels of aluminum in bone when serum PTH values remain elevated (14, 80). Parathyroidectomy appears to enhance the rate of aluminum accumulation in bone in patients undergoing long-term dialysis, and this disturbance may adversely affect bone formation and skeletal mineralization (63, 114). However, low serum levels of PTH may aggravate the toxic effect of existing levels of aluminum in bone rather than serving as a factor that promotes its accumulation of aluminum in bone. In studies in the rat, both the production of bone collagen and the mineralization of osteoid are impaired to a greater degree in animals parathyroidectomized before the start of aluminum loading than in parathyroid-intact rats given equal amounts of aluminum parenterally (28, 109, 110). These effects are not solely attributable to the extent of aluminum deposition in bone (28, 109).

Experimental evidence that aluminum loading diminishes the secretion of PTH *in vivo* is limited (77, 82, 83). Reductions in serum PTH levels were reported in rats that developed osteomalacia after repeated injections of aluminum (82), but the results of several other studies indicate that the adverse effects of aluminum on the formation of bone and the mineralization of osteoid can occur in the absence of changes in serum PTH levels of (28, 77, 83, 109). Although reductions in bone and matrix formation during aluminum loading may not be mediated by aluminum-induced decreases in the secretion of PTH, differences in the serum levels of PTH can modify the skeletal response to aluminum deposition *in vivo*. Additional experimental work is required to define more precisely the interactions between PTH and aluminum on the metabolism of bone.

REFERENCES

1. Alfrey, A. C. (1986) Kidney Int. (1986) 29:S8.
2. Alfrey, A. C. (1980) Neurotoxicology 1:43.
3. Alfrey, A. C., LeGendre, G. R., Kaehny, W. D. (1976) N. Eng. J. Med. 294:184.
4. Platts, M. M., Goods, G. C., Hislop, J. S. (1977) Br. Med. J. 2:657.
5. Ward, M. K., Feest, T. G., Ellis, H. A., Parkinson, I. S., Kerr, D. N. S. (1978) Lancet 1:841.
6. Parkinson, I. S., Feest, T. G., Ward, M. K., Fawcett, R. W. P., Kerr, D. N. S. (1979) Lancet 1:406.
7. Pierides, A. M., Edwards, Jr. W. G., Cullu, Jr. U.S., McCall, J. T., Ellis, H. A. (1980) Kidney Int. 18:115.
8. Boyce, B. F., Fell, G. S., Elder, H. Y., Junor, B. J., Elliot, H. L., Beastall, G., Fogelman, I., Boyle, I. T. (1982) Lancet II:1009.
9. Ott, S. M., Maloney, N. A., Coburn, J. W., Alfrey, A. C., Sherrard, D. J. (1982) N. Engl. J. Med. 307:709.
10. Hem, J. D. (1986) Kidney Int. 29:S3.
11. Trapp, G. A. (1986) Kidney Int. 29:S12.
12. Burnatowska-Hledin, M., Mayor, G. H. (1985) Am. J. Kidney Dis. 5:283.
13. Alfrey, A. C., Hegg, A., Craswell, P. (1980) Am. J. Clin. Nutr. 33:1509.
14. Coburn, J. W., Norris, K. C., Nebeker, H. G. (1986) Seminars in Nephrology 6:68.
15. King, S. W., Savory, J., Wills, M. R. (1982) J. Clin. Lab. Sci. 12:143.

16. Henry, D. A., Goodman, W. G., Nudelman, R. K., DiDomenico, N. D., Alfrey, A. C., Slatopolsky, E., Coburn, J. W. (1984) Kidney Int. 25:362.

17. Berlyne, G. M., Ben-Ari, J., Pest, D., Wemberger, J., Stern, M., Gilmore, G. R., Levine, R. (1970) Lancet II:494.

18. Klein, G. L., Ott, S. M., Alfrey, A. C., Sherrard, D. J., Hazlet, T. K., Miller, N. L., Maloney, N. A., Berquist, W. E., Ament, M. E., Coburn, J. W. (1982) Trans. Assoc. Am. Phys. 95:155.

19. Graf, H., Stummvol, H. K., Meisinger, V., Kovarik, J., Wolf, A., Pinggera, W. F. (1981) Kidney Int. 19:587.

20. Kovalchik, M. T., Kaehny, W. D., Hegg, A. P., Jackson, J. T., Alfrey, A. C. (1978) J. Lab. Clin. Med. 92:712.

21. Stummvoll, H. K., Graf, H. (1985) Am. J. Kidney Dis. 5:293.

22. Trapp, G. A. (1983) Life Science 33:311.

23. Markesbery, W. R., Ehmann, W. D., Hossain, T. I. M., Alauddin, M., Goodin, D. T. (1981) Ann. Neurol. 10:511.

24. Cann, C. E., Prussin, S. G., Gordan, G. S. (1979) J. Clin. Endocrinol. Metab. 49:543.

25. Elliott, H. L., MacDougall, A. I. (1978) Proc. Eur. Dial. Transplant. Assoc. 15:157.

26. Mayor, G. H., Sprague, S. M., Hourani, M. R., Sanchez, T. V. (1980) Kidney Int. 17:40.

27. Mayor, G. H., Burnatowska-Hledin, M. A. (1983) Fed. Proc. 42:2979.

28. Alfrey, A. C., Sedman, A., Chan, Y. K. (1985) J. Lab. Clin. Med. 105:227.

29. Chan, Y., Alfrey, A. C., Posen, S., Lissner, D., Hills, E., Dunstan, C., Evans, R. (1983) Calcif. Tissue Int. 23:344.

30. Llach, F., Felsenfeld, A. J., Coleman, M. D., Pederson, J. A. (1984) In: Robinson, R. R. (ed) Nephrology, Proceedings of the Ninth International Congress of Nephrology. Vol. II. New York: Springer-Verlag, p. 1375.

31. Hodsman, A. B., Sherrard, D. J., Alfrey, A. C., Ott, S., Brickman, A. S., Miller, M. L., Maloney, N. A., Coburn, J. W. (1982) J. Clin. Endocrinol. Metab. 54:539.

32. Hodsman, A. B., Sherrard, D. J., Wong, E. G. C., Brickman, A. S., Lee, D. B. N., Alfrey, A. C., Singer, F. R., Norman, A. W., Coburn, J. W. (1981) Ann. Intern. Med. 94:629.

33. Maloney, N. A., Ott, S. M., Alfrey, A. C., Miller, N. L., Coburn, J. W., Sherrard, D. J. (1982) J. Lab. Clin. Med. 99:206.

34. Schreeder, M. T., Favero, M. S., Hughes, J. R., Peterson, N. J., Bennett, P. H., Maynard, J. E. (1983) J. Chron. Dis. 36:581.

35. Arieff, A. I., Cooper, J. D., Armstrong, D., Lazarowitz, C. (1979) Ann. Intern. Med. 90:741.

36. Parsons, V., Davies, C., Goode, C., Ogg, C., Siddiqui, J. (1971) Br. Med. J. 4:273.

37. Sorenson, J. R. J., Campbell, I. R., Tepper, L. B., et al. (1974) Environ. Health Perspect. 8:3.

38. Gorsky, J. E., Dietz, A. A., Spencer, H., Osis, D. (1979) Clin. Chem. 25:1739.

39. Greger, J. L., Baier, M. J. (1983) Food Chem. Toxicol. 21:473.

40. Clarkson, E. M., Luck, V. A., Hynson, W. V., Baily, R. R., Eastwood, J. B., Woodhead, J. S., Clements, V. R., O'Riordan, J. L. H., DeWardener, H. E. (1972) Clin. Sci. 43:519.

41. Cam, J. M., Luck, V. A., Eastwood, J. B., DeWardener, H. E. (1976) Clin. Sci. Molec. Med. 51:407.

42. Ott, S. M. (1985) Am. J. Kidney Dis. 5:297.

43. Andreoli, S. P., Bergstein, J. M., Sherrard, D. J. (1984) N. Eng. J. Med. 310:1079.
44. Felsenfeld, A., Gutman, R. A., Llach, F., Harrelson, J. M. (1982) Am. J. Neph. 2:147.
45. Cannata, J. B., Briggs, J. D., Junor, B. J. R. (1983) Br. Med. J. 286:1937.
46. Salusky, I. B., Coburn, J. W., Paunier, L., Sherrard, D. J., Fine, R. N. (1984) J. Pediatr. 105:717.
47. Lam, M., Ricanati, E. S., Alfrey, A. C., Coburn, J. W. (1983) Kidney Int. 23:129. (abstr)
48. Ihle, B. U., Becker, G. L. (1985) Am. J. Kidney Dis. 5:302.
49. Fienroth, M., Fienroth, M. V., Berlyne, G. M. (1982) Miner Electrolyte Metab. 8:29.
50. Adler, A. J., Berlyne, G. M. (1985) Am. J. Physiol. 249:G209.
51. Henry, H. L., Norman, A. W. (1985) Calcif. Tissue Int. 37:484.
52. Cannata, J. B., Suarez-Suarez, C., Cuesta, V., et al. (1984) Proc. Eur. Dial. Transplant. Assoc. 21:354.
53. Angle, C. R., McIntire, M. S. (1982) Adv. Pediatr. 29:3.
54. Kaehny, W. D., Hegg, A. P., Alfrey, A. C. (1977) N. Engl. J. Med. 296:1389.
55. Burnatowska-Hledin, M. A., Mayor, G. H., Lau, K. (1985) Am. J. Phys. 249:F192.
56. Klein, G. L., Alfrey, A. C., Miller, N. L., et al. (1982) Am. J. Clin. Nutr. 35:1425.
57. Galle, P. (1983) In: *Advances in Nephrology,* vol. 12. Hamburger, J., Crosnier, J., Maxwell, M. H., (eds) Chicago: Year Book Medical Publishers, p. 85.
58. Ott, S. M., Maloney, N. A., Klein, G. L., Alfrey, A. C., Ament, M. E., Coburn, J. W. (1983) Ann. Intern. Med. 98:910.
59. Boukari, M., Jaudon, M. C., Rottembourg, M. (1978) Lancet II:1044.
60. Dreuke, T., Lacour, B., Touam, M., Basile, C., Bourdon, R. (1985) Nephron 39:10.
61. Alfrey, A. C., Hegg, A., Miller, N., Berl, T., Berns, A. (1979) Miner Electrolyte Metab. 2:81.
62. Norris, K. C., Crooks, P. W., Nebeker, H. G., Hercz, G., Milliner, D. S., Gerszi, K., Slatopolsky, E., Andress, D. L., Sherrard, D. J., Coburn, J. W. (1985) Am. J. Kidney Dis. 6:342.
63. Andress, D. L., Ott, S. M., Maloney, N. A., Sherrard, D. J. (1985) N. Eng. J. Med. 312:468.
64. Alfrey, A. C. (1985) Am. J. Kidney Dis. 5:309.
65. Mayor, G. H. (1985) Am. J. Kidney Dis. 5:306.
66. Sherrard, D. J. (1986) Seminars in Nephrology 6:56.
67. Kaehny, W. D., Alfrey, A. C., Holman, R. E., Schorr, W. J. (1977) Kidney Int. 12:361.
68. Rozas, U. V., Port, F. K., Easterling, R. E. (1978) J. Dialysis 2:459.
69. Gacek, E. M., Balss, A. L., Uvelli, D. A. (1979) Trans. Am. Soc. Artif. Intern. Organs 25:409.
70. Ricanati, E. S., Ott, S. M., Klein, K. L., Alfrey, A. C., Sherrard, D. J., Coburn, J. W. (1982) Kidney Int. 21:176. (abstr)
71. Hercz, G., Salusky, I. B., Milliner, D. S., et al. (1985) Kidney Int. 27:180. (abstr)
72. Cumming, A. D., Simpson, G., Bell, D., Cowie, J., Winney, R. J. (1982) Lancet 1:103.
73. Hercz, G., Milliner, D. S., Shinaberger, J. H., Nissenson, A. R., Cutler, R. E., Goodman, W. G., Gentile, D. E., Kraut, A. P., Coburn, J. W. (1984) Kidney Int. 25:257.

74. Kaye, M. (1983) Clin. Nephrol. 20:208.
75. Slatopolsky, E. R., Cagler, S., Pennell, J. P. (1971) J. Clin. Invest. 50:492.
76. Ihle, B., Buchanan, M., Stevens, B., et al. (1981) Am. J. Kidney Dis. 2:255.
77. Goodman, W. G., Gilligan, J., Horst, R. (1984) J. Clin. Invest. 73:171.
78. Goodman, W. G. (1984) J. Lab. Clin. Med. 103:749.
79. Goodman, W. G. (1985) Proc. Soc. Exp. Biol. Med. 179:509.
80. Quarles, L. D., Gitelman, H. J., Drezner, M. K. (1986) Seminars in Nephrology 6:90.
81. Ellis, H. A., McCarthy, J. H., Herrington, J. (1979) J. Clin. Pathol. 32:832.
82. Robertson, J., Felsenfeld, A., Haygood, C., and Llach, F. (1983) Kidney Int. 23:327.
83. Goodman, W. G., Henry, D. A., Horst, R., Nudelman, R. K., Alfrey, A. C., Coburn, J. W. (1984) Kidney Int. 25:370.
84. Quarles, L. D., Dennis, V. W., Gitelman, H. J., Harrelson, J. M., Drezner, M. K. (1985) J. Clin. Invest. 75:1441.
85. Sherrard, D. J., Baylink, D. J., Wergedal, J. E., Maloney, N. A. (1974) J. Clin. Endocrinol. Metab. 39:119.
86. Charhon, S. A., Chavassieau, P. M., Chapuy, M. C., Boivin, G. Y., Meunier, P. J. (1985) J. Lab. Clin. Med. 106:123.
87. Kerr, D. N. S., Walls, J., Ellis, H., et al. (1979) J. Bone Joint Surg. 51B:578.
88. Ellis, H. A. (1983) Nieren- und Hochdruckkhraneit 12:S198.
89. Coburn, J. W., Brickman, A. S., Sherrard, D. J., et al. (1977) Proc. Eur. Dial. Transplant Assoc. 14:442.
90. Pierides, A. M., Ellis, H. A., Simpson, W., Dewar, J. H., Ward, M. K., Kerr, D. N. S. (1976) Lancet 1:1092.
91. Siddiqui, J. Y., Simpson, W., Ellis, H. A., Kerr, D. N. S. (1971) Proc. Eur. Dial. Transplant Assoc. 8:149.
92. Pierides, A. M., Ward, M. K., Kerr, D. N. S. (1976) Lancet 1:1234.
93. Hodsman, A. B., Wong, E. G. C., Sherrard, D. J., Brickman, A. S., Lee, D. B. N., Singer, F. R., Norman, A. W., Coburn, J. W. (1983) Am. J. Med. 74:407.
94. Ott, S. M., Andress, D. L., Nebeker, H. G., Milliner, D. S., Maloney, N. A., Coburn, J. W. (1986) Kidney Int. 29:S108.
95. Malluche, H. H., Smith, A. J., Abreo, K., Faugere, M. C. (1984) N. Eng. J. Med. 311:140.
96. Cournot-Witmer, G., Zingraff, J., Plachot, J. J., Escaig, F., Lefevre, R., Boumati, P., Bourdeau, Garabedian, M., Galle, P., Bourdon, R., Drueke, T., Balsan, S. (1981) Kidney Int. 20:375.
97. Frost, H. M. (1963) Can. J. Biochem. Phys. 41:31.
98. Frost, H. M. (1983) In: Recker, R. R. (ed) *Bone Histomorphometry: Techniques and Interpretation.* Boca Raton, FL: CRC Press, p. 109.
99. Frame, B., Parfitt, A. M. (1978) Ann. Int. Med. 89:966.
100. Baylink, D. J., Stauffer, M., Wergedal, J., Rich, C. (1970) J. Clin. Invest. 49:1122.
101. Stauffer, M., Baylink, D., Wergedal, J., Rich, C. (1973) Am. J. Physiol. 225:269.
102. Evans, R. A., Flynn, J., Dunstan, C. R., George, C. R. P., McDonnell, G. D. (1982) Miner. Electrolyte Metab. 7:207.
103. Miyahara, T., Hayashi, M., Kozuki, H. (1984) Toxicol Letters 21:247.
104. Liu, C. C., Howard, G. A. (1984) Clin. Res. 32:50A.
105. Blumenthal, N. C., Posner, A. S. (1984) Calcif. Tiss. Int. 36:439.
106. Meyer, J. L., Thomas, W. C. R., Jr. (1982) J. Urol. 128:1372.
107. Thomas, W. C., Jr. (1982) Proc. Soc. Exp. Biol. Med. 170:321.

108. Hodsman, A. B., Anderson, C., Leung, F. Y. (1984) Miner. Electrolyte Metab. 10:309.

109. Goodman, W. G., (1987) Kidney Int. 31:923.

110. Lewis-Finch, J., Bergfeld, M., Martin, K., Chan, Y. L., Teitelbaum, S., Slatopolsky, E. (1986) Kidney Int. 30:318.

111. Kraut, J. A., Shinaberger, J. H., Singer, F. R., Sherrard, D. J., Saxton, J., Miller, J. H., Kurokawa, K., and Coburn, J. W. (1983) Kidney Int. 23:725.

112. Andress, D. L., Voights, A., Felsenfeld, A., Llach, F. (1983) Kidney Int. 24:364.

113. Felsenfeld, A. J., Harrelson, J. M., Gutman, R. A., Wells, S. A. Jr., Drezner, M. K. (1982) Ann. Intern. Med. 96:34.

114. De Vernejoul, M. C., Marchais, S., London, G., et al. (1985) Kidney Int. 27:785.

115. Sedman, A. B., Alfrey, A. C., Miller, N. L., Goodman, W. G. (1987) J. Clin. Invest. 79:86.

116. Teitelbaum, S. L., Bergfeld, M. A., Freitag, J., Hruska, K. A., Slatopolsky, E. (1980) J. Clin. Endocrinol. Metab. 51:247.

117. Morrissey, J., Rothstein, M., Mayor, G., Slatopolsky, E. (1983) Kidney Int. 23:699.

118. Howard, G. A., Baylink, D. J. (1980) Miner. Electrolyte Metab. 3:44.

119. Cannata, J. B., Briggs, J. D., Junor, B. J. R., Fell, G. S., Beastall, G. (1983) Lancet 1:501.

120. Salusky, I. B., Goodman, W. G., Brill, J., Foley, J., Slatopolsky, E., Fine, R. N., Coburn, J. W. (1986) J. Bone Mineral Res. (Suppl 1) 534 (abstr.).

121. Posner, A. S., Blumenthal, N. C., Boskey, A. L. (1986) Kidney Int. 29:S17.

122. Meyer, J. L., Thomas, W. C. (1986) Kidney Int. 29:S20.

123. Martin, R. B. (1986) Clin. Chem. 32:1797.

124. Bertholf, R. L., Wills, M. R., Savory, J. (1984) Biochem. Biophys. Res. Commun. 125:1020.

125. Mladenovic, J. (1988) J. Clin. Invest. 81:1661.

126. Coburn, J. W., Robertson, J. A., Norris, K. C., Salusky, I. B., Goodman, W. G. (1989) Kidney Int. 35:398 (abstr.).

127. Mischel, M. G., Salusky, I. B., Goodman, W. G., Coburn, J. W. (1989) Kidney Int. 35:399 (abstr.).

128. Froment, D. H., Molitoris, B. A., Alfrey, A. C. (1989) Kidney Int. 35:398 (abstr.).

129. Bakir, A. A., Hryhorczuk, D. O., Berman, E., Dunea, G. (1986) Trans. Am. Soc. Artif. Intern. Organs 32:171.

130. Ittel, T. H., Buddington, B., Miller, N. L., Alfrey, A. C. (1987) Kidney Int. 32:821.

131. Williams, J. W., Vera, S. R., Peters, T. G., et al. (1986) Ann. Intern. Med. 104:782.

132. Slatopolsky, E., Weerts, C., Finch, J., et al. Kidney Int. 29:226 (abstr.).

133. Salusky, I. B., Coburn, J. W., Brill, J. et al. (1988) Kidney Int. 33:975.

134. Smith, G. D., Winney, R. J., McLean, A., Robson, J. S. (1987) Kidney Int. 32:96.

135. Andress, D. L., Maloney, N. A., Coburn, J. W., Endres, D. B., Sherrard, D. J. (1987) J. Clin. Endocrinol. Metab. 65:16.

136. Andress, D. L., Nebeker, H. G., Ott, S. M., et al. (1987) Kidney Int. 31:1344.

137. Ott, S. M., Feist, E., Andress, D. L., et al. (1987) J. Lab. Clin. Med. 109:40.

138. Hercz, G., Norris, K. C., Miller, J. H., Shinaberger, J. H., Coburn, J. W. (1986) Kidney Int. 29:215 (abstr.).

139. Hercz, G., Salusky, I. B., Norris, K. C., Fine, R. N., Coburn, J. W. (1986) Kidney Int. 30:944.

14

Fluoride Metabolism
and the Osteoporotic Patient

M. R. MARIANO-MENEZ, G. K. WAKLEY,
S. M. FARLEY, AND D. J. BAYLINK

Recently, there has been increasing interest in fluoride and its therapeutic role in osteoporosis, a condition characterized by reduced bone mass and increased risk for fractures, particularly in the spine, hip, and wrist. This chapter will describe fluoride with respect to its metabolism, toxicology, and effects on bone and other tissues. The bulk of the chapter will be devoted to the clinical application of fluoride in osteoporosis.

Fluoride is the ionic form of elemental fluorine, a member of the halogen family. It is the 13th most abundant element on the earth's crust, occurring naturally in limestone, sandstone, coral deposits, rocks, and water. The natural fluoride content of water depends on the geological formation (i.e., rock strata, volcanic area), its source (deep wells contain higher fluoride levels than surface water), and the amount of rainfall and water evaporation as rainwater absorbs fluoride from the atmosphere (1).

Drinking water, however, is not the only source of fluoride in the human body. The widespread industrial use of fluoride has contributed significantly to airborne fluoride, which can be absorbed through the respiratory system. Since fluoride is well distributed in the environment, humans are exposed to the element in a wide range of concentrations from water, soil, atmosphere, vegetation, livestock, the food chain (from the use of fluoridated water in commercial food processing), dental products, and drugs.

Clinical interest in fluoride emerged in the 1930s following observations of a reduction in the incidence of dental caries in communities with naturally fluoridated water supplies (2). This led to fluoridation of drinking water in many countries, with the optimum fluoride concentration established at 0.7–1.2 ppm (3). In the United States, it is estimated that most untreated wells contain less than 0.5 ppm fluoride (1).

In the meantime, skeletal effects from drinking water containing excessive fluoride and from industrial exposure were reported from different geographical areas. Various investigators (4–10) described osteosclerosis, marginal osteophytes, and ossification of the ligaments in the lumbar spine. In the long bones, thickening of the cortex, obliteration of the medullary cavity, and periosteal new bone formation were noted. Furthermore, Leone et al. (10, 11) reported in 1955 and 1960 a higher incidence of osteoporosis among residents of Cameron, Texas, and Framingham, Massachusetts, where the drinking water contained only traces of fluoride. This was in marked contrast to the lower incidence of osteoporosis observed in other areas of Texas, where there was high fluoride content in the water. Bernstein (12) reported similar findings in which the prevalence of col-lapsed vertebrae was much lower and increased less rapidly with age in women residents of a high-fluoride area in North Dakota compared to a low-fluoride area.

It was not until 1961 that Rich and Ensinck (13, 14) initiated the use of flu-oride in patients with osteoporosis to promote subclinical osteosclerosis. The ob-jective was to use fluoride long enough, and at doses that were well tolerated, to strengthen the skeleton without affecting the ligaments and muscular attachments.

METABOLISM AND TOXICOLOGY OF FLUORIDE

Pertinent to the use of fluoride to increase bone mass with minimal adverse effects are the absorption, distribution, retention, and excretion of the ion (Fig. 14-1). The plasma fluoride concentration, measured using a fluoride ion-specific elec-trode, is influenced by these different metabolic processes. Beyond certain fluo-ride levels, the risk of adverse effects is increased.

Under ordinary conditions, the absorption of fluoride from the gastrointestinal tract is rapid, and the bioavailability (fraction that reaches the circulation) is al-most 90–100 percent (2, 15–18, 20). The absorptive mechanism is by simple diffusion of the undissociated molecule hydrogen fluoride (HF) across the gastric and upper intestinal mucosa. No active transport mechanism is involved. Fluoride is detectable in the blood within 10 min after it is ingested (provided that soluble fluorides are administered), reaches a peak concentration in 30–60 min and has a plasma half-life that ranges from 2 to 9 hrs. Several factors, however, can affect the bioavailability of fluoride, including:

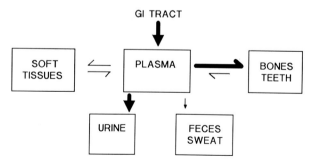

Fig. 14-1 An overview of fluoride metabolism.

1. Solubility of fluoride. While soluble fluoride preparations are rapidly absorbed, slow-release and enterocoated fluoride pills that have an insoluble matrix show lower peak serum levels and less bioavailability (19).
2. Gastric acidity (pH). The rate of fluoride absorption is directly related to gastric acidity. Studies on animals pretreated with atropine or cimetidine to reduce gastric acid secretion revealed lower fluoride absorption (8, 15, 20). Similar results are reported by Franke et al. on subjects with achlorhydria (21).
3. Nature of food and beverage. Dietary sources of fluoride can influence the serum level. Regarding animal sources, fish is richest in fluoride, the calcium content of the bones and skin attracting fluoride from seawater. Regarding plant sources of fluoride, tea leaves are a rich source. Foods rich in calcium or protein, on the other hand, tend to bind fluoride, causing less absorption from the gastrointestinal tract (15, 22).
4. Presence of other ions. Aluminum, calcium, magnesium, and chloride present in food or water reduce fluoride absorption, whereas sulfate increases fluoride uptake (15, 22).
5. Renal status. The kidney is the major organ of fluoride excretion in the body; thus, impaired renal function will cause higher fluoride retention. Ekstrand (16) showed that the fluoride clearance was 40 ml/min at a urinary flow of 0.6 mg/min and was increased to 80 ml/min at a flow of 1.2 mg/min. Fluoride excretion is also pH-dependent, a low urine pH being associated with low fluoride clearance (2, 17, 23).
6. Previous fluoride exposure from other sources. The serum fluoride level is linearly related to its concentration in drinking water and the duration of exposure; the longer the exposure to fluoride, the higher the serum level due to cumulative retention in tissues until a steady-state level is achieved (2).

Following absorption and passage to the blood, fluoride is distributed to the different tissues of the body but is deposited mostly in hard tissues (i.e., bones and teeth). Fluoride has a specific affinity with the hydroxyapatite of bony tissue, being incorporated directly into the crystalline mineral phase to replace the hydroxyl ion, thereby forming fluoroapatite (17, 24). This process occurs more rapidly in the trabecular portion of the bone than the cortex, where the fluoride induces new bone formation. Interestingly, in vitro work suggests that fluoride is a bone cell-specific mitogen, which could account for the observed bony changes (25). However, the exact mechanism of the fluoride effects on bone has not been established.

In general, of the fluoride that is ingested by a relatively unexposed individual, about 50 percent is retained in tissues, almost exclusively in bones. Longer exposure to large doses of fluoride results in less fluoride being retained (i.e., bone is more saturated) (2, 17, 26). The amount that is not retained is eliminated, mainly through the kidneys and less through the feces, sweat, and saliva. Reduction in the serum fluoride concentration produces a back-diffusion of fluoride from the bone crystallite into the blood. After stopping fluoride completely, the half-life for elimination of fluoride from the bones is as long as 8 years (27).

TOXICOLOGY

Because fluoride is a potentially toxic agent, careful dosing and monitoring of the serum levels are important. The "normal" steady-state level of serum fluoride is 0.2–0.4 µM in healthy subjects living in areas with low fluoride content, and about 0.5–1.0 µM in areas with fluoridated water (17, 28). When a subject is exposed regularly to large doses of fluoride, either as drug therapy for osteoporosis or from environmental exposure, a new steady-state level is reached in plasma that is dependent on the dose, the amount of fluoride deposited in bones, and on the renal excretion rate (2). Serum fluoride levels in our patients receiving the recommended dose of 1–1.5 mg/kg fluoride has usually been in the range of 10–20 µM (41).

Although the lethal dose of fluoride in humans is not precisely known, it lies in the range of 15–30 mg/kg body weight (up to 5–10 g NaF) (17, 18). With these massive doses, the functions of many enzymes in the body are inhibited, and nausea, vomiting, abdominal cramps, respiratory failure, and ultimately death may occur within several hours (18). Fortunately, such acute intoxication is very rare and usually accidental in nature. Deserving of greater attention are the possible adverse effects following chronic fluoride exposure from water containing naturally excessive fluoride levels that occur in certain areas, from industrial emissions, and from the long-term use of fluoride as a treatment for osteoporosis. Because of fluoride's affinity for hydroxyapatite, the main target organs are teeth and bones; the soft tissues are much less affected.

Teeth

Although fluoride is considered the cornerstone of modern preventive dentistry because of its cariostatic property, excessive doses can produce dental or enamel fluorosis. The incidence of dental caries depends on the fluoride intake, falling sharply as the concentration of fluoridated water approaches 1.0 ppm. However, at higher concentrations, there is little further reduction in caries, and higher doses are in fact associated with adverse dental effects (8, 17, 18, 30). Thus, water supplies are either fluoridated or defluoridated to meet the optimum concentration of 0.7–1.2 ppm. Dental fluorosis may become a public health concern when water fluoride concentrations exceed 1.8 ppm. It is only during the first 10–12 years of life, when the permanent teeth are being formed, i.e., the enamel-building cells are active, that the teeth are susceptible to the effects of excessive fluoride (10, 17, 18, 29). The first sign of dental fluorosis is "mottling," which consists of small whitish or brownish spots on the surface of the teeth. This may progress to formation of grooves, deformation of teeth, and destruction of enamel.

Bones

Skeletal involvement is one of the basic diagnostic criteria in fluorosis. The changes in the bone occur very gradually, and it may take 10–20 years of continuous intake of excessive amounts of fluoride before these become radiographically detectable (8, 29).

In 1931, Moller and Gudjonsson (5) were the first to describe the skeletal changes that occurred in factory workers after several years of exposure to cryolite dust (a compound consisting of sodium aluminum fluoride). Similar skeletal changes were later reported by other investigators, not only from fluoride-emitting industries but also from endemic exposure in communities with naturally fluoridated water supplies (4, 6–8, 10). The most severe cases were observed in the Indian province of Punjab, where fluoride in water was 0.2–40.0 ppm, mostly 2–5 ppm (30). It remains an enigma, however, that although all the people in the area were exposed to the same water source, not everyone developed osteosclerosis, and those who did presented considerable variability in the degree of manifestations.

The initial symptom of skeletal fluorosis was arthalgia, usually involving the back, elbows, or shoulders. As the condition became worse, joint stiffness ensued, causing a marked restriction of movement in the spine, especially in the thoracic and lumbar regions, and in large joints, especially in the hip (7, 18, 30).

Radiographically, the changes were always more pronounced in the vertebral column and the pelvis than in the peripheral skeleton. An increase in bone density became detectable by X-ray when fluoride in dry bone exceeded 4,000 ppm (18, 31). The most frequent radiographic changes were increased density and lack of sharpness in the contour of the thoraco-lumbar spine, pelvis, ribs, and clavicles. In severe cases, there was almost absolute white opacity in the vertebrae. Later, the ligaments and fibrocartilaginous attachments at the posterior ends of the ribs, iliac crest, and ischial bones became opacified. In the extremities, the cortices were much thickened, and the marrow cavities narrowed. Less commonly, periosteal new bone formation and free intra-articular bodies were noted (5–8, 10, 18, 30).

Histologically, coarsening and condensation of the trabecular bone, subperiosteal formation of fibrous bone, thickening of the cortices and irregular matrix formation were described as a result of the chronic high fluoride exposure (8, 30). In addition, it has been demonstrated that the fluoride content of bones in industrial workers exposed chronically to fluoride is significantly higher than in an age-matched control group (8, 24). Various studies have indicated a bone fluoride content of 2,000 ppm as representing the upper limit of normal.

Soft Tissues

Although bones and teeth are the major target organs for fluoride, soft tissue organs can also be affected. This was first recognized in 1931, when Moller described gastrointestinal symptoms in cryolite workers including nausea, vomiting, lack of appetite, excessive salivation, and obstipation (5). Roholm, in 1937, described other nonskeletal manifestations, including neurological (dizziness, sleepiness, headaches, tiredness), cardiorespiratory (shortness of breath, cough, palpitations), and dermatologic symptoms (32).

Reports on the effects of chronic fluoride exposure to the kidneys are conflicting. Some investigators observed impaired kidney function (i.e., reduced urea clearance and rate of filtration) in persons drinking highly fluoridated water (5–16 ppm) in India (30). In contrast, a U. S. Public Health Service survey (33) reported no loss of kidney function in persons drinking fluoridated water (8 ppm) compared to a control group. Sometimes it may be difficult to determine whether a pre-existing kidney dysfunction precipitated excessive fluoride storage in the body or a coexisting kidney problem is the result of long-term fluoride intake.

There has been no convincing experimental or epidemiological evidence to support theories regarding possible carcinogenic and mutagenic effects of fluoride (18, 33).

FLUORIDE IN OSTEOPOROSIS

The ideal treatment for osteoporosis is not a program that would merely prevent or retard bone loss; rather, it is one that would stimulate bone formation to increase spinal bone density to the extent that the osteoporotic patient is no longer at risk for spinal fracture. The level of spinal bone density below which the risk of developing spontaneous fracture significantly increases is referred to as the fracture threshold, and has been calculated by quantitative computed tomography (QCT) to be 100 mg/cm^3 in women and about 130 mg/cm^3 in men (35). Of all the agents that have been used to treat osteoporosis, only fluoride has definitely been shown to stimulate osteoblast proliferation and activity (21, 36), and increase spinal bone density above the fracture threshold (37).

Several clinical studies have been conducted to determine the efficacy and safety of fluoride in the treatment of osteoporosis. To evaluate patient response to fluoride, several indices have been monitored, including one or a combination of the following: relief of back pain, level of activity, serum alkaline phosphatase, spinal radiography, spinal bone density using QCT or dual-photon absorptiometry (DPA), distal radial bone density using single-photon absorptiometry (SPA), femoral neck or hip bone density using DPA, bone histomorphometry, and fracture rate.

Pain and Activity Response

Several investigators using various doses and durations of fluoride therapy have reported 50–100 percent of osteoporotic patients showing a reduction in back pain with a significant increase in activity (21, 36, 38–40). In our previous studies, 93% of patients (37/40) who had chronic back pain and limited activity prior to treatment reported improvement in symptoms after 20 (± 16) months of sodium fluoride (NaF) at doses of 66–88 mg/day (41). Forty percent eventually had complete disappearance of pain and full resumption of activities. Although most of the above-mentioned studies were uncontrolled, we feel they represent strong subjective evidence for an osteogenic response to fluoride. Subjective symptoms, however, are not a sufficient criterion of effectiveness, especially since osteoporosis may be characterized by spontaneous remissions and exacerbations.

Biochemical Effects

Serum alkaline phosphatase (SALP) activity has often been noted to increase in response to fluoride therapy. This response was frequently dose dependent and usually observed with doses greater than 50 mg of NaF per day; studies using smaller doses have reported no change (36–38, 40–44, 51, 52). The SALP response was confirmed in our studies where 87 percent (46/53) of osteoporotics treated with 66–88 mg of NaF showed a significant increase in their serum levels (41). Although there was marked interpatient variation in the onset and peak increase of SALP, the half-time for the increase was 9 months, and SALP remained elevated after 2 years of fluoride therapy. The increase in SALP was shown to correlate with the following: (1) decreased back pain; (2) increased bone density on spinal radiographs and, on bone biopsy, (3) increased trabecular bone volume; and (4) increased osteoid length, reflecting the osteogenic action of fluoride. Consistent with these *in vivo* findings, *in vitro* studies have shown that fluoride directly stimulates proliferation and ALP activity of bone-forming cells (25).

A decreased rate of excretion of calcium in the urine has occasionally been observed with fluoride therapy, suggesting a positive calcium balance effect (13, 14, 42). Most clinical studies report no significant change in the serum calcium, phosphorus, and parathyroid hormone levels (38, 42, 43, 45).

Radiographic Changes

Lateral films of the thoracic and lumbar spine that are taken both prior to and during therapy can be useful in determining any fluoridic changes in the skeleton (Fig. 14-2). These changes include coarsening of the trabecular markings, increase in trabecular width, and thickening of the vertebral end plates (36, 42, 45–47). However, there may be wide interobserver variation in the interpretation of radiolucency and trabecular structure.

Clinical studies indicate that at least 1 year of treatment is required before any unambiguous improvement can be detected radiographically (42, 46–48). The mean time for the onset of radiographic response is 3 years. Although the radiographic changes increase in direct proportion to the duration of therapy, only one-third to two-thirds of patients given long-term fluoride medication have been observed to present increased vertebral trabeculation (42, 45, 48). Riggs (45, 48) reported that patients with a radiographically demonstrable increase in bone density had a markedly lower vertebral fracture rate than those without radiographic response.

Densitometric Changes

Since the effect of fluoride to increase bone formation occurs earlier and to a larger magnitude in trabecular than in cortical bone (36, 49–51), the most effective skeletal sites monitored to determine response to therapy are the spine (75% trabecular bone), proximal femur (hip) especially the highly trabecular Ward's triangle, and the distal radius (35% trabecular bone at a site 1.5–2 cm proximal to the radial styloid). Methods have been devised to quantitate the bone mass in these specific areas of interest (49, 50, 53).

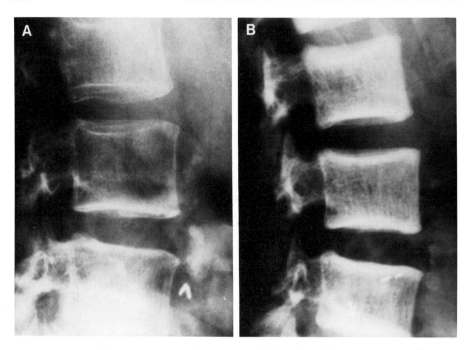

Fig. 14-2 Lateral lumbar X-rays of a 60-year-old female with postmenopausal osteo-porosis (A) before and (B) after 3 1/2 years of treatment with fluoride 40 mg/day. Reprinted from Baylink et al. (1983) with permission from Caries Res. (36).

Most studies report no significant change in the radial bone density as measured by bone mineral analysis (BMA) using single-photon absorptiometry (36, 38, 39, 45). The reason for this may be the lower metabolic activity in the radius since it has a greater amount of cortical bone. Furthermore, the radius is non-weight-bearing, and it has been shown that the peripheral effects of fluoride are observed most frequently in weight-bearing bones (44, 51). Thus, the radius is not a good site to monitor the positive effect of fluoride therapy.

The spine, on the other hand, is very metabolically active and capable of large changes in bone mass (5–10%/year) (49, 50) and is therefore the most sensitive site for monitoring the skeletal response discovered so far. QCT and dual-photon absorptiometry (DPA) were developed to quantitate the bone changes directly in the spine (49, 50, 53). The DPA can also be applied to measure the proximal femur and several other anatomical sites. Since QCT and DPA have been used only in the past few years, there are few data available on bone density changes in response to fluoride therapy utilizing these methods.

We report here data from our own experience with QCT in fluoride-treated patients. Nineteen female osteoporotics treated with 77 mg/day NaF for at least 2 years had significantly higher spinal bone density when compared to (1) their predicted pretreatment values, and (2) age- and sex-matched untreated osteoporotic patients (54). In another study (44), 21 osteoporotics treated with NaF 77 mg/day and calcium 1,500 mg/day demonstrated significant increases in spinal bone density as measured by QCT after 6 and 12 months. The QCT values and serum ALP were positively correlated ($r = .84$) at 12 months. Long-term studies involving a larger number of patients are now being conducted to determine the magnitude of the skeletal response to fluoride as a function of time using these precise and sensitive methods.

Bone Histomorphometry

Pretreatment and posttreatment transiliac bone biopsies were done in some studies to evaluate histologically the effect of fluoride. The dose of NaF ranged from 45 to 120 mg/day, and repeat biopsies were performed at least 1–2 years after initiating therapy. Most of these studies (36, 38–40, 43, 47, 55, 56) clearly demonstrated a significant increase in bone volume (trabecular volume and thickness) and bone formation parameters (trabecular osteoid volume, osteoid surface, osteoblast-covered osteoid, and osteoid seam thickness). The marked increase in bone formation compared to bone resorption thus led to an overall positive skeletal balance. These histologic changes appeared to be dose- and time-dependent.

Another effect of fluoride on bone that has caused some concern is inhibition of mineral deposition causing an osteomalacic appearance histologically, a change seen despite normal levels of serum calcium and phosphorus (36, 38, 39, 47, 55, 56). The mineralization lag time (the time between deposition of osteoid and onset of mineralization in this osteoid) when evaluated by tetracycline labeling is increased, thereby widening the osteoid width. Reutter and Olah (47) have demonstrated that the mineralization defect ultimately corrects itself with time. Our own studies (56) confirmed this finding where, in the course of time on therapy, the lamellae formed eventually became mineralized. Some studies (45, 55) indicate that concurrent administration of calcium and/or vitamin D prevented or minimized the occurrence of osteomalacia and any increase in bone resorption. However, the prevention of fluoride-induced osteomalacia was not confirmed in other studies (38, 39, 47).

Effects on Vertebral Fracture

Since the major complication from osteoporosis is fracturing, perhaps the most relevant measure of therapeutic efficacy would be that the increase in bone mass resulting from fluoride stimulation of bone formation would prevent fracture. Several studies (36, 38, 39, 45, 47, 48) report that the augmented bone mass is indeed accompanied by a significant decrease in the rate of new vertebral fractures. This usually required 1–2 years of treatment, and the rate continued to improve with time on therapy. Fluoride-treated osteoporotic patients who showed increases in vertebral bone mass radiographically had only one-seventh the fracture rate of other non-fluoride-treated osteoporotic patients (45, 48). A controlled study conducted by Riggs' group (48) showed a significantly lower fracture rate in a fluoride-treated group than in a placebo group or a conventionally treated group (i.e., one given calcium with or without vitamin D). Thus, there appears to be a fluoride-responsive subpopulation of osteoporotics that exhibits an increase in bone mass attended by a lower fracture rate.

Side Effects

The major side effects experienced with fluoride therapy are gastrointestinal irritation (nausea, vomiting, pain, and, rarely, gastrointestinal bleeding) and ar-
thralgic/periarthralgic pains, usually involving the ankles, knees, or hips. The
incidence of side effects varies among investigators and ranges from zero to 50
percent (36–43, 47, 48), depending on the dose and formulation of fluoride administered. In our study of 120 osteoporotic patients given NaF 66–88 mg/day,
43 percent of patients experienced GI discomfort, and this usually occurred within
a few weeks or months of therapy, while 38 percent of patients complained of
periarticular pain which usually became manifest after several months to a year
of therapy. Thirty-seven percent of patients reported no adverse reactions (52).

The side effects were readily managed, and rarely required discontinuing fluoride therapy. In the majority of cases, the GI symtoms could be resolved by
switching to an intestinal- or slow-release formulation of fluoride. In other cases,
withholding fluoride for 1 to 3 weeks and then resuming at the same or lower
dose, or addition of a histamine H2 antagonist resulted in relief of discomfort.
Complaints of periarticular pain were managed by discontinuing fluoride for 2 to
4 weeks until all symptoms dissipated. Fluoride was then resumed at the same or
lower dose, or switched to a slow release formulation. In only 3 percent of patients
was fluoride permanently discontinued because of the side effects (52).

CONCLUSIONS

The bulk of evidence suggests that fluoride is an effective treatment for osteoporosis capable of restoring bone mass and preventing further fracturing. It is a
relatively safe form of treatment with side effects that ordinarily can be easily
managed and reversed. However, at least 1–2 years of treatment is required before
a substantial increase in bone mass can be achieved, and a small subgroup of
patients do not respond or respond poorly. Further studies are needed to determine
the reasons for the poor responders and the means by which the response can be
hastened and enhanced. If these disadvantages can be overcome, fluoride may
become the most important therapeutic advance for osteoporosis.

REFERENCES

1. Waldbott, G. L., Burgstahler, A. W., McKinney, H. L. (1978) In: *Fluoridation,
The Great Dilemma*. Kansas: Coronado Press, p. 28.
2. Ekstrand, J. (1977) In: *Studies on the Pharmacokinetics of Fluoride in Man* (Thesis).
Stockholm, p. 7.
3. U.S. Public Health Service Drinking Water Standards (1962) PHS Pub. No. 956
Washington D.C. U.S. Govt Printing Office, p. 8.
4. Morris, J. W., (1965) Am. J. Roentgenol Radium Ther. Nucl. Med. 94:608.
5. Moller, P. F., Gudjonsson, S. W. (1932) Acta. Radiol. 13:269.

6. Azar, H. A., Nucho, C. K., Bayyuk, S. I., Bayyuk, W. (1961) Ann. Intern. Med. 55:193.

7. Czervinski, E., Lankosz, W. (1978) In: Courvoisier, B., Donath, A., Baud, C. A. (eds) *Fluoride and Bone*. Bern: Hans Huber, p. 144.

8. Franke, J., Runge, H., Fengler, F. (1978) In: Courvoisier, B., Donath, A., Baud, C. A. (eds) *Fluoride and Bone*. Bern: Hans Huber, p. 129.

9. Jolly, S. S. (1970) In: *Fluoride in Medicine*. Bern: Hans Huber, p. 106.

10. Leone, N. C., Stevenson, C. A., Hilbish, T. F., Sosman, M. C. (1955) Am. J. Roentgenol Radium Therapy Nucl. Med. 74:874.

11. Leone, N. C., Stevenson, C. A., Besse, B. et al., (1960) Arch. Indust. Health 21:326.

12. Bernstein, D. S., Sadowsky, N., Hegsted, D. M., Guri, C. D., Stare, F. J. (1966) J. Am. Med. Assoc. 198:499.

13. Rich, C., Ensinck, J. (1961) Nature 191:185.

14. Rich, C., Ensinck, J., Ivanovich, P. (1964) J. Clin. Invest. 43:545.

15. Waldbott, G. L., Burgstahler, A. W., McKinney, H. L. (1978) In: *Fluoridation The Great Dilemma*. Kansas: Coronado Press, p. 47.

16. Ekstrand, J., Ehrnebo, M., Boreus, L. O. (1978) Clin. Pharmacol. Ther. 23:329.

17. Whitford, G. M. (1983) Dental Hygiene 57:16.

18. Schlatter, C. (1978) In: Courvoisier, B., Donath, A., Baud, C. (eds) *Fluoride and Bone*. Bern: Hans Huber, p. 1.

19. Hasvold, O., Ekren, T. (1981) Eur. J. Clin. Pharmacol. 19:225.

20. Whitford, G. M., Pashley, D. H. (1984) Calcif. Tissue Int. 36:302.

21. Franke, J., Rempel, H., Franke, M. (1974) Acta. Orthop. Scand. 45:1.

22. Rao, G. S. (1984) Ann. Rev. Nutr. 4:115.

23. Whitford, G. M., Pashley, D. H., Stringer, G. I. (1976) Am. J. Physiol. 230:527.

24. Bang, S., Baud, C. A., Boivin, G., et al., (1978) In: Courvoisier, B., Donath, A., Baud, C. A. (eds) *Fluoride and Bone*. Bern: Hans Huber Pub., p. 168.

25. Farley, J. R., Wergedal, J. E., Baylink, D. J. (1983) Science 222:330.

26. Weatherell, J. A. (1969) In: Barltrop., D., Burland, W. L. (eds) *Mineral Metabolism in Paediatrics*. Oxford, Edinburgh: Blackwell Scien. Pub., p. 53.

27. Largent, E. J. (1959) In: Muhler, J. C., Hine, M. K. (eds) *Fluorine and Dental Health*. Bloomington: Indiana Univ. Press, p. 132.

28. Hodge, H. C., Taves, D. R. (1970) In: *Fluoride and Human Health*. Geneva: World Health Organization Monograph Series, 59:254.

29. Waldbott, G. L., Burgstahler, A. W., McKinney, H. L. (1978) In: *Fluoridation the Great Dilemma*. Kansas: Coronado Press, p. 98.

30. Singh, A., Jolly, S. S., Bansal, B. C., Mathus, C. C. (1963) Medicine 42:229.

31. Dinman, B. D., Backentose, D. L., Carter, R. P., et al., (1976) J. Occup. Med. 18:17.

32. Roholm, K. (1937) In: *Fluorine Intoxication: A Clinical-Hygienic Study*. London: H. K. Lewis & Co., 1:364.

33. Leone, N. C., Shimkin, M. B., Arnold, F. A. Jr., et al., (1954) Public Health Rep. 69:925.

34. Hodge, A. C., Smith, F. A. (1977) J. Occup. Med. 19:12.

35. Odvina, C. V., Wergedal, J. E., Libanati, C. R., Schulz, E. E., Baylink, D. J. (1988) Metabolism 37:221.

36. Baylink, D. J., Duane, P. B., Farley, S. M., Farley, J. R. (1983) Caries Res. 17(S1):56.

37. Mariano-Menez, M. R., Tudtud, L. A., Bock, M. B., Farley, S. M., Baylink, D. J. (1988) Clin. Res. (In press).

38. Briancon, D., Meunier, P. J. (1981) Ortho Clinics of N. America 12:629.

39. Lane, J. M., Healey, J. H., Schwartz, E., et al., (1984) Ortho. Clinics of N. America 15:729.

40. Ringe, J. D., Kruse, H. P., Kuhlencordt, (1978) In: Courvoisier, B., Donath, A. (eds) *Fluoride and Bone*. Bern: Hans Huber, p. 228.

41. Farley, S. M., Wergedal, J. E., Smith, L. C., et al., (1987) Metabolism 36:211.

42. Dambacher, M. A., Lauffenburger, T., Lammle, B., Haas, H. C. (1978) In: Courvoisier, B., Donath, A. (eds) *Fluoride and Bone*. Bern: Hans Huber, p. 238.

43. Jowsey, J., Riggs, B. L., Kelly, P. J., Hoffman, D. L. (1972) Amer. J. Med. 53:43.

44. Farley, S. M., Libanati, C. R., Schulz, E. E., et al., (1984) Calcif. Tissue Int. 36:A41.

45. Riggs, B. L., Hodgson, S. F., Hoffman, D. L., et al., (1980) JAMA 243:446.

46. El-Khoury, G. Y., Moore, T. E., Albright, J., Huang, H. K., Martin, R. K. (1982) AJR 139:39.

47. Reutter, F. W., Olah, A. J. (1978) In: Courvoisier, B., Donath, A., Baud, C. A. (eds) Fluoride and Bone. Bern: Hans Huber, p. 249.

48. Riggs, B. L., Seeman, E., Hodgson, S. F., Taves, D. R., O'Fallon, W. M. (1982) N. Engl. J. Med. 306:446.

49. Wahner, F. W., Dunn, W. L., Riggs, B. L. (1983) Seminars Nucl. Med. 13 (282).

50. Ruegsegger, P., Stebler, B., Dambacher, M. (1982) Earlwood Scientific Symposium 57:96.

51. Schulz, E. E., Libanati, C. R., Farley, S. M., Kirk, G. A., Baylink, D. J. (1984) J. Nucl. Med. 25:651.

52. Mariano-Menez, M. R., Farley, S. M., Tudtud, L. A., et al., (1987) Clin. Res. 35:155A.

53. Mazess, R. B., Peppler, W. W., Chesney, R. W., et al., (1984) Calcif. Tissue Int. 36:8.

54. Farley, S. M., Libanati, C. R., Smith, L., et al., (1985) In: 67th Annual Meeting Endo. Soc. Abstr., p. 254.

55. Baylink, D. J., Bernstein, D. S. (1967) Clin. Orthop. 55:51.

56. Lundy, M., Wergedal, J., Baylink, D. J. (1987) Clin. Res. 35:154A.

15
Tin

JANET L. GREGER

Tin has no known function in the growth or maintenance of bone. In fact, it is doubtful that tin is an essential element. However, tin may affect bone metabolism in two primary ways. First, excess tin in the body tends to accumulate in bone, but the functional consequences are not known. Second, the ingestion of tin can depress the absorption and alter the utilization of several essential minerals, particularly calcium and zinc, that are needed for bone growth and maintenance.

SOURCES OF TIN EXPOSURE

Dietary Exposure to Tin

Typical Western diets have been reported to contain 1–50 mg tin daily (1–4). Differences in estimates primarily reflect differences in the amounts of canned foods, particularly foods packed in unlacquered cans, included in diets.

Most foods contain only small of tin naturally (1, 4). Although stannous chloride is on the FDA's list of Generally Recognized as Safe (GRAS) food additives, the average American consumed only 2.7 mg stannous chloride daily in 1977 (5). Several organotin compounds are used as polymerization aids in plastics, but little tin from these compounds is believed to actually enter the food supply (6). Similarly, despite many industrial sources of tin, little of this tin remains in water supplies, because most tin salts are insoluble in water (7). Thus most fresh, frozen, and bottled foods contain less than 1 μg Sn/g food.

The tin content of canned foods can vary greatly. Foods packed in cans that are totally coated with lacquer generally contain less than 4 μg Sn/g food (2). Foods (e.g., pineapple, grapefruit and orange juices, applesauce, tomato sauce) that are often packed in cans not coated with lacquer have been found to contain 40–150 μg Sn/g food when the cans were opened (2, 4).

Storage conditions will affect the amount of tin in canned foods. Canned foods, particularly those with high nitrate and acid levels, accumulate tin when stored for several months (8). Moreover, foods stored in opened cans in the refrigerator for 3–7 days can accumulate very high (>250 μg/g) levels of tin (2, 9).

Most Americans and Europeans consume a limited amount of canned foods. Canned vegetables and fruits currently account for less than 5 percent (w/w) of the food included in the British Total Diet Study menu (4), and foods canned in tin-plated cans account for less than 5 percent (w/w) of the food included in the U.S. Total Diet Study menu (11). It is possible, however, to identify individuals who utilize more canned foods. Low-income individuals and institutions, such as nursing homes and schools, often select canned fruits, vegetables, and juices because of economy and ease of storage. Mothers sometimes leave the juice in opened cans in the refrigerator for their children's snacks. Individuals who routinely consume canned fruits, vegetables, and juices from unlacquered cans could ingest 50 to more than 200 mg tin daily (2).

Exposure to Tin in Dental and Medical Products

A number of tin-containing compounds, especially stannous fluoride, have been used in toothpastes and mouth rinses (11). Mouth rinses containing .1 percent stannous fluoride contain about 750 μg Sn/ml (12). The actual ingestion of tin from these products is difficult to estimate, because the percentages of these products swallowed by individuals vary greatly.

Tin is an essential component of many nuclear diagnostic kits used in skeletal and cardiac imaging. The reducing power of the tin makes it possible to label a variety of ligands with technetium-99m (13, 14). Patients are frequently injected with milligram quantities of tin during these diagnostic tests (13, 14).

METABOLISM OF INORGANIC TIN

Absorption and Urinary Excretion

Generally both animals (15–18) and humans (19, 20) fed moderate ($\approx$100 μg Sn/g dry weight) or large doses of tin have found to excrete more than 90 percent of the tin in feces. However, human subjects fed very low levels of tin (.11 mg Sn/day) lost only 50 percent of their tin intake in feces (20).

Little is known about factors that affect the absorption of tin. Tin II may be absorbed somewhat better than tin IV (2.5 vs. .64%) (15). Absorption of tin does not appear to be sensitive to changes in the anion component of tin salts or to the presence of a number of other dietary factors (15, 16). However, Johnson and Greger (18) observed that three-fold increases in dietary zinc levels resulted in greater fecal losses of tin when animals were fed 100–200 μg Sn/g diets.

Some tin lost in the feces may be of endogenous origin (14, 15). Hiles (15) noted that 12.1 percent of a single IV dose of [113]Sn II appeared in the feces whereas only 3.1 percent of a single IV doses of [113]Sn IV appeared in the feces of rats.

Little tin is excreted in the urine of men or animals (3, 15, 16, 20). However, urinary losses of tin will reflect large difference in tin intake. Eight human subjects excreted four times as much tin (122 vs. 29 μg Sn/day) in urine when fed 50 mg rather than 0.11 mg tin daily (20).

Retention of Tin in Tissues

Although the absorption and overall apparent retention of tin by human subjects in balance studies is low (3, 19, 20), tin has been found in at least trace amounts in most mammalian tissues (1). Rats fed diets supplemented with tin have been found to accumulate tin in their tibias, kidneys, and livers in proportion to their dietary intake of tin. Thus rats fed 2,000 μg Sn/g diet for only 21 days accumulated 46 μg Sn/g wet weight in their tibias (18). Johnson and Greger (18) found that the concentrations of tin in the tibias of rats fed diets supplemented with 200 μg Sn/g diet were more than five times greater than the concentrations of tin in kidneys and nearly 20 times greater than the concentrations of tin in livers. Other investigators have also observed that animals fed tin accumulated more tin in bone than in soft tissues (15, 17, 21, 22).

Similarly, Srivastava et al. (13) and Oster et al. (23) have reported that tin injected in a variety of forms (tin II or tin IV bound to pyrophosphate, ethylidenehydroxy disodium phosphonate, methylene diphosphonate, and diethylenetriaminepentacetic acid) tended to accumulate more tin in bone than in soft tissues. Gouaillardou and Conti (24) have demonstrated that bone uptake of ^{99m}Tc-Sn-phosphate complexes is dependent on the charges of the complexes which reflect the tin/ligand ratios.

BENEFICIAL EFFECTS OF TIN

Many experts doubt that tin is an essential nutrient (1, 25, 26). In 1970 Schwarz et al. (27) reported that low levels of tin (.5–2 μg Sn/g diet) promoted growth in suboptimally growing rats fed purified amino acid-based diets and housed in plastic isolator systems. These observations have not been confirmed (25).

A number of investigators have studied the cariostatic properties of tin in diets, dentifrices, and mouth washes with rat models and human subjects (12, 28–32). The results have not been consistent. However, several investigators have noted that stannous fluoride had slightly more cariostatic activity than other fluoride compounds, because the tin compound more effectively reduced plaque accumulation and gingivitis (12, 31, 32).

TOXIC EFFECTS OF TIN

Toxic Effects of Organic Tin

A variety of extremely toxic organic tin compounds are used commercially (33–35). The toxicity of these compounds depends on the organic constituents of the tin compounds, the manner of exposure, and the animal species studied. Generally these compounds affect the central nervous system, liver, and immune system (34, 35). Little has been published on their effects in bone, so this will not be discussed here.

Toxic Effects of Acute Exposure to Inorganic Tin

Animals and humans are fairly resistant to single large oral doses of tin (36–38). Generally the symptoms of acute toxicity to oral doses of inorganic tin include nausea, abdominal cramping, diarrhea, and vomiting; symptoms usually occur after the consumption of canned juices or acidic punches contaminated with 500–2,000 μg Sn/ml. Other factors besides tin in these beverages may have exacerbated the local irritation of the gastrointestinal tract in these cases.

Several investigators have reported the effects of a single injection of tin in animal models. Many of the injected doses were extremely large, and their relevance to any real situation could be questioned, but some of the injected doses were within 10-fold of the injected doses (10–40 μg/kg body weight) of tin administered routinely with radiopharmaceuticals to humans (13, 24, 39–43).

Zareba et al. (39) demonstrated that 18 hours after an i.p. dose, $SnCl_2$ (2 mg/kg) depressed activity of δ-amino levulinic acid dehydratase by 60 percent. Kappas and Maines (40) demonstrated that an injection of only 25 μmole Sn/kg body weight induced kidney heme oxygenase levels; larger doses (250 μmoles/kg) induced both liver and kidney heme oxygenase activity and depressed liver and kidney ethylmorphine N-dimethylase and cytochrome P-450 levels but did not affect δ-amino levulinic synthetase activity. Burba (41) demonstrated that a single injection (200 μg Sn/kg) of stannous chloride depressed hepatic azo-reductase and aromatic hydroxylase activity and reduced hepatic cytochrome P-450 levels.

Dwivedi et al. (42, 43) observed that partially hepatectomized rats injected with very large doses of tin (20–30 mg Sn/kg body weight) had depressed activity of δ-amino levulenic acid dehydratase, δ-amino levulinic acid synthetase and elevated activity of heme oxygenase in the liver. The practical ramifications of this work are now being considered (43). Heme oxygenase activity can be inhibited *in vivo* for extended periods subsequent to binding to zinc or tin protoporphyrins. Thus, metalloporphyrins are being suggested as a means of suppressing bilirubin production.

Toxic Effects of Chronic Exposure to Inorganic Tin

Growth Depression and Changes in Cellular Function

Some of the effects of tin on growth and cell function may be indirect and due to interactions between tin and essential minerals such as zinc, calcium, copper, iron, and selenium; some of the effects may be direct. McLean et al. (44) have found that *in vitro* tin II but not tin IV was readily taken up by ovary cells and damaged the DNA in the cells.

Several investigators have observed that the effects of inorganic tin on growth are dependent on the doses and the form of the tin salts fed. Growth of rats was usually depressed when dietary tin levels were elevated above 500 μg Sn/g (45–48).

The activity of some enzymes was affected not only by injections of tin but also by ingestion of tin. Generally animals given tin orally had less dramatic responses to tin than animals injected with tin. This reflected differences in the size of doses and the effectiveness of the gut as a barrier. Ingestion of tin has been demonstrated to depress the activity of serum alkaline phosphatase and serum lactic dehydrogenase (21, 47). Johnson and Greger (18) demonstrated that very high levels of dietary tin (>2,000 μg Sn/g diet), but not moderate levels of dietary tin (≈200 μg Sn/g diet), inhibited blood δ-amino levulinic acid dehydratase activity in rats. Zinc partially reversed *in vitro* the inhibition of this enzyme by tin (49), but ingesting additional zinc did not counteract the effect of tin on δ-amino levulinic acid dehydratase activity in rats (18).

Interactions with Zinc and Selenium

Potentially some of the effects of tin on growth and enzyme levels can be explained on the basis of interactions between tin and zinc or selenium. It is well established that growth depression is a common symptom of zinc deficiency (26). Several of the enzymes affected by tin are zinc metalloproteins.

Rats fed ≥500 μg Sn/g diet have depressed levels of zinc in bone and soft tissues (17, 48). Tibia zinc levels were even sensitive to moderate doses of tin (100–200 μg Sn/g diet). At least part of this effect is due to the effect of dietary tin on apparent absorption of zinc. Johnson et al. (50) found that human subjects lost an additional 2 mg of zinc daily in the feces when fed 50 mg tin rather than .1 mg tin daily; this resulted in significantly poorer overall retention of zinc by these subjects. Valberg et al. (51) confirmed these results and found that inorganic tin depressed the absorption by humans of ^{65}Zn from a turkey test meal. However, Solomons et al. (52) could not demonstrate a tin–zinc interaction in subjects fed load doses of both tin and zinc.

The mechanism by which tin affects zinc absorption appears to depend on the dose. When rats were fed high levels of tin (≈2,000 μg Sn/g diet), their gastrointestinal tracts were hypertrophied, and endogenous losses of zinc in the feces were significantly increased (48). When moderate levels of tin (≈200 and 500 μg Sn/g diet) were fed, endogenous losses of zinc in the feces were constant, but the true absorption of zinc tended to be depressed.

Less is known about the interaction between tin and selenium. Hill and Matrone (53) showed that high dietary levels of tin depressed the apparent absorption of selenium from chick intestinal segments. Greger et al. (54) demonstrated that human subjects fed 50 mg versus .11 mg tin daily apparently absorbed significantly less selenium. Chiba et al. (55) found that the simultaneous injection of sodium selenite with tin prevented a decrease in δ-amino levulinic acid dehydratase activity in mice.

Anemia and Interactions with Copper and Iron

The ingestion of high levels of dietary tin can induce anemia in rats (45–47). One potential mechanism involves copper. Generally ingestion of ≥200 μg Sn/g diet has been found to depress copper levels in soft tissues (17, 18). The plasma copper levels of animals fed high levels of tin (500 and 2,000 μg Sn/g diet) were depressed to less than 20 percent of the levels found in control animals. It is well established that copper deficiency can induce anemia (26). Moreover deGroot (45) demonstrated that the addition of copper to the diets of rats eliminated the anemia induced by feeding 150 μg Sn/g diet.

Schäfer and Forth (56) have demonstrated that very concentrated solutions of tin decreased the net absorption of fluid and ^{59}Fe from rat jejunal segments. However, poor absorption of iron is probably not a major cause of anemia in rats fed tin, because soft tissue (kidney and liver) levels of iron are not depressed in animals fed tin (17, 18). Ingestions of high levels of dietary tin ($>1,000$ µg Sn/g diet), but probably not moderate levels, may induce anemia in other ways too (18), because tin can alter the activity of at least two enzymes involved in heme metabolism, δ-amino levulinic acid dehydratase and heme oxygenase (40, 57).

Although all of these factors may affect the development of anemia in laboratory animals that are fed high levels of tin, their significance to humans fed moderate levels of tin is questionable. Johnson et al. (50) found that the addition of 50 mg tin daily (equivalent to about 100 µg Sn/g dry diet) to the diets of human subjects for 20 days had no effect on the apparent absorption of copper or iron or on plasma copper, ceruloplasmin, or ferritin levels. Similarly, no changes in iron metabolism were observed in rats fed only 100 µg Sn/g diet (18).

Changes in Bone and Calcium Metabolism

There are a number of potential mechanisms by which tin affects bone metabolism. Tin adversely affects certain enzymes. Japanese workers have observed that oral exposure to tin depressed the activity of acid and sometimes alkaline phosphatases not only in serum and the duodenal mucosa (21, 58, 59) but also in bone (21, 22, 60). Rats fed as little as 200 µg Sn/g diet for 90 days had significantly depressed acid phosphatase activity in femoral epiphyses (60). Rats orally dosed with 2 mg Sn/kg body weight for only 3 days had depressed levels of acid and alkaline phosphatase activity in their femoral diaphyses and epiphyses (22).

These Japanese workers have also found that oral exposure to tin depressed calcium levels in bone (21, 22, 59, 60), serum (59, 61), and the duodenal mucosa (58) but elevated calcium levels in kidneys of rats (62). Oral exposure to tin affected calcium levels more in the femoral epiphyses than in the femoral diaphyses (29, 59, 60). Ingestion of diets that contained as little as 50 µg Sn/g diet for 90 days significantly depressed the calcium levels in serum and femoral epiphyses of rats (60). Johnson and Greger (18) also observed that low levels of dietary tin ($\approx$100 µg Sn/g diet) depressed the calcium content (but not concentration) of tibias, but they observed no changes in plasma calcium levels.

Serum and bone phosphorus levels were not sensitive to dietary tin in most studies (21, 22, 50), but serum phosphorus levels were depressed in one study (60).

The mechanisms by which calcium levels in serum and bone are affected by tin are not clear. Yamaguchi and his associates in a series of studies with rats found that oral tin exposure increased biliary volume and calcium content (61) that IP injections of tin decreased the volume and total acidity of gastric contents (63) and that oral tin exposure decreased calcium absorption and decreased the calcium-binding capacity of duodenal mocusal homogenates to one-quarter (58). However, in a later study Yamaguchi et al. (64) found that oral doses of tin depressed the calcium content of the femoral epiphyses of rats without affecting fecal or urinary losses of calcium. Similarly Johnson and Greger (20) observed no changes in fecal or urinary losses of calcium when human subjects were fed 50 mg rather than .11 mg tin daily. These differences in data reflect differences in the doses of tin administered, the routes of administration, and the calcium and phosphorus contents of diets.

Although the mechanism by which tin and calcium interact is unclear, it appears that the depressed levels of calcium and elevated levels of tin in the bones of animals administered tin orally may have practical consequences. Yamaguchi et al. (65) observed in rats that the hydroxyproline content of femoral epiphysis was decreased and that *in vitro* collagen synthesis, as judged by the incorporation of ^{3}H-proline into collagen hydroxyproline, was depressed among rats given tin orally. Ogoshi et al. (66) observed that the compressive strength of femurs of rats given tin (300 μg Sn/ml) in their drinking water was significantly decreased.

CONCLUSIONS

Most Americans consume only small amounts of tin daily. Some individuals, however, regularly ingest moderately large doses of tin daily (i.e., 50–200 mg) through the use of canned foods; some of these individuals may be injected occasionally with radiopharmaceuticals that contain tin.

Generally tin is fairly nontoxic. Hence exposure to these amounts of tin probably would be important only to individuals who consume low levels of essential elements (e.g., zinc, copper, and perhaps calcium) that interact with tin. For example, many elderly individuals and some children routinely consume less than two-thirds of the recommended daily allowances (RDA) for zinc (67, 68). Most women in the United States consume less than two-thirds of the RDA for calcium (69). Chronic consumption of moderately high doses of tin may lead to a deterioration in nutritional status and perhaps functional consequences for some of these individuals.

REFERENCES

1. Schroeder, H. A., Balassa, J. J., Tipton, I. H. (1964) J. Chron. Dis. 17:483.
2. Greger, J. L., Baier, M. (1981) J. Food Sci. 46:1751.
3. Tipton, I. H., Steward, P. L., Dickson, J. (1969) Health Phys. 16:455.
4. Sherlock, J. C., Smart, G. A. (1984) Food Additives and Contaminants 1:277.
5. Committee on the GRAS List Survey—Phase III (1979) The 1977 Survey of Industry on the Use of Food Additives. Washington DC: National Academy of Sciences, p. 1789.
6. Kumpulainen, J., Koivistoinen, P. (1977) Residue Rev. 66:1.
7. Safe Drinking Water Committee 1977. *Drinking Water and Health.* Washington DC: National Academy of Sciences, p. 292.
8. Nagy, S., Rouseff, R., Ting, S. V. (1980) J. Agric. Food Chem. 28:1166.
9. Capar, S. G., Boyer, K. W. (1980) J. Food Safety 2:105.
10. Pennington, J. A. T. (1983) J. Am. Dietet. Assoc. 82:166.
11. Schäfer, S. G., Femfert, U. (1984) Regul. Toxicol. & Pharmacol. 4:57.
12. Leverett, D. H., McHugh, W. D., Jensen, Ø. E. (1984) J. Dent. Res. 63:1083.

13. Srivastava, S. C., Meinken, G. E., Richards, P., Som, P., Oster, Z. H., Atkins, H. L., Brill, A. B., Knapp, F. F. Jr., Butler, T. A. (1985) Int. J. Nucl. Med. Biol. 12:167.

14. Francis, M. D., Tofe, A. J., Hiles, R. A., Birch, C. G., Beran, J. A., Grabenstetter, R. J. (1981) Int. J. Nucl. Med. Biol. 8:145.

15. Hiles, R. A. (1974) Toxicol. & Appl. Pharmacol. 27:366.

16. Fritsch, P., deSaint Blanquat, G., Derache, R. (1977) Food Cosmet. Toxicol. 15:147.

17. Greger, J. L., Johnson, M. A. (1981) Food Cosmet. Toxicol. 19:163.

18. Johnson, M. A., Greger, J. L. (1985) J. Nutr. 115:615.

19. Calloway, D. H., McMullen, J. J. (1966) Am. J. Clin. Nutr. 18:1.

20. Johnson, M. A., Greger, J. L. (1982) Am. J. Clin. Nutr. 35:655.

21. Yamaguchi, M., Saito, R., Okada, S. (1980) Toxicology 16:267.

22. Yamaguchi, M., Sugii, K., Okada, S. (1981) J. Pharm. Dyn. 4:874.

23. Oster, Z. H., Som, P., Srivastava, S. C., Fairchild, R. G., Meinken, G. E., Tillman, D. Y., Sacker, D. F., Richards, P., Atkins, H. L., Brill, A. B., Knapp, F. F. Jr., Butler, T. A. (1985) Int. J. Nucl. Med. Biol. 12:175.

24. Gouaillardou, D., Conti, M. L. (1987) Appl. Radiat. Isotop. 38:103.

25. Nielsen, F. H. (1980) In: *Inorganic Chemistry in Biology and Medicine*. Washington DC: American Chemical Society, p. 23.

26. Underwood, E. J. (1977) *Trace Elements in Human and Animal Nutrition*. New York: Academic Press, pp. 56, 196, 449.

27. Schwarz, K., Milne, D. B., Vinyard, E. (1970) Biochem. Biophys. Res. Comm. 40:22.

28. McDonald, J. L. Jr., Stookey, G. K. (1973) J. Nutr. 103:1528.

29. Stookey, G. K., McDonald, J. L. Jr. (1974) J. Dental Res. 53:1398.

30. Stookey, G. K., McDonald, J. L., Hughes, S. B., Smith, R. E., Stange, R. D. (1974) Arch. Oral. Biol. 19:107.

31. Tinanoff, N., Brady, J. M., Gross, A. (1976) Caries Res. 10:415.

32. Ferretti, G. A., Tanzer, J. M., Tinanoff, N. (1982) Caries Res. 16:298.

33. Kimbrough, R. D. (1976) Env. Health Perspectives 14:51.

34. Krigman, M. R., Silverman, A. P. (1984) Neuro. Toxicol. 5:129.

35. Cook, L. L., Stine, K. E., Reiter, L. W. (1984) Toxicol. & Appl. Pharmacol. 76:344.

36. Warburton, S., Udler, W., Ewert, R. M., Haynes, W. S. (1962) U.S. Public Health Rep. 77:798–800.

37. Benoy, C. J., Hooper, P. A., Schneider, R. (1971) Food Cosmet. Toxicol. 9:645.

38. Barker, W. H. Jr., Runte, V. (1972) Am. J. Epidemiol. 96:219.

39. Zareba, G., Chmielnicka, J., Kustra, G. (1986) Ecotoxicol. Environ. Safety 11:144.

40. Kappas, A., Maines, M. D. (1976) Science 192:60.

41. Burba, J. V. (1983) Toxicol. Lett. 18:269.

42. Dwivedi, R. S., Kaur, G., Srivastava, R. C., Murti, C. R. K. (1985) Industr. Health 23:1.

43. Maines, M. D. (1988) FASEB J. 2:2557.

44. McLean, J. R. N., Blakey, O. H., Douglas, G. R., Kaplan, J. G. (1983) Mutation Res. 119:195.

45. deGroot, A. P. (1973) Food Cosmet. Toxicol. 11:955–962.

46. deGroot, A. P., Feron, V. J., Til, H. P. (1973) Food Cosmet. Toxicol. 11:19.

47. Dreef-Van Der Meulen, H. C., Feron, V. J., Til, H. P. (1974) Path Europ. 9:185.

48. Johnson, M. A., Greger, J. L. (1984) J. Nutr. 114:1843.

49. Chiba, M., Kikuchi, M. (1984) Toxicol. & Appl. Pharmacol. 73:388.

50. Johnson, M. A., Baier, M. J., Greger, J. L. (1982) Am. J. Clin. Nutr. 35:1332.

51. Valberg, L. S., Flanagan, P. R., Chamberlain, M. J. (1984) Am. J. Clin. Nutr. 40:536.

52. Solomons, N. W., Marchini, J. S., Duarte-Favaro, R. M., Vannuchi, H., Dutra de Oliveira, J. E. (1983) Am. J. Clin. Nutr. 37:566.

53. Hill, C. H., Matrone, G. (1970) Federation Proceed. 29:1474.

54. Greger, J. L., Smith, S. A., Johnson, M. A., Baier, M. J. (1982) Biol. Tr. Element Res. 4:269.

55. Chiba, M., Fujimoto, N., Kikuchi, M. (1985) Toxicol. Lett. 24:233.

56. Schäfer, S. G., Forth, W. (1983) Ecotoxicol. & Environ. Safety 7:87.

57. Chiba, M., Ogihara, K., Kikuchi, M. (1980) Arch. Toxicol. 45:189–195.

58. Yamaguchi, M., Kubo, Y., Yamamoto, T. (1979) Toxicol. & Appl. Pharmacol. 47:441.

59. Yamaguchi, M., Kitade, M., Okada, S. (1980) Toxicol. Lett. 5:275.

60. Yamaguchi, M., Sugii, K., Okada, S. (1981) Toxicol. Lett. 9:207.

61. Yamaguchi, M., Yamamoto, T. (1978) Toxicol. & Appl. Pharmacol. 45:611.

62. Yamamoto, T., Yamaguchi, M., Sato, H. (1976) J. Toxicol. & Env. Health 1:749.

63. Yamaguchi, M., Naganawa, M., Yamamoto, T. (1976) Toxicol. & Appl. Pharmacol. 36:199.

64. Yamaguchi, M., Sugii, K., Okada, S. (1982) Toxicol. Lett. 10:7.

65. Yamaguchi, M., Sugii, K., Okada, S. (1982) J. Pharm. Dyn. 5:388.

66. Ogoshi, K., Kurumatani, N., Aoki, Y., Moriyama, T., Nanzai, Y. (1981) Toxicol. Appl. Pharmacol. 58:331.

67. Hambidge, K. M., Walravens, P. A., Brown, R. M., Webster, J., White, S., Anthony, M., Roth, M. L. (1976) Am. J. Clin. Nutr. 29:734.

68. Sandstead, H. H., Henriksen, L. K., Greger, J. L., Prasad, A., Good, R. A. (1982) Am. J. Clin. Nutr. 36:1046.

69. Science and Education Administration (1980) Nationwide Food Consumption Survey 1977–78, Preliminary Rep. No. 2, U.S. Dept. of Agriculture, Washington DC, p. 75.

16

Zinc

JAMES C. WALLWORK AND HAROLD H. SANDSTEAD

Zinc was first reported to be essential for a living organism (*Aspergillus niger*) in 1869 by Raulin (1). Subsequently its requirement by higher plants was established (2, 3). Because of the difficulties with preparation of diets and appropriate husbandry, it was not until 1934 that Todd et al. (4) reported its requirement by the rat. Suggestions of its need by humans included reports by Eggleton (5, 6) and Vallee et al. (7). Finally, Prasad et al. (8–10) described zinc deficiency in human adolescents. Subsequent research and factorial calculations (11, 12) suggested provisional requirements for persons at different stages of the life cycle. More recent research refined these suggestions and established times in life when persons are probably at greatest risk of deficiency [reviewed by Sandstead et al. (13), Hambridge et al. (14)]. All species are at greatest risk of deficiency during intervals of rapid growth. Thus for humans, the fetus, young child, and adolescent are at greatest risk. Others at risk are individuals who are repairing injured tissues, as occurs during wound healing.

The importance of zinc for bone growth was suggested by the findings of Follis et al. (15), who reported narrower epiphyseal cartilage in long bones from young zinc-deficient rats than among zinc-adequate controls. The smaller femurs of the zinc-deficient rats had a zinc concentration (95 μg/g ash) that was only 40 percent of control values. Subsequently, abnormalities of skeletal growth associated with zinc deficiency have been reported in birds (16–18), calves (19), and pigs (20). Supplementation with adequate zinc in these deficiency studies was associated with an increased bone growth and bone age toward normal levels. Thus it seemed clear that adequate zinc nutriture is essential for bone growth and that zinc deficiency is reflected by bone zinc content.

ZINC, GROWTH, NUCLEIC ACID, AND PROTEIN METABOLISM

Many of the manifestations of zinc deficiency such as growth depression (3), dermatitis (21–23), poor wound healing (24–29), depressed immune response (30–34), teratology (35, 36), and hypogonadism (9, 37–39) are probably mediated, at least in part, through impairment of nucleic acid synthesis and repair, suppressed expression of the genetic code, and suppressed synthesis of proteins. Insufficient zinc may also be present for binding to enzymes, hormones, or other proteins so as to influence their tertiary structure, biological activity, or receptivity.

Development and function of the cellular matrix of cartilage and bone including chondrocytes, osteoblasts, and osteoclasts may be adversely influenced by poor zinc nutriture. This effect is accentuated in growing animals. Special attention to zinc nutriture may be required at other times of stress (e.g., during aging and/or disease, and at times of bone fractures at any age).

The presence of zinc in the cell nucleus, nucleolus, and chromosomes (40) was suggestive of a role for this metal in cell turnover. Since then, zinc has been implicated in several reactions or events that may be related to cell division and differentiation.

Impaired synthesis of nucleic acids in zinc-deficient animals and tissues (41–43) is probably caused by decrease in activity of the enzymes that mediate nucleic acid synthesis and repair. Zinc deficiency has been reported adversely to affect two alternative pathways of synthesis for deoxythymidine monophosphate, a precursor of DNA. Tissues from zinc-deficient rats have subnormal activities of thymidine kinase (EC 2.7.1.21), which catalyzes the synthesis of deoxythymidine monophosphate from deoxythymidine (44, 45), and thymidylate synthetase (EC 3.1.3.35), which catalyzes the conversion of deoxyuridyl monophosphate to deoxythymidine monophosphate (46, 47). Because the action of thymidine kinase has been suggested to be the rate-limiting step in DNA biosynthesis, the effect of zinc deficiency may be mainly at this step (47).

Lieberman et al. (48) reported depressed activity of DNA polymerase in rat kidney cells cultured in zinc-deficient medium. In addition, decreased thymidine incorporation has been observed in tissues from zinc-deficient rats (41, 42). This depression was rapidly reversible upon administration of zinc. Similarly, zinc deficiency depressed thymidine incorporation in 12-day-old rat embryos (49), in skin wound healing (27), and in sponges implanted under the skin (44). Perhaps related to these findings, the activity of purified calf thymus deoxynucleotidyl transferase, inhibited with chelating agents, was restored by zinc, indicating that it may be a zinc-activated enzyme (50). Subsequently, DNA polymerases (EC 2.7.7.7) from several species (*Escherichia coli,* sea urchin, bacteriophages T4 and T7) were reported to contain stoichiometric amounts of zinc (51–53). However, recent studies have shown that zinc was present in much lower concentrations than stoichiometric levels in purified active samples of *E. coli* DNA polymerase I (54–56) and bacteriophage T7 DNA polymerase (57), with the conclusion that these enzymes are not zinc metalloenzymes. Furthermore, the addition of zinc tended to inhibit the activity of these purified enzymes. Consequently, the function of zinc in DNA polymerase, if any, needs to be carefully reevaluated.

RNA-dependent DNA polymerases (or reverse transcriptases) are found in type C oncogenic RNA viruses, and they catalyze the synthesis of the DNA complement from the RNA genome. Reverse transcriptases from several sources (avian myeloblastosis virus, murine leukemia, type C viruses) have been reported to be zinc metalloenzymes (58, 59).

The degradative pathway of DNA metabolism has also been reported to be affected by zinc nutriture. Nucleoside phosphorylase (EC 3.1.3.5) is an integral plasma membrane enzyme of most mammalian cells and has been widely used as a membrane marker (60). The activity of this enzyme, which cleaves phosphate from nucleoside 5-phosphates (i.e., converts inosine, deoxyinosine, and deoxyguanosine to hypoxanthine, guanosine, and xanthine, respectively) has been reported to be depressed in zinc-deficient tissues (61). Chelation studies of nucleoside phosphorylase isolated from either bacterial or mammalian cells indicate that this enzyme may require zinc for activity (62, 63). Prasad and Rabbani (61) suggested that one function of this enzyme is in the regulation of deoxyguanosine, which may be toxic to T lymphocytes. Zinc deficiency may also lead to the accumulation of the substrates of nucleoside phosphorylase in the cellular matrix of cartilage and bone.

There was about 50 percent depression in the activity of DNA-dependent RNA synthesis in *in vitro* incubation of nuclei isolated from the liver (43) or forebrain (64) of rats suckled to zinc-deficient dams. Synthesis of RNA was also depressed in cultures of (*Rhodotorula gracilis* grown in a medium low in zinc (65), whereas it was unchanged in *Mycobacterium smegmatis* grown in a medium low in zinc (66). The sequential assembly of four ribonucleoside triphosphates into RNA in the presence of DNA template and an extrinsic divalent metal ion, Mg, is catalyzed by DNA-dependent RNA polymerase (EC 2.7.7.6). The effect of zinc deficiency on RNA synthesis has been studied extensively in *Euglena gracilis* by Vallee and colleagues (67–69). Zinc deficiency alters the composition of mRNA in this organism. Normal cells of *E. gracilis* contain three types of RNA polymerase (I, II, III), unlike the zinc-deficient cells, which contain only one RNA polymerase, different in composition from RNA polymerases I, II, or III. Histones (classes H1, H2A, H2B, H3, and H4) were completely absent from the *E. gracilis* cells grown in zinc-deficient medium, in contrast to cells grown in zinc-adequate medium, which contained a normal complement of histones. An unusual group of arginine- and asparagine-rich polypeptides was associated with chromatin in zinc-deficient *E. gracilis* cells. These compounds could not be detected when zinc was added to the medium.

Since RNA polymerase from *E. coli* was first shown to be a zinc metalloenzyme containing 2 mole of zinc per mole of enzyme (70), RNA polymerases from a number of organisms have been reported to contain stoichiometric amounts of zinc (71).

Eukaryotic cells contain three nuclear RNA polymerases (I, II, and III) which transcribe different classes of cellular genes. tRNA and 5S rRNA are the most abundant transcription products of RNA polymerase III. Several auxiliary transcription factors have been described that direct the polymerase to the target gene (72). One of these transcription factors (TF III A, or factor A), isolated from *Xenopus laevis,* contains two tightly bound zinc ions, which are involved in the regulation of 5S RNA synthesis (73), and has been reported to be a zinc metalloenzyme (74). A similar zinc-containing transcription regulatory protein has been isolated for a specific gene from yeast cells (75). The structures of these proteins (zinc-finger proteins) have been partially elucidated; they contain repetitive zinc-containing domains with two pairs of cysteines and histidines, the most common ligands for zinc. This structure would explain how these small proteins can bind to the long internal control region of the 5S RNA gene and stay bound during the passage of an RNA polymerase molecule (76).

The activity of an RNA-degradative enzyme, ribonuclease, is increased in zinc-deficient tissues (77, 78), suggesting that the catabolism of RNA may be regulated by zinc.

The synthesis and activity of these enzymes and many others may be diminished by the adverse effects of zinc deficiency on protein synthesis (77, 79–84). Abnormalities related to zinc nutriture that might contribute to depression of protein synthesis are abnormal formation or stability of polyribosomes (85–88) and possibly the production of an unusual RNA polymerase that can change the base content of the RNA produced (*E. gracilis*) (89). Recently Hicks and Wallwork (84), in studies of cell-free systems isolated from the livers of zinc-deficient rats, presented evidence that suggested that zinc is involved in protein synthesis at the translational level. This study indicates that the activities of some aminoacyl-tRNA synthetases from rat liver may be zinc-dependent. The zinc content and sensitivity to zinc of a series of prokaryotic aminoacyl-tRNA synthetases have been explored (90–92). *E. coli* tyrosyl-tRNA synthetase (EC 6.1.1.1) and phenylalanyl-tRNA synthetase (EC 6.1.1.20) do not appear to contain tightly bound zinc. However, *E. coli* isoleucyl-tRNA synthetase (EC 6.1.1.5) and *E. coli* and *Bacillus stearothermophilis* methionyl-tRNA synthetase (EC 6.1.1.10) contain tightly bound zinc, and tRNA aminoacylation is reversibly inhibited by addition of o-phenanthroline (92). Furthermore, Vallee and Falchuk (93) reported that the elongation factor I from rat liver, which is involved in the synthesis of protein, is a zinc metalloprotein.

Besides being a requirement for cellular protein synthesis in general, zinc has been shown to be essential for the synthesis of histones in the rat (81, 83) and in *E. gracilis* (68). Recent observations in rats have revealed decreases in H1^O histones in liver from zinc-deficient rats (94). H1^O histones appear to play a critical role in the linking of DNA to nucleosomes, in the higher-order coiling of DNA, and perhaps in the expression of the genetic code (95–99).

ZINC, TERATOGENESIS, AND BONE DEVELOPMENT

The requirement of zinc for nucleic acid synthesis and genomic function may influence the occurrence of the teratology associated with zinc deficiency in experimental animals (100). Although the precise role of zinc in cell division and differentiation is undefined, Record (101) speculates that it is required for DNA unwinding, replication, and reassociation. Research that supports this concept includes observations of a variety of chromosomal abnormalities in rapidly dividing fetal liver cells (102) from a zinc-deficient rat dam and a report that DNA synthesis is apparently more severely affected by zinc deficiency in embryonic rat brain than in other parts of the body during early fetal life (103). A high incidence of external cranofacial anomalies such as cleft palate, micrognathia, agnathia, micropthalmia, and hydrocephalus has been recorded in zinc-deficient rat fetuses (36, 104, 105). Hickory et al. (257) reported terata that were limited mainly to vertebrae, ribs, and long bones as a consequence of Zn deficiency in rats. In addition, calcification of cranial and long bones appeared delayed. Similar terata of the skeletal system were observed in offspring from rat dams that had been subjected to streptozotocin-induced diabetes prior to mating. Styrud et al (267) pointed out that sacral dysgenesis was a teratogenic feature associated with maternal diabetes and zinc deficiency in the rat. Dietary zinc supplementation of the pregnant streptozotocin-induced diabetic rat dam improved the growth, development, and skeletal ossification in these pups, suggesting that this condition may have mimicked, in part, zinc deficiency-induced teratology (106, 107). In the guinea pig, humeral zinc concentrations increased with gestational age before term and showed a marked decline during the neonatal period (268). The rat, however, mainly accumulates skeletal zinc during postnatal development (269).

Recently, Hunt et al. (270) reported that lactational zinc deficiency in rat pups, despite postlactational zinc repletion, induced long-term imbalances in adult bone mineral metabolism. When compared to pair-fed controls at 150 days of age, these animals exhibited increased bone levels of P and Mg and decreased bone K.

ZINC, COLLAGEN, AND MUCOPOLYSACCHARIDE METABOLISM

The effects of zinc on collagen synthesis have usually been studied in the skin. Zinc deprivation has been reported to impair collagen biosynthesis in rats and to interfere with the cross-linking of peptides within the collagen structure (108–110). The latter may be responsible for the less dense appearance and abnormal staining of such collagens in histologic section. The collagen formed in zinc-deficient rats also appeared to contain a higher than normal proportion of "ground substance" and fewer fibroblastic nuclei (25). One would anticipate that zinc deficiency might produce a similar abnormality in bone collagen biosynthesis.

The biosynthesis of subcutaneous collagen and noncollagenous protein was depressed in zinc-deficient young rats (108). McClain et al. (110) reported that the incorporation of $[2\text{-}^{14}C]$glycine into alpha-1 and alpha-2 chains and L-$[U\text{-}^{14}C]$proline into the salt-soluble collagen fraction was depressed in skin from zinc-deficient rats. Suwarnasarn et al. (111) and others (112) also reported that proline incorporation into tibial epiphyseal plate was impaired in such animals. The effect of zinc nutriture on collagen cross-linking remains to be clarified. McClain and co-workers (110) reported that zinc deficiency appeared to enhance the formation of covalent intramolecular cross-links in skin collagen, because the content of beta components was increased, and the salt-soluble collagen pools contained an increased titer of aldehyde groups. They also showed that zinc deficiency apparently inhibited intermolecular covalent cross-linking, because there was a reduction in the amount of collagen that could be extracted with dilute acid solutions, and this collagen is biologically "older" than the salt-soluble moieties. However, Fernandez-Madrid et al. (108) disputed these conclusions and stated that such a cross-linking defect could only be established in zinc deficiency by determining the cross-linking profiles of collagen from zinc-deficient tissue.

Zinc deficiency appeared to influence other aspects of amino acid and protein metabolism in bones. Histidine supplementation partially alleviated bone defects that occurred in zinc-deficient chicks (113). Neilsen et al. (114) found depressed *in vivo* ^{35}S incorporation into the epiphyseal plate and the primary spongiosa of zinc-deficient chicks. Zinc deficiency also depressed *in vivo* ^{35}S incorporation into the epiphyseal plate of young rat femurs (112). There is a general consensus, then, that zinc deficiency alters the metabolism of sulfate and consequently the status of the mucopolysaccharides in the regions of bone elongation. Hsieh and Navia (115) and Bolze et al. (271) also reported that zinc deficiency interferes with glycosaminoglycan metabolism in the bone formed within alveolar implants in the guinea pig and in rib cartilage of rats, respectively. These effects of zinc deficiency on proteoglycan synthesis appear to be mediated by alterations in tissue sulfation factors, the somatomedins. The sulfation factor(s), or somatomedins, are peptides of low molecular weight that are regulated by the growth hormone. Daughaday et al. (116) reported that growth hormone produces growth indirectly through generation of a serum factor, somatomedin, which acts directly to produce cartilage proliferation and linear skeletal growth. Somatomedin increases growth of cartilage by increasing the incorporation of sulfate into chondroitin sulfate, thymidine into DNA, proline into hydroxyproline of collagen, and uridine into RNA. Cossack (117) and Bolze (271) reported a depression in plasma somatomedin-C in zinc-deficient rats as compared to zinc-adequate controls. Some of these differences may be attributable to decreased food intake in severe zinc deficiency. Subsequently, Cossack (118) found that the level of plasma somatomedin-C was inversely correlated with the zinc concentration in the tibia and with body weight gains, and concluded that the growth retardation associated with zinc deficiency relates, at least in part, to the effect of zinc deficiency on somatomedin-C.

ZINC, CARBONIC ANHYDRASE, AND COLLAGENASE

Carbonic anhydrase (EC 4.2.1.1), a zinc-dependent enzyme (119, 120), has a role in bone resorption and remodeling (121–123). Its activity in bone is believed to be mediated via parathyroid hormone (265). However, bone carbonic anhydrase activity was not reduced by zinc deficiency in rats (124). Another enzyme, which is involved in bone remodeling, is collagenase (EC 3.4.24.3). Findings of Seltzer et al. (125) suggest that rat collagenase is a zinc-containing enzyme. An adverse effect of zinc deficiency on bone collagenase activity and collagen turnover in chicks was reported by Starcher et al. (126).

ZINC AND ALKALINE PHOSPHATASE

Alkaline phosphatase (EC 3.1.3.1) is a zinc-containing enzyme, and its concentrations in bone appear to be related to osteoblastic activity (collagen and proteoglycan synthesis). The enzyme is also thought to play a role in the calcification of newly deposited bone matrix, because it carries out the nonspecific hydrolysis of phosphate monoesters in the cell. This role remains a controversial subject, since calcification can proceed in its absence (127). Dietary zinc deficiency in a number of species has been associated with a depression in the activity of alkaline phosphatase in different tissues including bone (10, 128–135). Weismann and Høyer (136) reported an inverse relationship between the activity of alkaline phosphatase and zinc concentrations in serum from a number of subjects including a young patient with zinc depletion syndrome and several individuals with acrodermatitis enteropathica. Under carefully controlled conditions in the Clinical Research Unit at the Human Nutrition Research Center in Grand Forks, North Dakota, the serum activity of alkaline phosphatase and plasma zinc concentrations from normal male volunteers fed a controlled diet were also found to be directly associated ($N = 225, r = .2487, p = .0143$) (Sandstead et al., unpublished data).

ZINC, FATTY ACIDS, AND PROSTAGLANDINS

Recently, it has been proposed that zinc is needed for the activity of the 6 and 5 desaturase enzymes which act in sequence on linoleic acid to produce γ-linoleic and arachidonic acids, as well as in several reactions in the synthesis of prostaglandins (137, 138). Odutuga (139) also reported abnormalities in fatty acid profiles of bones and teeth from zinc-deficient rats. He postulated a role for zinc in prostaglandin biosynthesis from essential fatty acids that could influence bone or tooth mineralization. Because tissue prostaglandin levels have been implicated in both bone formation and bone resorption, a deficit in its biosynthesis would be expected to reduce connective tissue synthesis and turnover in the skeleton (140–143). The effects of prostaglandins are concentration dependent causing bone resorption at high concentration and stimulation of bone formation *in vivo* when they are administered chronically to rats (277).

ZINC NUTRITURE AND BONE ZINC CONTENT

As predicted from the findings of Follis et al. (15), the zinc content of bone reflects the zinc status of growing animals. This relationship has been shown by several observers (144). Demonstration of this relationship is shown in Fig. 16-1 (145). Findings from this study suggest that the zinc requirement for optimal growth in Fisher 344 rats is about 6 $\mu g/g$ in a diet based on spray-dried egg white protein (20% by weight) that provides at least 140 percent of NRC requirements for minerals (145). The experiment showed that excess dietary zinc (above 6 $\mu g/$ g of diet) caused the accumulation of zinc in the bones of young rats independent of growth. This finding is in agreement with earlier observations on rats (147, 148), Japanese quail (149), and carp (150).

The availability of bone zinc for metabolism of other tissues has been the subject of several studies the results of which appear to be controversial. Brown et al. (151) found that the lower total bone zinc and bone zinc concentrations of severely zinc-deficient growing rats were apparently independent from their bone calcium and phosphorus turnovers. They suggested that bone zinc mobilized during periods of dietary zinc deficiency was distributed to other tissues in growing animals. Giugliano and Millward (272) studied severe zinc deficiency in immature male rats and concluded that bone slowly gives up zinc to support minimal muscle growth. Harland et al. (149) found that zinc supplementation prior to zinc restriction resulted in improved growth of Japanese quail. In general, then, (excess) bone

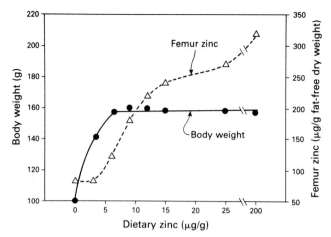

Fig. 16-1 Body weights and femur zinc concentrations of growing rats fed increasing levels of zinc in a 20 percent egg white diet for 28 days. Thirty-day-old male rats were fed 20 percent spray-dried egg white diets enriched with biotin for 28 days. The mineral mix was formulated to provide at least 140 percent of the NRC requirements for rats (84). Different levels of zinc were added to the diet and fed to eight groups of animals. These include unsupplemented (0.4 µg Zn/g diet) and 3, 6, 9, 12, 15, 25, and 200 µg Zn/g diet. Six animals were used in each dietary group. Femur zinc was measured according to the procedure described by Wallwork et al. (146).

zinc stores in growing animals can be mobilized during periods of zinc deprivation, and the same proviso for withdrawal-upon-demand appears to pertain to fetal guinea pig bone (268). However, zinc release from bone is probably negligible in the absence of active bone turnover, a phenomenon that is most clearly demonstrable during growth or in a calcium-deficient state (100, 152). Murray and Messer's (152) studies in growing zinc-deficient rats indicated that bone zinc is only released in a "passive manner"; zinc deficiency did not increase the rate of bone resorption as measured by the release of ^{3}H-tetracycline. Consistent with this interpretation, we (Wallwork and Sandstead, unpublished data) observed only a small difference (5–6%) between femur zinc concentrations from adult male rats subjected to either a severely zinc-deficient or a zinc-supplemented diet for an extended period of 85 days (Table 16-1). Similar findings were reported by Hurley and Tao (153), who found that very little zinc was released from the skeleton of mature pregnant rats unless their dietary intake of calcium was severely restricted. Murray et al. (154) point out that the increased availability of zinc during conditions of simultaneous zinc and calcium deficiencies appears to be strictly secondary to bone resorption, and under the influence of parathyroid hormone in response to calcium deficiency rather than zinc deficiency directly promoting bone absorption.

The effect of bone resorption on the release of zinc from the skeleton may be important during lactation. This situation is particularly true in the rat, where a significant amount of skeletal mineral must be released to maintain the high calcium content of that species' milk. Lactational mineral mobilization, then, could be viewed, in part, as an adaptation required for the nutriture of the large number

Table 16-1 Body Weights and Femur Zinc Concentration for Adult Long-Evans Male Rats Maintained on a Zinc-Deficient Diet With and Without Zinc Supplementation (25 ppm Zn) in the Drinking Water for 85 Days (mean ± SD)[a]

Dietary regimen	Number of rats in group	Starting weight (g)	Final weight (g)	Weight change (g)	Femur zinc[b]
Zinc-deficient	9	606 ± 90	532 ± 77	−75 ± 46[a]	431 ± 22[a]
Zinc-adequate Pair-fed	9	596 ± 89	520 ± 23	−76 ± 57[a]	466 ± 23[b]
Ad libitum-fed	5	573 ± 29	616 ± 34	43 ± 18[b]	454 ± 16[b]

[a]Values not sharing a common postscript letter are significantly different—$p < .05$.
[b]Fat-free dry weight (μg/g).

of pups in a normal litter. Maternal dietary calcium intake during this period is also critical. Very low dietary calcium levels result in about a 50 percent loss of skeletal mineral during lactation (155–158), but such losses are much less when dietary calcium levels are adequate. Animals fed a normal rat chow (Ca = 1.2%) during gestation and lactation will lose about 15–35 percent of their skeletal mineral (159–161). On a comparative basis, maternal rats lose dramatically more bone calcium and phosphorus per kilogram than lactating humans (162). For example, a 300-g rat secretes 190–225 mg Ca/kg/day through the breast milk (163), whereas a 60-kg woman loses only 4–6 mg Ca/kg/day through the breast milk (650–1,000 ml/day) (164). Greer et al. (165) reported that lactating women appeared able to compensate for loss of calcium and phosphorus during the early months of lactation. These findings appeared to conflict with earlier reports of loss of bone mineral during the first 3 months of lactation in humans (166–168). In addition, Wardlaw and Pike (169) reported that even though women consumed the RDA for calcium, long-term lactation (i.e., three or four infants for intervals of approximately 11 months for each child) caused a 15 percent depletion of the ultradistal bone mass in the forearm.

Murray et al. (154) also observed that zinc-adequate but calcium-deficient growing rats had femur zinc concentrations that were nearly double the levels in zinc-adequate, calcium-adequate controls. This finding might indicate that the zinc accumulated in the noncalcified matrix that was formed in response to zinc deficiency. Some of this zinc was probably present in alkaline phosphatase, which is increased under such circumstances (170).

ZINC NUTRITURE AND BONE HISTOLOGY

The essentiality of zinc for bone formation is further suggested by several studies. Haumont (171) found high concentrations of zinc at the sites of calcification in the long bones of dogs. Skeletal abnormalities were a conspicuous feature of zinc deficiency in growing birds (16–18). In the epiphyses of zinc-deficient chicks, the chondrocytes nearest the blood vessels were apparently histologically normal. However, the cells remote from blood vessels were shaped differently; they resided in a more cellular matrix and stained with a lower than normal intensity for alkaline phosphatase (16), and their patterns of differentiation/maturation were delayed and erratic (172). This picture is consistent with a pattern of impaired chondrogenesis (16, 173) and bone calcification (174) (see also effect of Zn deprivation on ^{35}S incorporation, p. 555). Osteoblastic activity in the body collar of the long bones was also depressed. In zinc-deficient pullets, the long bones were shortened and thickened, and these changes occurred in proportion to the degree of zinc deficiency (18).

Rats appear to respond to zinc deficiency in a fashion similar to that of avian species. An impairment in chondrogenesis and calcification of cartilage was shown by the failure of the growth plates to thin with age (111). Zinc-deficient rats also fail to form a normal thickness of circummetaphyseal compact bone as viewed by scanning electron microscopy (Fig. 16-2). These deficits compromised the biomechanical competence of the tissue. Experiments showed that the force required to displace the epiphysis of zinc-deficient weanling rats was consistently less than that required for their pair-fed controls (Fig. 16-3).

ZINC AND NUTRIENT INTERACTIONS: EFFECT ON BONE GROWTH AND DEVELOPMENT

Zinc and Protein

Protein malnutrition has been reported to reduce bone growth in pigs, rhesus monkeys, and rats (175–177). Zinc deficiency may be associated with human protein energy malnutrition (178, 179) and may be exacerbated during recovery, when the growth rate is rapid (180, 181). In such children, multiple factors contribute to impaired bone growth. Among these factors is protein deficiency, which results in fewer amino acids being available for glycoprotein and collagen synthesis (see

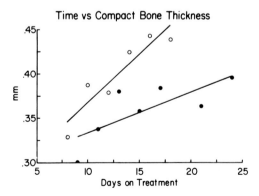

Fig. 16-2 Relationship between compact bone thickness and time of treatment O—O, zinc-restricted rats, y = 0.26 + 0.01x; ●—●, zinc-adequate pair-fed control rats, y = 0.29 + 0.005x. The two lines are significantly different (p < .005). After x = 13.2 days, the compact bone thicknesses for the zinc-deficient rats are significantly (p < .05) greater than those representing the pair-fed rats. (From Suwarnasarn et al. (111), with permission.]

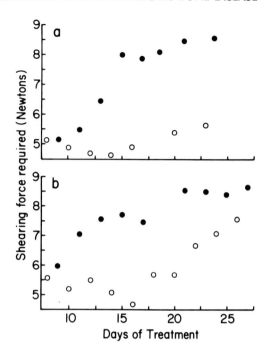

Fig. 16-3 Relationship between the shearing force required to displace the epiphysis and time of treatment for both zinc-deficient (○—○) and pair-fed control (●—●) male rats from (a) the first trial and (b) the second trial. (From Suwarnasarn et al. (111), with permission.]

p. 549). Furthermore, zinc deficiency prevents effective utilization of amino acids for protein synthesis (77, 79–84).

Wallwork et al. (148) reported an example of the interaction between zinc and protein nutriture as it affected bone zinc content in rats. When dietary protein was 6 percent and zinc 6 μg/g, mean (± SD) femur zinc concentration was 139 (± 28) μg/g dry fat-free weight. When zinc was held at 6 μg/g but the protein content increased to 11.3 and 15.0 percent, femur zinc levels were reduced to 61 percent (85 ± 19 μg/g) and 54 percent (75 ± 5μg/g), respectively. The lower growth rate of the protein-deprived (6% dietary protein) rats probably accounted for these differences.

Zinc, Calcium, and Phosphorus

The essentiality of calcium for bone and tooth development and repair is well documented. Recently the practice of calcium supplementation of women of all ages for the prevention of osteoporosis has been a subject of controversy (182–186). Such supplementation may influence intestinal absorption and/or homeostasis of several minerals including zinc. This interaction is exemplified by a high positive correlation between the circadian changes in serum zinc and ionized calcium concentrations (six healthy adult men) (187). This study suggested that a common regulator may control the serum biorhythms. In experimental animals the adverse effect of dietary calcium on intestinal absorption of zinc (188–192) was attributed to excess phytic acid in the diet (193–195). However, a direct effect of a high calcium intake, in the absence of phytic acid, on absorption and retention of ^{65}Zn was shown in rats (196). The addition of phosphorus to experimental diets further enhanced the adverse effect of calcium on zinc retention (197). More recently, however, in an exhaustive study Greger and colleagues (266) could find little effect of calcium supplementation in several forms (including calcium phosphate dibasic, calcium lactate, calcium carbonate with and without supplemental iron and vitamins, dolomite, oyster shell, and nonfat dry milk) on the utilization of zinc by rats.

Similar findings were obtained in humans. Using calcium gluconate as a source of calcium, Spencer et al. (198) found that a 10-fold increase in calcium intake did not impair ^{65}Zn absorption of men. More recently, they reported that great variation in dietary calcium and phosphorus did not influence the zinc balance of 36 adult men under controlled conditions (199). Similar findings, using calcium carbonate and hydroxyapatite as the calcium source, were observed in studies of ^{65}Zn absorption in 13 postmenopausal women (200). On the basis of these studies it does not appear that calcium supplements, as commonly consumed, impair zinc nutriture.

On the other hand, the effects of dietary constituents may be another matter. Studies by Pecoud et al. (201) have shown that dairy products and calcium- and phosphorus-rich foods caused reduced intestinal absorption of zinc. There is no ready explanation for this effect. It has been suggested that the binding of zinc by phosphorylated bovine casein submits causes depressed bioavailability (202). In addition, metabolic studies of 45 normal men indicated that increased dietary phosphorus and protein were associated with reduced zinc retention (203, 204). This finding is consistent with experimental findings of Greger and Snedeker (205). Further analysis of the data by regression analysis suggested that an interaction between dietary calcium and phytate and the level of dietary protein (nitrogen) influences zinc retention. The equation that described this relationship is: Zinc retention $= -0.66 + 0.40$ (diet zinc) $- 0.14$ (diet nitrogen) $- 10.49$ (diet calcium $\times$ diet phytate); $r^2 = .20$, $p < .0001$, $N = 195$. This finding in humans is consistent with the above-noted interaction of calcium and phytate that impaired calcium retention of experimental animals (206). Solomons et al. (207) demonstrated an inhibitory effect of tortillas and frijoles on absorption of zinc from oyster. We interpret these findings as indicating that habitual consumption of such foods that are rich in dietary fiber, Maillard browning products, phytic acid, and calcium (from the lime-soaked corn) might adversely affect zinc nutriture over the long term and, thus, might contribute to growth retardation.

Parfitt (208) considered zinc to be a dietary component that could be an important factor in bone loss. In support of this concept, Freudenheim et al. (209) found a positive association between dietary zinc and change in mineral content of the radius in postmenopausal women who were not supplemented with zinc (i.e., high levels of zinc intake correlated with slower loss of bone mineral). On the other hand, Murray and Messer (152) could find no relationship between zinc status, bone resorption, and the rate of zinc deposition in rat bone under conditions of either passive bone turnover or accelerated bone loss induced by a calcium-deficient diet.

Zinc has been reported to stimulate differentiated cell functions—the ability of osteoblasts to synthesize and export collagen (273). Using roller tube cultures of embryonic chick femurs, Kaji et al. (274) showed that excess Zn caused a tenfold increase in medium alkaline phosphatase. They suggested that excess Zn inhibited physicochemical calcification and induced osteomalacia. Feeding unphysiologically high levels of dietary zinc (1,000–2,000 ppm) has been reported to cause reduced weight and ash content of bones from growing rats (262–264). This osteopenic effect was not observed in thyroparathyroidectomized (TPTX) rats (264), indicating that high intakes of zinc stimulated bone resorption through the actions of parathyroid hormone. From a study of TPTX rats, Chausmer et al. (210) reported that parathyroid hormone caused an increased accumulation of ^{65}Zn in certain soft tissues and bone by an apparent nonspecific effect, whereas calcitonin appeared to have specific influences on zinc homeostasis.

Zinc and Vitamin D

1,25-Dihydroxycalciferol increases intestinal absorption of calcium and phosphate, epiphyseal plate calcification, and percent femur ash in rats (211). Vitamin D nutriture has also been linked to zinc utilization. Several apparently conflicting reports have appeared in the literature, so the nature of this interaction is unclear. However, it may be species-specific or related to age and growth.

In the chick, the effect of dietary vitamin D on zinc absorption or utilization appears somewhat more controversial. Wasserman (212) could find no difference in ^{65}Zn absorption from ligated duodenum segments in either rachitic or cholecalciferol-supplemented chicks. In a similar experimental model, Koo et al. (213) found that neither cholecalciferol nor 1,25-dihydroxycalciferol appeared to affect zinc absorption directly. Nevertheless, when cholecalciferol was added to a diet deficient in both vitamin D and calcium, chicks showed a significant improvement in the skeletal uptake of ^{65}Zn (214, 215). The apparent interaction probably took place during intestinal absorption, since cholecalciferol administered by subcutaneous injection failed to influence ^{65}Zn uptake by bone (215). The skeletal incorporation of radiozinc in the chick appears to be inversely related to dietary calcium levels. Supplements of cholecalciferol to chicks reared on calcium-adequate/zinc-deficient and calcium-adequate/zinc-adequate diets decreased radiozinc deposition into tibial bone (214). Yet, these relationships may not pertain to the adult bird. Keinholz et al. (216) observed that an eightfold increase in dietary cholecalciferol caused a twofold increase in adult hen femur zinc.

In swine, vitamin D decreased zinc absorption when dietary zinc intake was low but had no affect when dietary zinc was adequate (217). In rats, Becker and Hoekstra (218) reported that vitamin D caused an increase in zinc absorption from the intestine when zinc-supplemented diets were fed. This effect was not found when zinc-deficient diets were fed or when ^{65}Zn was injected. Vitamin D also appeared to increase zinc deposition in bone but not soft tissues. The findings suggested that deposition of zinc in the skeleton was secondary to the effect of vitamin D on bone growth. Chang et al. (219) also found that vitamin D caused an increase in the bone zinc of rats when the diets contained either 9 percent or 18 percent protein. They concluded that the effect of vitamin D on bone deposition of zinc was not a secondary event that occurred with calcification and growth. Their interpretation was based on the finding of increased bone calcification when dietary protein was increased, whereas there was no significant increase in femur zinc when dietary zinc was increased. Recently, the active form of vitamin D, $1,25(OH)_2D_3$ was shown to have a marked inhibitory effect on bone resorption and appeared to enhance the accumulation of Zn and Ca in bone of young adult female rats (275).

More recently Leek et al. (220) reported delayed bone growth and defective mineralization in infant rhesus monkeys that had been subjected to a marginally zinc-deficient diet from conception to age 3 years. The retardation in skeletal maturation was persistent during this time, but bone mineralization began to recover after 6 months and was only slightly subnormal at 3 years (276). Some of these skeletal abnormalities appeared to resemble symptoms of rickets observed in humans (e.g., bowing and fracture formations). Unfortunately, vitamin D measurements were not performed in this study.

Perhaps related to these observations is a report in which the bone and dentine of rats fed a high intake of zinc (4240 μg/g diet) accumulated zinc four- to six-fold when there was concomitant calcium deficiency (221). The rate, extent of uptake, and subsequent release of this sequestered zinc appeared less when vitamin D was added to the diet (222). In addition, an interaction between zinc and vitamin D was suggested by Sivakumar and Belavady (223), who reported that a concomitant zinc deficiency exacerbated the low calcium absorption that was associated with vitamin D deficiency in weanling rats.

In summary, there appears as yet to be no general, well-characterized consistent effect of vitamin D on zinc metabolism. Perhaps species or age play a role in this interaction.

ZINC DEFICIENCY IN HUMANS

The first evidence of zinc deficiency in man was in a report concerning Chinese subjects with protein deficiency (5, 6). Since then chronic zinc deficiency has been reported in adolescents in Egypt and Iran (8–10, 224). These male subjects displayed severely stunted growth and hypogonadism (9) that was responsive to zinc treatment (225). The main contributing factors to this deficiency were probably the high intake of bread prepared from whole-meal wheat flour and very infrequent intake of red meat or other sources of readily bioavailable zinc. The consumption of whole-meal unleavened wheat bread, as is common among villagers in Egypt and Iran, results in high intakes of dietary fiber, lignin, phytate, and products of Maillard browning. Such foods have been shown to impair zinc retention by humans (226–229). Subjects in Egypt were often infested with hookworm and schistosomiasis and thus had chronic blood loss. Subjects in Iran were clay eaters, which presumably sequestered zinc in the intestine and prevented its absorption (224). Clay contains negatively charged ions, which tend to bind positively charged metal ions such as zinc and iron. Consequently, these dietary components fail to be absorbed from the intestine and are excreted in the feces. The high calcium content of clay may also play a role, because the predominant food of these people is cereal, which has a high phytate concentration, and this could lead to the formation of insoluble complexes of calcium, zinc, and phosphate. Zinc would again be lost to the body and excreted in the feces. The zinc deficiency syndrome has since been described from Turkey (230, 231) and China (232).

Infants and children suffering from protein–energy malnutrition are at risk from zinc deficiency (179). Those children being treated by food supplementation and showing signs of recovery from protein–energy malnutrition display signs of zinc deficiency if not supplemented (180, 181). Severe zinc deficiency is less prevalent in the industrialized countries, but certain groups have been shown to be at risk. These include infants with acrodermatitis enteropathica (21, 233–235); inadequately fed, premature infants (236); persons given prolonged inadequate parenteral (237–239) or enteral (31) alimentation; patients with severe intestinal malabsorption (23, 240, 241), uremia (242), or sickle cell anemia (243); cases of alcoholism and cirrhosis of the liver (22, 244); and diabetic women and their offspring (245). Less severe zinc deficiency has been reported in infants (246, 247), young children (246, 248–252), adolescents (253, 254), and the elderly (23, 204, 255, 256, 258–260).

In these various zinc deficiency syndromes, abnormalities in bone that can be directly related to zinc nutriture, other than depressed growth, have not been clearly characterized. X-ray examination of the long bones of severely growth-retarded, zinc-deficient Egyptian male adolescents (aged 12–19 years) indicated that their bone age was approximately 60 percent of chronological age (261). This information confirmed the trends of the height and weight age determinations of these subjects (10, 225).

SUMMARY

In this review, we have addressed the role of zinc in skeletal development and mineral metabolism. *First,* zinc is essential for the prenatal and postnatal growth of bone and mineral metabolism. Nutritional zinc deprivation causes fetal skeletal abnormalities in several species, and it decreases linear and radial growth, collagen synthesis, and bone zinc levels in growing animals. The histology of the Zn-deficient epiphyseal growth plate becomes less well defined, and the biomechanical competence of the tissue suffers in the sense that lower than normal forces are required to displace the epiphyses. *Second,* evidence exists that it is difficult to correct the effects of chronic zinc deficiency. In previously zinc-deficient animals and man, nutritional repletion with adequate zinc for extended time periods does not completely reverse the abnormalities in mineral metabolism. *Third,* we have noted the controversy that exists about the availability of bone zinc stores for somatic and skeletal growth during episodes of zinc deficiency in humans and experimental animals. There is radiologic evidence that the epiphyses of zinc-deficient growth-stunted Egyptian children remain open for an extended time period. The role of zinc in all of these processes relates to knowledge that the element, as part of metalloenzymes, is required for DNA, RNA, and protein synthesis, and that it is also a structural component of finger proteins. Zinc metalloenzymes such as carbonic anhydrase and collagenase are important in bone resorption and remodeling. This larger picture involves the synthesis of growth factors (somatomedins, prostaglandins), mitogenesis and chondro-osseous matrix, as well as the interrelationships between zinc nutriture and several other nutrients such as protein, vitamin D, calcium, and phosphorus. Thus, zinc appears to be directly and indirectly involved in the interactive processes that influence bone modeling and remodeling.

REFERENCES

1. Raulin, J. (1869) Ann. Sci. Natl. Botan. Biol. Veg. 11:93–299.
2. Maze, P. (1914) Ann. Inst. Pasteur 28:21–69.
3. Sommer, A. L., Lipman, C. B. (1926) Plant Physiol. 1:231–249.
4. Todd, W. R., Elvehjem, C. A., Hart, E. B. (1934) Am. J. Physiol. 107:146–156.
5. Eggleton, W. G. E. (1939) Biochem. J. 33:403–406.
6. Eggleton, W. G. E. (1940) Biochem. J. 34:991–997.
7. Vallee, B. L., Wacker, W. E. C., Bartholomay, A. F., Robin, E. D. (1956) New Engl. J. Med. 255:403–408.
8. Prasad, A. S., Halsted, J. A., Nadimi, M. (1961) Am. J. Med. 31:532–546.
9. Prasad, A. S., Miale, A., Jr., Farid, Z., Sandstead, H. H., Schulert, A. R., Darby, W. J. (1963) Arch. Intern. Med. 111:407–428.
10. Prasad, A. S., Schulert, A. R., Miale, A., Jr., Farid, Z., Sandstead, H. H. (1963) Am. J. Clin. Nutr. 12:437–444.
11. Sandstead, H. H. (1973) Am. J. Clin. Nutr. 26:1251–1260.
12. World Health Organization (1973) Report of a WHO Expert Committee. WHO Technical Report Series No. 532. Geneva: World Health Organization, 63pp.
13. Sandstead, H. H. (1981) In: Bronner, F., Coburn, J. W. (eds) *Disorders of Mineral Metabolism*. New York: Academic Press, pp. 94–157.
14. Hambidge, K. M., Casey, C. E., Krebs, N. F. (1986) In: Mertz, W. (ed) *Trace Elements in Human and Animal Nutrition*. New York: Academic Press, pp. 81–89.
15. Follis, R. H., Jr., Day, H. G., McCollum, E. V. (1941) J. Nutr. 22:223–237.
16. O'Dell, B. L., Newberne, F. M., Savage, J. E. (1958) J. Nutr. 65:503–533.
17. Fox, M. R. S., Harrison, B. N. (1964) Proc. Soc. Exp. Biol. Med. 116:256–259.
18. Zeigler, T. R., Scott, M. L., McEvoy, R. K., Greenlaw, R. H., Huegin, F., Strain, W. H. (1962) Proc. Soc. Exp. Biol. Med. 109:239–242.
19. Miller, J. K., Miller, W. J. (1962) J. Nutr. 6:467–474.
20. Miller, E. R., Luecke, R. W., Ullrey, D. E., Baltzer, B. V., Bradley, B. L., Hoefer, J. A. (1969) J. Nutr. 95:278–286.
21. Moynahan, E. J. (1974) Lancet II:399–400.
22. Weismann, K., Roed-Petersen, J., Hjorth, N., Kopp, H. (1976) Int. J. Dermatol. 15:757–761.
23. Weismann, K., Wanscher, B., Krakauer, R. (1978) Acta Dermatovener (Stockholm) 58:157–161.
24. Sandstead, H. H., Shepard, G. H. (1968) Proc. Soc. Exp. Biol. Med. 128:687–689.
25. Sandstead, H. H., Lanier, V. C., Shepard, G. H., Gillespie, D. (1970) Am. J. Clin. Nutr. 23:514–519.
26. Oberleas, D., Seymour, J. K., Lenaglian, R., Hovanesian, J., Wilson, R. F., Prasad, A. S. (1971) Am. J. Surg. 121:566–568.
27. Hsu, T. H. S., Hsu, J. M. (1972) Proc. Soc. Exp. Biol. Med. 140:157–160.

28. Buerk, C. A., Chandy, M. G., Pearson, E., MacAuly, A., Soroff, H. S. (1973) Surg. Forum 24:101–103.

29. Haeger, K., Lanner, E. (1974) J. Vas. Dis. 3:77–81.

30. Fraker, P. J., Haas, S. M., Luecke, R. W. (1977) J. Nutr. 107:1889–1895.

31. Pekarek, R. S., Sandstead, H. H., Jacob, R. A., Barcome, D. F. (1979) Am. J. Clin. Nutr. 32:1466–1471.

32. Duchateau, J., Delespesse, G., Vereeke, P. (1981) Am. J. Clin. Nutr. 34:88–93.

33. Beach, R. S., Gershwin, M. E., Hurley, L. S. (1982) Science 218:469–471.

34. Dardenne, M., Pleau, J.-M., Nabarra, B., Lefrancier, P., Derrien, M., Choay, J., Bach, J.-F. (1982) Proc. Natl. Acad. Sci. USA 79:5370–5373.

35. Hurley, L. S., Swenerton, H. (1966) Proc. Soc. Exp. Biol. Med. 123:692–696.

36. Warkany, J., Petering, H. G. (1972) Teratology 5:319–334.

37. Barney, G. H., Orgebin-Crist, M. C., Macapinlac, M. P. (1968) J. Nutr. 95:526–534.

38. Underwood, E. J., Somers, M. (1969) Aust. J. Agric. Res. 20:889–897.

39. Abbasi, A. A., Prasad, A. S., Rabbani, P., DuMouchelle, E. (1980) J. Lab. Clin. Med. 96:544–550.

40. Fujii, T. (1954) Nature (Lond) 174:1108–1109.

41. Sandstead, H. H., Rinaldi, R. A. (1969) J. Cell. Physiol. 73:81–83.

42. Williams, R. B., Chesters, J. K. (1970) Br. J. Nutr. 24:1053–1059.

43. Terhune, M. W., Sandstead, H. H. (1972) Science 177:68–69.

44. Prasad, A. S., Oberleas, D. (1974) J. Lab. Clin. Med. 83:634–639.

45. Record, I. R., Dreosti, I. E. (1979) Nutr. Rep. Intern. 20:729–755.

46. Record, I. R., Dreosti, I. E., Smith, R. M. (1980) Proc. Aust. Biochem. Soc. 13:98.

47. Dreosti, I. E. (1984) In: Frederickson, C. J., Howell, G. A., Kasarskis, E. J. (eds) The Neurobiology of Zinc. Part A: Physiochemistry, Anatomy, and Techniques. New York: Alan R. Liss, pp. 1–26.

48. Lieberman, I., Abrams, R., Hunt, N., Ove, P. (1963) J. Biol. Chem. 238:3955–3962.

49. Swenerton, H., Shrader, R., Hurley, L. S. (1969) Science 166:1014–1015.

50. Chang, L. M. S., Bollum, F. J. (1970) Proc. Nat. Acad. Sci. USA 65:1041–1048.

51. Slater, J. P., Mildvan, A. S., Loeb, L. A. (1971) Biochem. Biophys. Res. Commun. 44:37–43.

52. Springgate, C. F., Mildvan, A. S., Abramson, R., Engle, J. L., Loeb, L. A. (1973) J. Biol. Chem. 249:5987–5993.

53. Mildvan, A. S., Loeb, L. A. (1979) CRC Crit. Rev. Biochem. 6:819–844.

54. Walton, K. E., Fitzgerald, P. C., Herrmann, M. S., Behnke, D. (1982) Biochem. Biophys. Res. Commun. 108:1353–1361.

55. Ferrin, L. J., Mildvan, A. S., Loeb, L. A. (1983) Biochem. Biophys. Res. Commun. 112:723–728.

56. Graham, D. R., Sigman, D. S. (1984) Inorg. Chem. 23:4188–4191.

57. Slaby, I., Lind, B., Holmgren, A. (1984) Biochem. Biophys. Res. Commun. 122:1410–1417.

58. Auld, D. S., Kawaguchi, H., Livingston, D. M., Vallee, B. L. (1974) Proc. Nat. Acad. Sci. USA 71:819–844.

59. Poiesz, B. J., Seal, G., Loeb, L. A. (1974) Proc. Nat. Acad. Sci. USA 71:4892–4896.

60. Solyom, A., Trams, E. G. (1972) Enzyme 13:329–372.

61. Prasad, A. S., Rabbani, P. (1981) Trans. Assoc. Am. Physicians 94:314–321.

62. Dvorak, H. F., Heppel, L. A. (1968) J. Biol. Chem. 243:2647–2653.

63. Pilz, R. B., Willis, R. C., Seegmiller, J. E. (1982) J. Biol. Chem. 257:13544–13549.

64. Fosmire, G. J., Al-Ubaidi, Y. Y., Halas, E., Sandstead, H. H. (1974) In: Frieden, E. (ed) *Advances in Experimental Medicine and Biology*. Vol. 48. New York: Plenum, pp. 329–343.

65. Cocucci, M. C., Rossi, G. (1972) Arch. Mikrobiol. 85:267–279.

66. Harris, A. B. (1969) J. Gen. Microbiol. 56:27–33.

67. Stankiewicz, A. J., Falchuk, K. H., Vallee, B. L. (1983) Biochem. 22:5150–5156.

68. Mazus, B., Falchuk, K. H., Vallee, B. L. (1984) Biochem. 23:42–47.

69. Falchuk, K. H., Mazus, B., Ber, E., Ulpino-Lobb, L., Vallee, B. L. (1985) Biochem. 24:2576–2580.

70. Scrutton, M. C., Wu, C. W., Goldthwait, D. A. (1971) Proc. Nat. Acad. Sci. USA 68:2497–2501.

71. Wu, F. Y.-H., Wu, C.-W., (1987) Ann. Rev. Nutr. 7:251–272.

72. Shastry, B. S., Ng, S.-Y., Roeder, R. G. (1982) J. Biol. Chem. 257:12979–12986.

73. Wu, C.-W. (1986) In: Bertini, I., Luchinet, C., Maret, W., Zeppezauer, M. (eds) *Zinc Enzymes*. Boston: Birkhauser, pp. 563–573.

74. Hanas, J. S., Hazuda, D. J., Wu, C.-W., (1985) J. Biol. Chem. 260:13316–13320.

75. Blumberg, H., Eisen, A., Sledziewski, A., Bader, D., Young, E. T. (1987) Nature (London) 328:443–445.

76. Miller, J., McLachlan, A. D., Klug, A. (1985) EMBO J. 4:1609–1614.

77. Somers, M., Underwood, E. J. (1969) Aust. J. Biol. Sci. 22:1277–1282.

78. Prasad, A. S., Oberleas, D. (1973) J. Lab. Clin. Med. 82:461–466.

79. Hsu, J. M., Anthony, W. L., Buchanan, P. J. (1969) J. Nutr. 99:425–432.

80. Grey, P., Dreosti, I. E. (1972) J. Comp. Pathol. 82:223–228.

81. Duerre, J. A., Ford, K. M., Sandstead, H. H. (1977) J. Nutr. 107:1082–1093.

82. Fosmire, G. J., Sandstead, H. H. (1977) Proc. Soc. Exp. Biol. Med. 154:351–355.

83. Wallwork, J. C., Duerre, J. A. (1985) J. Nutr. 115:252–262.

84. Hicks, S. E., Wallwork, J. C. (1987) J. Nutr. 117:1234–1240.

85. Tal, M. (1969) Biochim. Biophys. Acta 195:76–86.

86. Prask, J. A., Plocke, J. A. (1971) Plant Physiol. 48:150–155.

87. Sandstead, H. H., Terhune, M. W. (1974) In: Pories, W. J., Strain, W. H., Hsu, J. M., Woosley, R. W. (eds) *Clinical Applications of Zinc Metabolism*. Springfield, IL: Charles C. Thomas, pp. 9–18.

88. Fosmire, G. J., Fosmire, M. A., Sandstead, H. H. (1976) J. Nutr. 106:1152–1158.

89. Falchuk, K. H., Hardy, C., Ulpino, L., Vallee, B. L. (1977) Biochem. Biophys. Res. Commun. 77:314–319.

90. Posorske, L. H., Cohn, M., Yanagisawa, N., Auld, D. S. (1979) Biochim. Biophys. Acta 576:128–133.

91. Igloi, G. L., von der Haar, F., Cramer, F. (1980) Biochem. 19:1676–1680.

92. Mayaux, J.-F., Blanquet, S. (1981) Biochem. 20:4647–4654.

93. Vallee, B. L., Falchuk, K. H. (1981) Phil. Trans. R. Soc. Lond. B294:185–197.

94. Castro, C. F., Alvares, O. F., Sevall, J. S. (1986) Nutr. Rep. Intern. 34:67–74.

95. Thoma, F., Koller, T., Klug, A. (1979) J. Cell. Biol. 83:403–427.

96. Boulikas, T., Wiseman, J. M., Garrard, W. T. (1980) Proc. Natl. Acad. Sci. USA 77:127–131.

97. Smith, B. J., Johns, E. W. (1980) Nucleic Acids Res. 8:6069–6079.

98. Gjerset, R., Gorka, C., Hasthorpe, S., Lawrence, J. J., Eisen, H. (1982) Proc. Natl. Acad. Sci. USA 79:2333–2337.

99. Lennox, R. W. (1984) J. Biol. Chem. 259:669–672.

100. Hurley, L. S. (1981) Physiol. Rev. 61:249–295.

101. Record, I. R. (1987) Neurotoxicol. 8:369–378.

102. Bell, L. T., Branstrator, M., Roux, C., Hurley, L. S. (1975) Teratology 12:221–226.

103. Eckhert, C. D., Hurley, L. S. (1977) J. Nutr. 107:855–861.

104. Hurley, L. S., Gowan, J., Swenerton, H. (1971) Teratology 4:199–204.

105. Dreosti, I. E., Grey, P. C., Wilkins, P. J. (1972) S. Afr. Med. J. 46:1585–1588.

106. Uriu-Hare, J. Y., Stern, J. S., Reaven, G. M., Keen, C. L. (1985) Diabetes 34:1031–1040.

107. Uriu-Hare, J. Y., Stern, J. S., Keen, C. L. (1987) Fed. Proc. 46:595 (abstr).

108. Fernandez-Madrid, F., Prasad, A. S., Oberleas, D. (1973) J. Lab. Clin. Med. 82:951–961.

109. McClain, P. E. (1977) In: Friedman, M. (ed) *Protein Crosslinking-B Nutritional and Medical Consequences*. New York: Plenum, pp. 603–618.

110. McClain, P. E., Wiley, E. R., Beecher, G. R., Anthony, W. L., Hsu, J. M. (1973) Biochim. Biophys. Acta 304:457–465.

111. Suwarnasarn, A., Wallwork, J. C., Lykken, G. I., Low, F. N., Sandstead, H. H. (1982) J. Nutr. 112:1320–1328.

112. Lema, O., Sandstead, H. H. (1970) Fed. Proc. 29:297 (abstr).

113. Nielsen, F. H., Sunde, M. L., Hoekstra, W. G. (1967) Proc. Soc. Exp. Biol. Med. 124:1106–1110.

114. Nielsen, F. H., Dowdy, R. P., Ziporin, Z. Z. (1970) J. Nutr. 100:903–908.

115. Hsieh, H. S., Navia, J. M. (1980) J. Nutr. 110:1581–1588.

116. Daughaday, W. H., Hall, K., Raben, M. S., Salmon, W. D., Jr., Van den Braude, J. L., Van Wyk, J. J. (1972) Nature (London) 235:107.

117. Cossack, Z. T. (1984) Experientia 40:498–500.

118. Cossack, Z. T. (1986) Br. J. Nutr. 56:163–169.

119. Keilin, D., Mann, T. (1940) Biochem. J. 34:1163–1176.

120. Riordan, J. F., Vallee, B. L. (1976) In: Prasad, A. S., Oberleas, D. (eds) *Trace Elements in Human Health and Disease*. New York: Academic Press, pp 227–256.

121. Gay, C. V., Mueller, W. J. (1974) Science 183:432–434.

122. Anderson, R. E., Schraer, H., Gay, C. V. (1982) Anat. Rec. 204:9–20.

123. Vaananen, H. K., Parvinen, E. K. (1983) Histochemistry 78:481–485.

124. Huber, A. M., Gershoff, S. N. (1970) J. Nutr. 103:1175–1181.

125. Seltzer, J. L., Jeffrey, J. J., Eisen, A. Z. (1977) Biochim. Biophys. Acta 485:179–187.

126. Starcher, B. C., Hill, C. H., Madaras, I. G. (1980) J. Nutr. 110:2095–2101.

127. Genge, B. R., McLean, F. M., Sauer, G. R., Wuthier, R. E. (1987) J. Bone Min. Res. 2 (Suppl. 1): abstr. 173.

128. Prasad, A. S., Oberleas, D. (1971) J. Appl. Physiol. 31:842–846.

129. Prasad, A. S., Oberleas, D., Miller, E. R., Luecke, R. W. (1971) J. Lab. Clin. Med. 77:144–152.

130. Davies, M. I., Motzok, I. (1972) Comp. Biochem. Physiol. 42B:345–356.

131. Lease, J. G. (1972) J. Nutr. 102:1323–1330.

132. Norrdin, R. W., Krook, L., Pond, W. G., Walker, E. F. (1973) Cornell, Vet. 63:264–290.

133. Agergaard, N., Palludan, B. (1974) Aarsberetin Inst. Sterilitetsforsk Kgl. Vet. Landbohoejsk 17:47–59.

134. Lease, J. G. (1975) J. Nutr. 105:385–392.

135. Prasad, A. S., Rabbani, P., Abbasii, A., Bowersox, E., Spivey Fox, M. R. (1978) Ann. Intern. Med. 89:483–490.

136. Weismann, K., Høyer, H. (1985) Am. J. Clin. Nutr. 41:1214–1219.

137. Cunnane, S. C., Huang, Y. S., Horrobin, D. F., Davignon, J. (1981) Prog. Lipid Res. 20:157–160.

138. Cunnane, S. C., Horrobin, D. F., Manku, M. S. (1984) Proc. Soc. Exp. Biol. Med. 177:441–446.

139. Odutuga, A. A. (1982) Comp. Biochem. Physiol. 71A:383–388.

140. Jee, W. S. S., Ueno, K., Deng, Y. P., Woodbury, D. M. (1985) Calcif. Tissue Int. 37:148–157.

141. Wientroub, S., Wahl, L. M., Feuerstein, N., Winter, C. C., Reddi, A. H. (1983) Biochem. Biophys. Res. Commun. 117:746–750.

142. Chyun, Y. S., Raisz, L. G. (1984) Prostaglandins 27:97–103.

143. Sato, K., Fujii, Y., Kasono, K. I., Saji, M., Tsushima, T., Shizume, K. (1966) Biochem. Biophys. Res. Commun. 138:618–624.

144. Momcilovic, B., Belonje, B., Giroux, A., Shah, B. G. (1975) Nutr. Rep. Intern. 12:197–203.

145. Beguin, D. P., Theall, C., Wallwork, J. C. TEMA-6 Meeting, Asilomar, CA., June 1987.

146. Wallwork, J. C., Fosmire, G. J., Sandstead, H. H. (1981) Br. J. Nutr. 45:127–146.

147. Calhoun, N. R., McDaniel, E. G., Howard, M. P., Smith, J. C., Jr. (1978) Nutr. Rep. Intern. 17:299–306.

148. Wallwork, J. C., Johnson, L. K., Milne, D. B., Sandstead, H. H. (1983) J. Nutr. 113:1307–1320.

149. Harland, B. F., Spivey-Fox, M. R., Fry, B. E., Jr. (1975) J. Nutr. 105:1509–1518.

150. Jeng, S. S., Sun, L. T. (1981) J. Nutr. 111:134–140.

151. Brown, E. D., Chan, W., Smith, J. C., Jr. (1978) Proc. Soc. Exp. Biol. Med. 157:211–214.

152. Murray, E. J., Messer, H. H. (1981) J. Nutr. 111:1641–1647.

153. Hurley, L. S., Tao, S.-H. (1972) Am. J. Physiol. 222:322–325.

154. Murray, E. J., Langhaus, B., Messer, H. H. (1981) Nutr. Res. 1:107–115.

155. Ellinger, G. M., Duckworth, J., Dalgarno, A. C., Quenoville, M. H. (1952) Br. J. Nutr. 6:235–253.

156. Winter, F. R. de., Steendijk, R. (1975) Calcif. Tissue Res. 17:303–316.

157. Rasmussen, P. (1977) Calcif. Tissue Res. 23:87–94.

158. Wong, K. M., Singer, L., Ophaug, R. H. (1980) Calcif. Tissue Int. 32:213–219.

159. Brommage, R., DeLuca, H. F. (1984) J. Nutr. 114:1377–1385.

160. Halloran, B. P., DeLuca, H. F. (1980) Endocrinol. 107:1923–1929.

161. Hefti, E., Trechsel, U., Bonjour, J.-P., Fleisch, H., Schenk, R. (1982) Clin. Sci. 62:389–396.

162. Toverud, S. U., Boass, A. (1979) Vitam. Horm. 37:303–347.

163. Toverud, S. U., Harper, C., Munson, P. L. (1976) Endocrinol. 99:371–378.

164. Fomon, S. J. (1974) *Infant Nutrition* Philadelphia: WB Saunders, pp. 363–380.

165. Greer, F. R., Tsang, R. C., Search, J. E., Levin, R. S., Steichen, J. J. (1982) Am. J. Clin. Nutr. 38:431–437.

166. Sorenson, J. A., Cameron, J. R. (1967) J. Bone Joint Surg. 49-A:481–497.

167. Atkinson, P. J., West, R. R. (1970) J. Obstet. Gynecol. Br. 77:555–560.

168. Lamke, B., Brundin, J., Moberg, P. (1977) Acta Obstet. Gynecol. Scand. 56:217–219.

169. Wardlaw, G. M., Pike, A. M. (1986) Am. J. Clin. Nutr. 44:283–286.

170. Haumont, S., McClean, F. C. (1966) In: Prasad, A. S. (ed) *Zinc Metabolism.* Springfield, ILL.: Charles C. Thomas, pp. 169–186.

171. Haumont, S. (1961) J. Histochem. Cytochem. 9:141–145.

172. Hoekstra, W. G. (1969) Am. J. Clin. Nutr. 22:1268–1277.

173. Young, R. J., Edwards, H. M., Jr., Gillis, M. B. (1958) Poultry Sci. 37:1100–1104.

174. Westmoreland, N. (1971) Fed. Proc. 30:1001–1024.

175. Platt, B. S., Stewart, R. J. C. (1962) Br. J. Nutr. 16:483–496.

176. Ramalingaswami, V., Deo, M. G. (1968) In:McCance, R. A., Widdowson, E. M. (eds) *Calorie Deficiencies and Protein Deficiencies,* London: J. A. Churchill, pp. 265–275.

177. Nakamoto, T., Miller, S. A. (1977) J. Nutr. 107:983–989.

178. Smit, Z. M., Pretorius, P. J. (1964) J. Trop. Pediat. 9:105–112.

179. Sandstead, H. H., Shukry, S., Prasad, A. S., Gabr, M. K., El Hefney, A., Mokhtar, N., Darby, W. J. (1965) Am. J. Clin. Nutr. 17:15–26.

180. Golden, B. E., Golden, M. H. N. (1981) Am. J. Clin. Nutr. 34:892–899.

181. Golden, M. H. N., Golden, B. E. (1981) Am. J. Clin. Nutr. 34:900–908.

182. Anonymous (1985) Nutr. Rev. 43:345–346.

183. Spencer, H., Kramer, L. (1986) J. Nutr. 116:316–319.

184. Gordan, G. S., Vaughan, C. (1986) J. Nutr. 116:319–322.

185. Hegsted, D. M. (1986) J. Nutr. 116:2316–2319.

186. Marcus, R. (1987) J. Nutr. 117:631–635.

187. Markowitz, M. E., Rosen, J. F., Mizuchi, M. (1985) Am. J. Clin. Nutr. 41:689–696.

188. Hoekstra, W. G., Lewis, P. K., Phillips, P. H., Grummer, R. H. (1956) J. Animal Sci. 15:752–764.

189. Lewis, P. K., Hoekstra, W. G., Grummer, R. H. (1957) J. Animal Sci. 16:578–588.

190. Berry, R. K., Bell, M. C., Grainger, R. B., Buescher, R. G. (1961) J. Animal Sci. 20:433–439.

191. Forbes, R. M. (1960) Fed. Proc. 19:643–647.

192. Forbes, R. M., Yohe, M. (1960) J. Nutr. 70:53–57.

193. O'Dell, B. L., Savage, J. E. (1960) Proc. Soc. Exp. Biol. Med. 103:304–306.

194. Oberleas, D., Muhrer, M. E., O'Dell, B. L. (1962) J. Animal Sci. 21:56–61.

195. Davies, N. T., Nightingale, R. (1975) Br. J. Nutr. 34:243–258.

196. Heth, D. A., Hoekstra, W. G. (1965) J. Nutr. 85:367–374.

197. Heth, D. A., Becker, W. M., Hoekstra, W. G. (1966) J. Nutr. 88:331–337.

198. Spencer, H., Vankinscott, V., Lewin, I., Samachson, J. (1965) J. Nutr. 86:169–177.

199. Spencer, H., Kramer, L., Norris, C., Osis, D. (1984) Am. J. Clin. Nutr. 40:1213–1218.

200. Dawson-Hughes, B., Seligson, F. H., Hughes, V. A. (1986) Am. J. Clin. Nutr. 44:83–88.

201. Pecoud, A., Donzel, P., Schelling, J. L. (1975) Clin. Pharmacol. Ther. 17:469–474.

202. Allred, J. B., Kratzer, F. N., Porter, J. W. G. (1964) Br. J. Nutr. 18:575–582.

203. Sandstead, H. H., Klevay, L., Jacob, R., et al. (Book of abstracts), San Diego, CA: XII Internation. Congress of Nutrition, August 16–21, 1981:84.

204. Sandstead, H. H., Henriksen, L. K., Greger, J. L., Prasad, A. S., Good, R. A. (1982) Am. J. Clin. Nutr. 36:1046–1054.

205. Greger, J. L., Snedeker, S. M. (1980) J. Nutr. 110:2243–2253.

206. O'Dell, B. L. (1969) Am. J. Clin. Nutr. 22:1315–1322.

207. Solomons, N. W., Jacob, R. A., Pineda, O., Viteri, F. (1979) J. Lab. Clin. Med. 94:335–343.

208. Parfitt, A. M. (1983) Lancet II:1181–1184.

209. Freudenheim, J. L., Johnson, N. E., Smith, E. L. (1986) Am. J. Clin. Nutr. 44:863–876.

210. Chausmer, A. B., Stevens, M. D., Zears, R. (1980) Metabolism 29:617–623.

211. Sjoden, G., Lindgren, J. U., DeLuca, H. F. (1984) J. Nutr. 114:2043–2046.

212. Wasserman, R. H. (1962) J. Nutr. 77:69–80.

213. Koo, S. I., Fullmer, C. S., Wasserman, R. H. (1980) J. Nutr. 110:1813–1818.

214. Martin, W. G., Patrick, H. (1961) Poultry Sci. 40:1004–1009.

215. Worker, N. A., Migicovsky, B. B. (1961) J. Nutr. 75:222–224.

216. Kienholz, E. W., Sunde, M. L., Hoekstra, W. G. (1964) Poultry Sci. 43:667–675.

217. Whiting, F., Bezeau, L. M. (1958) Can. J. Animal Sci. 38:109–117.

218. Becker, W. M., Hoekstra, W. G. (1966) J. Nutr. 90:301–309.

219. Chang, I. H., Harrill, I., Gifford, E. D. (1969) Metabolism 28:625–629.

220. Leek, J. C., Vogler, J. B., Gershwin, M. E., Golub, M. S., Hurley, L. S., Hendrickx, A. G. (1984) Am. J. Clin. Nutr. 40:1203–1212.

221. Huxley, H. G., Leaver, A. G. (1966) Arch. Oral Biol. 22:1337–1344.

222. Leaver, A. G. (1967) Arch. Oral Biol. 12:773–775.

223. Sivakumar, B., Belavady, B. (1975) Ind. J. Biochem. Biophys. 12:386–388.

224. Halsted, J. A., Ronaghy, H. A., Abadi, P., Haghschenass, M., Amirhakemi, G. H., Barakat, R. M., Reinhold, J. G. (1972) Am. J. Med. 53:277–284.

225. Sandstead, H. H., Prasad, A. S., Schulert, A. R., Farid, Z., Miale, A., Jr., Bassilly, S., Darby, W. J. (1967) Am. J. Clin. Nutr. 20:422–442.

226. Reinhold, J. G. (1971) Am. J. Clin. Nutr. 24:1204–1206.

227. Reinhold, J. G., Nasr, K., Lahimgarzadeh, A., Hedayati, H. (1973) Lancet I:283–288.

228. Sandstead, H. H. (1982) In: Prasad, A. S. (ed) *Clinical and Public Health Significance of Trace Minerals in the World Population.* New York: Alan R. Liss, pp. 83–102.

229. Lykken, G. I., Mahalko, J., Johnson, P. E., Milne, D., Sandstead, H. H., Garcia, W. J., Dintzis, F. R., Inglett, G. E. (1986) J. Nutr. 116:795–801.

230. Cavdar, A. O., Arcasoy, A. (1972) Clin. Pediat. 11:215–223.

231. Cavdar, A. O., Arcasoy, A., Cin, S. (1977) Am. J. Clin. Nutr. 30:833–834.

232. Xue-Cun, C., Tai-An, Y., Jin-Sheng, H., Qui-Yan, M., Zhi-Min, H., Li-Xiang, L. (1985) Am. J. Clin. Nutr. 42:694–700.

233. Neldner, K. H., Hambidge, K. M. (1975) New Engl. J. Med. 292:879–882.

234. Hambidge, K. M., Nelder, K. H., Walravens, P. A., Weston, W. L., Silverman, A., Sabol, J. L., Brown, R. M. (1978) In: Hambidge, K. M., Nichols, B. L. (eds) *Zinc and Acrodermatitis Enteropathica.* New York: Spectrum, pp. 81–89.

235. Arlette, J. P. (1983) Pediat. Clin. N. Am. 30:583–596.

236. Shaw, J. C. L. (1979) Am. J. Dis. Child 133:1260–1268.

237. Arakawa, T., Tamura, T., Igarashi, Y., Suzuki, H., Sandstead, H. (1976) Am. J. Clin. Nutr. 29:197–204.

238. Tasman-Jones, C., Kay, R. G., Lee, S. P. (1978) Surg. Annu. 10:23–52.

239. Allen, J. I., Kay, N. E., McClain, C. J. (1981) Ann. Int. Med. 95:154–157.

240. McClain, C. J., Cuotor, C., Zieve, L. (1980) Gastroenterology 79:272–279.

241. Crofton, R. W., Glover, S. C., Ewen, S. W. B., Aggett, P. J., Mowat, N. A. G., Mills, C. F. (1983) Am. J. Clin. Nutr. 38:706–712.

242. Mahajan, S. K., Prasad, A. S., Rabbani, P., Briggs, W. A., McDonald, F. D. (1979) J. Lab. Clin. Med. 94:693–698.

243. Warth, J. A., Prasad, A. S., Zwas, F., Frank, R. N. (1981) J. Lab. Clin. Med. 98:189–194.

244. McClain, C. J., van Thiel, D. H., Parker, S., Badzin, L. K., Gilbert, T. H. (1979) Alcoholism 3:135–141.

245. Keen, C. L., Hurley, L. S. (1987) Neurotoxicol. 8:379–388.

246. Hambidge, K. M., Hambidge, C., Jacobs, M., Baum, J. D. (1972) Pediat. Res. 6:868–874.

247. Walravens, P. A., Philip, A., Hambidge, K. M. (1976) Am. J. Clin. Nutr. 29:1114–1121.

248. Hambidge, K. M., Walravens, P. A., Whate, S., Anthony, M. L., Roth, M. L. (1976) Am. J. Clin. Nutr. 29:734–738.

249. Butrimovitz, G. P., Purdy, W. C. (1977) In: Meites, S. (ed) *Pediatric Clinical Chemistry. a Survey of Normals, Methods and Instrumentation with Commentary.* Washington DC: American Association for Clinical Chemistry, pp. 230–236.

250. Butrimovitz, G. P., Purdy, W. C. (1978) Am. J. Clin. Nutr. 31:1409–1412.

251. Buzina, R., Jusic, M., Colipp, P. J., Chen, S. Y., Cheruvanky, J., Maddaiah, V. T. (1981) Am. J. Dis. Child 13:322–325.

252. Hambidge, K. M., Krebs, N. F., Walravens, P. A. (1985) Nutr. Res. suppl. I:306–316.

253. Michaelsson, G., Vahlquist, A., Juhlin, L. (1977) Br. J. Dermatol. 96:283–286.

254. Michaelsson, G., Juhlin, L., Ljunghall, L. (1977) Br. J. Dermatol. 97:561–566.

255. Greger, J. L. (1977) J. Geront. 32:549–553.

256. Greger, J. L., Sciscoe, B. S. (1977) J. Am. Diabetes Assoc. 70:37–41.

257. Hickory, W., Nanda, R., Catalanotto, R. A. (1979) J. Nutr. 109:883–891.

258. Wagner, P. A., Krista, M. L., Bailey, L. B., Christakis, G. J., Jernigan, J. A., Araujo, P. E., Appledorf, H., Davis, C. G., Dinning, J. S. (1980) Am. J. Clin. Nutr. 33:1771–1777.

259. Bales, C. S., Stenman, L. C., Freeland-Graves, J. H., Stone, J. M., Young, R. K. (1986) Am. J. Clin. Nutr. 44:664–669.

260. Jacob, R. A., Russell, R. M., Sandstead, H. H. (1985) In: Watson, R. R. (ed) *CRC Handbook of Nutrition in the Aged,* Boca Raton, FL: CRC Press, pp. 77–88.

261. Sandstead, H. H. (1972) In: Patwardhan, V. N., Darby, W. J. (eds) *The State of Nutrition the Arab Middle East,* Nashville, TN: Vanderbilt Univ. Press, pp. 122–140.

262. Ferguson, H. W., Leaver, A. G. (1972) Calcif. Tiss. Res. 8:265–275.

263. Sadasivan, V. (1951) Biochem. J. 48:527–530.

264. Yamaguchi, M., Mochizuki, A., Okada, S. (1982) J. Pharm. Dyn. 5:501–504.

265. Waite, L. C. (1972) Endocrinol. 91:1160–1165.

266. Greger, J. L., Krzykowski, C. E., Khazen, R. R., Krashoc, C. L. (1987) J. Nutr. 117:717–724.

267. Styrud, J., Dahlström, E., Eriksson, U. F. (1986) Upsala J. Med. Sci. 91:29–36.

268. Lui, E. M. K. (1987) Comp. Biochem. Physiol. 86C:173–183.

269. Bakka, A., Samarawickrama, G. P., Webb, M. (1981) Chem. Biol. Interact. 34:161–171.

270. Hunt, C. D., Halas, E. S., Eberhardt, M. J. (1988) Biol. Trace Element Res. 16:97–114.

271. Bolze, M. S., Reeves, R. D., Lindbeck, F. E., Elders, M. J. (1987) Am. J. Physiol. 252:E21-E26.

272. Giugliano, R., Millward, D. J. (1984) Br. J. Nutr. 52:545–560.

273. Yamaguchi, M., Oishi, H., Suketa, Y. Biochem. Pharmacol. (1987) 36:4007–4012.

274. Kaji, T., Kawatani, R., Takata, M., Hoshino, T., Miyahara, T., Kozuka, H., Koizumi, F. (1988) Toxicol. 50:303–316.

275. Soares, J. H., Jr., Sherman, S., Sinha, R. (1987) Nutr. Res. 7:151–164.

276. Leek, J. C., Keen, C. L., Vogler, J. B., Golub, M. S., Hurley, L. S., Hendrickx, A. G., Gershwin, M. E. (1988) Am. J. Clin. Nutr. 47:889–895.

277. Jee, W. S. S., Ueno, K., Woodbury, D. M., Price, P., Woodbury, L. A. (1987) Bone 8:171–176.

V
ARCHAEOLOGICAL DIETARY CONSIDERATIONS

17

Archaeological Diets and Skeletal Integrity

STEPHEN MOLNAR

One of the major concerns of archaeologists is the subsistence base of prehistoric people. Food, and the technology to acquire it, composes a subsistence base that has vastly changed over time and that differs from environment to environment. In addition to the study of the technological remains, a most important challenge to archaeologists is the description of dietary changes. Every item of material remains has been considered as evidence for its potential to shed light on past living conditions or on subsistence. Plant remains in the form of seeds, pollen, fiber, or shell are collected and examined carefully. Likewise, animal bones are classified as to species, size, and nutritional value. Even the stomach contents of mummies and fecal material have been examined, as have the frozen tissues preserved in arctic regions. All such materials have provided some evidence of ancient diets and health of the extinct populations. More sophisticated techniques have been borrowed from chemistry and physics in recent years to assist in the analysis.

The results of these analyses describe, in broad categories, dietary changes over time and throughout the world's regions. These dietary influences, drawn from the scattered material remains, enable statements to be made about the gradual transformation from food gathering to simple horticulture to early agriculture. But, from this evidence alone, little can be said about the biological impact of a "revolution" in subsistence strategy. The best record of the impact of dietary change comes from the skeletal remains of the people who used the tools, who hunted the animals, and who collected or grew the plants. Fortunately, several aspects of dietary change influence the development and maintenance of bone—sometimes in a positive and sometimes in a negative way. Human skeletons preserved over time provide significant evidence of this past influence if the bone record is read correctly.

One of the earliest and most obvious changes that occurred was the reduction in skeletal size and robusticity. Human ancestors from the late Pleistocene period (35,000 years ago) were larger and had thicker bone than their descendants, who, though still hunters and gatherers of wild plants, had shifted their subsistence base to include a greater variety of animal and plant materials, especially the marine resources easily collected by the end of the Pleistocene. Further reduction in body size occurred with the advent of settled village life as *Homo sapiens* learned to domesticate plants and animals. This agricultural transition brought about many environmental changes establishing a newer, more complex human ecology. Such an ecological complex influenced growth and health, which is reflected in the skeletal remains of populations descendant over the following generations.

Studies of the Greek and Mycenaean Bronze Age remains by Angel (1) showed an average body size reduction and an increase in pathologies. Also, Saul's study (2) of Mayan skeletons in southern Mexico and Guatemala document physical and pathological changes within a few generations. His "osteobiographic" analysis attempted to interpret the evidence of changing diet and declining health as contributory factors to the collapse of the Mayan civilization. Armelagos and colleagues (3) also used osteological evidence to describe the influence of diet on skeletal development and health. The recovery of large quantities of burials from the Sudan, which spanned a broad time range, provided a population record encompassing this transition to food production. They compared Mesolithic preagricultural populations from 12,000 years ago to three groups of agriculturalists who had occupied the same region from 3400 B.C. to A.D. 550. An increase in pathologies, a higher death rate, and a decline in bone density were among the major changes to occur over time. These and many other studies provide evidence that outlines the influences of dietary changes and probable deficiencies. In fact, wherever the archaeological record of floral, faunal, and technological remains show a major transition in subsistence, there is evidence of change in the quality of the skeletal remains.

Several specific dietary factors have been implicated. The most important diet shift in the New World was the heavy dependence on maize, a dependence that exists to this day in parts of Latin America. Since maize is deficient in lysine, it was suggested that there may be an effect on the synthesis of collagen preventing the normal cross-linking of maturing collagen (4). The coarse-ground grains, the major dietary component in the Greek Bronze Age, would be high in phytates. This would bind with calcium and zinc, reducing their absorption (5). Growth would be retarded, as it was in recent times and is even today among populations eating unleavened bread high in bran content (6).

Because of the number of variables involved, there can only be speculation at this point about the causes of the health and growth changes. The crowding in permanent or semipermanent settlements would contribute to pollution and disease, as attested to by the many pathological lesions of bone that begin to appear in significant frequencies at about the time of the agricultural revolution (1, 2, 7). The narrowing of nutritional variety would reduce the chance of acquiring a balance of nutrients as observed in modern hunters when they shift to an agricultural economy. Robson (8) noted that, when such a shift has occurred in the last few decades, the actual counts of plants used showed a reduction in the variety of food plants from as many as 300 to 15 when former nomads began to grow their own food.

More specific detail on diet influence is required, and this can only come from the bone itself. The gross observations of bone pathologies, density, and size are not enough. Fortunately, several methods of microanalysis of individual trace elements have been applied to the study of prehistoric bone. These elements may provide a record of biological events or, according to Saul, an _____ly," because dietary variability can affect different elemental comp

Cereal grains and many vegetables are higher in manganese _____ molybdenum than meat. Zinc, copper, and selenium are more _____ animal flesh. Detection of ratios of these elements in bone cou_ diet. The most useful ratio for dietary deduction has proved __ __ strontium and calcium because of the discrimination of the mammalian biological system against strontium. Paleontologists comparing bone taken from animals at different feeding levels—grazers, browsers, and carnivores—noted a reduction in strontium at the higher tropic levels (9). Comparison of strontium levels among a variety of human populations showed subtle variations between the proportions of meat and vegetables in their diets. Strontium/calcium ratios have been compared so widely among humans by this time that concentrations above certain levels are taken to indicate diets high in animal flesh, while strontium is indicative of a vegetable diet. A recent study of bones from a Hellenistic cemetery showed a shift from high-strontium, low-zinc levels during the earliest periods to a condition of low levels of both strontium and zinc in the more recent burials which, according to the authors, was probably due to the addition of grains high in phytic acid (5).

Fortunately for paleodietary analysis, there is also another avenue of investigation. There is a discrimination against the heavier carbon isotopes by certain plants. As described below, the $^{13}CO_2$ is fixed into carbohydrates in a greater proportion by many tropical plant species, and several such species have become important in the human diet—for example, maize. It is thus possible to plot the spread of maize among North American Indians as it became an important part of their subsistence base. Another important diet source, seafood, also influences isotope ratios. Because of the high concentration of ^{13}C in marine carbonates, differentiation has even been made between terrestrial and seafood diets. The ancient Danish skeletons described by Tauber (10) showed a reduction in the concentration of ^{13}C over time. During the Mesolithic, just prior to adoption of agriculture, there was a high dependence on seafood. When diets shifted to contain more terrestrial foods, mostly grains low in the ability to fix $^{13}CO_2$, then the ^{13}C concentration declined proportiontely.

These trace elements and isotope ratios can provide important and effective tools to expand the scope of our knowledge of the bone biology of extinct populations. But there are numerous factors that may distort values and confound the analysis. The mixing of diet is one such factor; some substances may interfere with absorption of another dietary component. Another consideration is the possible uneven distribution throughout the skeletal system. Some bones, ribs for example, may have a greater or lesser concentration of an element. A major problem is always the state of preservation. Since the buried material sampled is infuenced by soil and water, there are numerous diagenic or postmortem exchanges that occur over time and that must be taken into account. Some elements are more subject to diagenesis than others, as will be considered below.

All of these factors contribute to the problem of prehistoric bone analysis. It is not now nor has it ever been an easy task to reconstruct those biological conditions of the past that relate to skeletal development and maintenance. But, if the methods of elemental analysis are carefully applied and adequate standards are used, then much may be said about the evolution of the human diet, about its effect on bone, and about bone as a record of metabolic events.

THE FOOD CHAIN AND THE HEAVIER ISOTOPES
OF CARBON AND NITROGEN

Biological systems may discriminate against the heavier isotopes during the absorption of nutrients. Different plant species take up varying proportions of carbon and nitrogen isotopes, for example. Plants that fix atmospheric nitrogen have less capacity to take up ^{15}N than plants that use soil components as a nitrogen source, and marine plants have a higher ^{15}N content than either. Variations in photosynthesis differentiate between plants in their carbon-fixing efficiencies. Tropical grasses and their domestic descendants incorporate a greater proportion of ^{13}C than temperate-zone plants. Animals that selectively feed on these plant resources will incorporate varying proportions of heavier carbon and nitrogen isotopes into their tissues. The feeding specializations of grazing or browsing animals may then be determined by the $^{13}C/^{12}C$ and $^{15}N/^{14}N$ ratios (11, 12). Further up the food chain, the carnivores will also have carbon and nitrogen ratios reflective of the herbivores upon which they feed. A small stepwise enrichment of the isotopes may contribute to an evaluation of the trophic level occupied by an organism (13).

In the case of the human diet, the same factors may apply, and the statement "You are what you eat" is clearly demonstrated by the isotope ratios of $^{13}C/^{12}C$ and $^{15}N/^{14}N$. Recent studies comparing contemporary East African agriculturists with their pastoral counterparts showed significant isotope ratio differences. The agriculturists dependent on plant foods had lower ^{15}N values than the pastoral people who consumed larger quantities of milk, meat, and blood of their domestic animals (14). Likewise, the relative abudance of plants of different carbon-fixing abilities is reflected in the ^{13}C levels.

These phenomena of plant and animal isotope discrimination have been applied in recent years to studies of dietary components of prehistoric populations. Since we are dealing with archaeological bone, our data source is limited to collagen and, to some degree, carbonate. As described below, collagen provides a record with minimal diagenic change, and several researchers have examined the isotope ratios from skeletal remains of many extinct populations. These remains represent peoples who have lived under diverse environmental conditions and were dependent on diverse diets. Carbon and nitrogen isotope ratios have proved useful as evidence of these diets.

Carbon Isotopes and the Food Chain

The worldwide average for the ratios of the stable isotopes of carbon, ^{12}C and ^{13}C, is 100:1.1, which is assumed to have remained unchanged over time, but there is a broad difference in the isotope ratio among organic materials. Marine limestones, for example, contain a high proportion of the heavier isotopes compared to the cellulose of wood and some grasses and in contrast to herbaceous plants. Throughout the plant kingdom, in fact, there are great differences in the $^{13}C/^{12}C$ ratios. The environment, as well as plant physiology, is influential. Aquatic plants in hard water have a higher ratio than those in soft water, and seawater plants have the highest ratio of all. There is even a difference among terrestrial plants, which is due to the type of photosynthesis process, some processes being more effective than others in the uptake and fixing of carbon dioxide. Animals, whose feeding habits cause them to specialize in certain parts of the plant kingdom, will have a corresponding carbon ratio in their tissues.

By convention, carbon isotope ratios are compared against a particular sample of marine carbonate, a cretaceous marine fossil, from the Peedee Formation in South Carolina. This sample was selected because it had the highest known $^{13}C/^{12}C$ ratio (15). It was assigned a value of zero (PDB standard) and, in comparison, most other-based materials have negative values. For example, carbon dioxide in the atmosphere has a value of -7, the difference between an air sample and the standard which is designated by δ in parts per thousand (0/00), the relative ^{13}C content. In contrast, an urban atmosphere heavily polluted with hydrocarbons from fossil fuels, has -8 0/00. Leaves from a common variety of peas have a δ ^{13}C of -26 compared to the -14 0/00 of maize.

Plant Dietary Sources

Distinctions can be made between plants in their δ ^{13}C values because of the different photosynthesis pathway used by certain varieties. During photosynthesis, plants will take up ^{12}C in preference over ^{13}C or ^{14}C. Those plants (C3) that fix three carbon atoms to a phosphoglycerate compound will discriminate to a greater degree than those that fix four carbon atoms in a dicarboxylic acid (C4 plants). The C3 process was first described in algae, spinach, and barley (16), and later a different process (C4) was identified in sugarcane (17). Other grasses of tropic origin were also noted to have a C4 process, whereas temperate zone plants were C3 types. The C4 plants are a highly efficient processor, using less time and less water in the tissue-building process.

A third class of plant photosynthesis is known, the CAM process. These plants, mostly succulents, can shift to a C3-like process that discriminates against the heavier carbon isotopes when there is ample moisture and growth is rapid. During dry periods, the plant follows a crassulacean acid metabolism (CAM), which discriminates less against ^{13}C than the C3 process.

The result is that the three processes of fixing carbon dioxide allow dietary inputs to be evaluated. Plants of economic importance to man fit mainly into either the C3 or C4 class. Wheat and barley are C3; maize, millet, and sorghum, descendants of tropical grasses, are C4 types. These are nonoverlapping in their relative ^{13}C concentrations and allow distinction to be made between major classes of food resources (18).

The particular sample used in determining δ ^{13}C values is most important because of the process of "fractionation." Different tissues of the organism will incorporate varying isotope ratios during their formation. Fat will have a lower relative ^{13}C value than the diet, for example, and collagen will be higher in its δ ^{13}C. Vogel (19) demonstrated a range of fractionation of the fat, flesh, hide, and bone collagen among African ungulates. Collagen favors ^{13}C by 3–5 0/00, and fat discriminates by roughly the same amount. Both fractionation and the rate of turnover of stable carbon isotopes may influence test results, particularly if an animal diet varies through time (12). Therefore, dietary interpretation can best be maximized by an analysis of bone collagen, soft tissue, and fecal or stomach contents. Except for bone collagen these sources are unavailable when dealing with recent or fossilized skeletal remains. How well these methods may work in dietary reconstruction was shown by the results reported by Jones and co-workers (20), who studied tissue changes of δ ^{13}C in response. to C4 and C3 feed grains. They noted that δ ^{13}C of feces of animals corresponded to their diets just as did the observed associations between δ ^{13}C of milk (21). Feeding cattle diets alternating between C4 and C3 plants also caused a shift in the δ ^{13}C in the hair of animals. Equilibrium values were reached in the hair over a 74- 120-day period. Using these data, Jones and co-workers suggested the measure of δ ^{13}C uptake by animal tissues as a method for the analysis of rate of uptake of carbon from the metabolic pool (22). The fractionation and selectively favoring of, or discriminating against, ^{13}C may be further confounded by the extent to which amino acids are spared, depending on the availability of carbon from other dietary sources (23).

The significance of δ ^{13}C ratios in diets and the resulting tissue fractionation offers a means of metabolic studies using "self labels," as the ^{13}C and ^{15}N isotopes might be called. Matthews and Bier (24) proposed that studies of glucose end products could be conducted by adding a small amount of ^{13}C-enriched glucose to natural glucose. They noted that diets of Europeans are derived mainly from C3 plant food chains, in contrast to the C4-rich diet of Americans. By adding the relatively ^{13}C-enriched corn sugar, [13]CO_2 rises and can quantify glucose oxidation during a conventional glucose tolerance test. These studies and many more demonstrate the feasibility of using ratios of stable carbon isotopes for dietary and metabolic analysis. However, because of the nature of prehistoric samples, the state of bone preservation, and age variables, the application of δ ^{13}C is a more limited but still useful tool for dietary reconstruction.

Diet and ^{13}C in Prehistoric Remains

One of the major changes, if not the most important one, in North American prehistory was the introduction of maize into the diets of native Americans. The arrival of maize as a major cultigen in the Mississippi Valley and eastern North America influenced profound population changes, as described below. The major evidence for the increasing importance of maize, besides the actual plant remains found in the archaeological sites, was the measure of dietary carbon. Maize, a C4 plant, introduced a high percentage of δ ^{13}C into the dietary carbon, which in turn incorporated more ^{13}C into the tissues.

By the late Woodland period of the Mississippi Valley (ca. A.D. 800–1000), approximately 24 percent of dietary carbon came from the maize source (25). The populations continued to expand in numbers and developed into the highly complex societies famous for their mound building and large urban centers. These cultures (the Mississippian A.D. 1000–1250) had increased their reliance on maize to the point where an estimated 50 percent of dietary carbon came from this source.

Another application of carbon isotope ratios to diet reconstruction was a study of prehistoric Indians of upstate New York (26). The researchers noted a significant difference between the hunting and gathering peoples and their descendants. With the introduction of maize, there was an appreciable rise in δ ^{13}C. During this period, around A.D. 1000, maize became an important part of the diet, and δ ^{13}C of skeletal collagen rose from a -21.4 0/00 to -12 0/00. The heavier isotope value represents an increase of C4 plants as dietary carbon sources from zero to about 70 percent. Such a rise of δ ^{13}C values provided substantial evidence for the appearance of maize as an important dietary constituent in that region of North America (18).

In addition to identifying the contribution of C4 plants to dietary carbon, the measure of δ ^{13}C in collagen has been used to differentiate between prehistoric populations who specialized in marine or in terrestrial food sources. Tests of collagen from Greenland Eskimo and British Columbia Indian bone samples showed consistently higher δ^{13}C values than did populations from Canadian Caribou Eskimos, who gained most of their subsistence from terrestrial sources. The Eskimo and British Columbia Indian had diets that emphasized marine sources, an average of 7 0/00 higher due to the difference between atmospheric and oceanic carbon (27). Terrestrial mammals average -25.5 0/00 and marine mammals -17.5 0/00 due to the differences in their primary carbon sources. These differences are reflected in the consumers. The enrichment of about 5 0/00 by collagen is reflected in the collagen samples.

As noted above, Tauber (10) used similar methods to compare prehistoric Danish populations. Humans from the Mesolithic period gained most of their food from marine sources, and their diets generally resembled that of latter-day Greenland Eskimos. The ^{13}C concentration differed significantly from the Neolithic population. The later-day peoples of the Neolithic (ca. 5000 B.C.) relied more on terrestrial food sources, largely cultivated plants like wheat and barley.

These studies suggest that δ ^{13}C measures are sensitive indicators of dietary specialization when there had been major differences in carbon sources. Some workers believe that the measure is even sensitive enough to evaluate the proportions of different dietary components. However, the application of δ ^{13}C values to dietary interpretation is not without its problems.

The question investigated by a number of authors is the degree of postmortem change that may cause shifts in δ ^{13}C values. Degradation of collagen and the addition of organic fractions from the soil in the form of fungi, bacteria, or carbonates are factors that will be described in detail later in the diagenesis section. Here I will note that such a problem exists and must be considered with checks made against appropriate reference materials. Fossil Pleistocene deer bone, when compared against fresh-killed, showed that there had been a greater percentage of C3 plants in their diet than is represented in modern deer feed. This may be explained by the existence of a wetter climate during the later Pleistocene, or the organic fraction had lost its "isotopic memory" (11).

Van der Merwe (18), who had been successful in differentiating between prehistoric native Americans of pre- and postagricultural periods, was not able to apply the same method to human skeletal remains from Egypt and the southern Sahara. He reasoned that the introduction of C3 cultigens (wheat and barley) into these regions of C4 plants (millets and sorghum) should be recorded by the lowering of the δ ^{13}C in bones of populations dating from the time of arrival of the plants several thousands of years ago. However, skeletal remains from desert sites were heavily mineralized, and the collagen was decomposed. Van der Merwe reasoned that this problem makes it unlikely that bone collagen will be a useful method of isotope studies under certain conditions of preservation.

Because of some questions of collagen preservation, investigators have tried to use carbonate from the bone apatite fraction. The small amount of carbonate retains its original isotope proportions and has a linear relationship of δ ^{13}C values with collagen. The major problem is the removal of that carbonate deposited postmortem in the form of precipitants in bone fissures and haversian canals. Some success has been reported by Sullivan and Krueger (28), who showed results from analysis of bone carbonate from specimens over 10,000 years old. They removed the secondary carbonate deposits by treatment with acetic acid. However, Schoeninger and DeNiro (29) reported results demonstrating that bone apatite carbonate undergoes postmortem carbon exchange, and this diagenesis may shift δ ^{13}C values as much as 12 0/00 (a wider range than collagen). They concluded that carbonate apatite can only be useful if a method is developed to demonstrate that it has remained unaltered in the postmortem environment. X-ray diffraction patterns were suggested by Land (11) to determine the integrity of apatite.

Nitrogen Isotopes and Diet

The ratio of the isotopes ^{15}N/^{14}N in the atmosphere is the standard against which other substances are compared. Plants that fix atmospheric nitrogen will have a δ ^{15}N (relative value) about zero (the same as the standard), or they may be slightly positive. In contrast, plants that use soil nitrates as a source have more positive values. Animals feeding on these plants will have a δ ^{15}N that relates to their diet. An early study showed the relation of tissue proteins in rats fed on two diets with different δ ^{15}N values. One group was fed on soya meal, and the other milk protein. Both groups showed an enrichment of δ ^{15}N over the dietary protein, but the group on the casein-based diet had a higher δ ^{15}N value than the group on the soya protein diet (30). DeNiro and Epstein (13) in a feeding experiment with mice showed whole-body and individual tissue enrichment of between 2 and 5 0/00 δ ^{15}N.

The enrichment of ^{15}N in the food chain is sufficient to indicate trophic level as well as dietary concentration. Ambrose and DeNiro (14) studied the δ ^{15}N of bone collagen from several East African populations, as noted above. Those groups most dependent on plant foods, the agriculturists, had δ ^{15}N values between +8 and +12 0/00. In contrast, the pastoral peoples consuming quantities of milk, meat, and blood of domestic cattle had higher δ ^{15}N values, ranging between +12 and +18 0/00. The nitrogen enrichment of the blood and milk, in fact, placed these pastoralists at a slightly higher level than several species of East African carnivores. Such a study demonstrated, as did the animal experiments, that the

δ ^{15}N values of animal tissues are closely correlated to the isotopic composition of the diet.

Marine organisms are generally higher in ^{15}N, and populations of prehistoric or historic humans using this food resource have greater δ ^{15}N values. The study of coastal populations, whose reliance on marine organisms had been demonstrated by ethnographic or archaeological methods, showed a higher δ ^{15}N than agriculturists. An exception was a group of Bahamian fisherman who had lower values than expected for marine-dependent populations. A possible explanation perhaps lies in the fact that they exploited reef fish, whose feeding on nitrogen-fixing algae gave them a lower δ ^{15}N (23, 31). Keegan and De Niro (32) described the lowered ^{15}N in the coral reef communities of the Bahamas. Bone samples of prehistoric Bahamians showed lower ^{15}N isotopes of the collagen which reflected a dependence on organisms from the shallow water reef communities.

In conclusion, the use of carbon and nitrogen isotopes for paleodietary reconstruction is a valuable addition to the study of human food use and adaptation in the past. In fact, at least one study argued that it may even be the most accurate method for determination of dietary composition. DeNiro and Epstein (13) noted the decline of the δ ^{15}N values in Tehuacan, Mexico, over a 7,000-year period and argued that the δ ^{15}N values plus the rise of δ ^{13}C gave evidence for the increasing use of maize and beans in the later occupation periods. However, there are problems associated with physiological fractionation and diagenesis that must be considered, as I shall now discuss.

TRACE ELEMENTS OF BONE AS DIETARY MARKERS

In recent years anthropologists have made effective use of sophisticated chemical analysis techniques to record the presence of minute quantities of certain trace elements in prehistoric bone. The elements zinc, magnesium, and strontium have been especially useful because of their uneven distribution in the food chain. The concentrations of these elements in bone were taken to indicate dietary specialization. Since the reports of tissue discrimination, strontium, especially, has played a major role in paleodietary reconstruction. Just as the stable isotope ratios of carbon would indicate certain plant types in the diet, strontium concentrations relative to calcium could be used to recognize dietary shifts through time (33, 35). Anthropologists have attempted to use such derived dietary differences to distinguish between cultures, age groups, sexes, and even social classes. These attempts have met with varying degrees of success because of the nature of bone mineral, trace element diversity in the food chain, and diagenic changes (the postmortem alteration of bone composition). These variables confound any comparisons made between faunal as well as between human remains, and the more cautious and careful workers take note of these difficulties.

Strontium and Calcium Ratios

Because the quantities of fallout from atomic tests in the 1950s deposited several radioactive elements in the food chain, many studies were directed toward understanding their uptake and biological activity. Considerable attention was directed toward the behavior of ^{90}Sr, one of the more dangerous of the bone-seeking isotopes. Among the many results from this attention was the clearer understanding of strontium behavior in mammalian physiology.

According to Gran and Nicolaysen (36), strontium is intimately connected with calcium metabolism. A more recent study even claims that strontium is essential to normal calcification in humans and probably plays a role in reducing dental caries (37). However, calcium is selectively favored at several physiological levels. The intestinal mucosa discriminates against the absorption of strontium, but the rate varies widely among individuals, depending on age and quantity of calcium present. The higher the concentration of calcium, the greater the dilution of strontium, and the greater the discrimination. The balance between absorption and discrimination rates of the two elements depends on those several variables that influence calcium concentration. The rate of flow of digestive juices and the quantity of dietary calcium are among the principal factors. In addition, there is a greater excretion of strontium in the urine because of the lower rate of resorption in the kidney. The results of this selective absorption, excretion, or reabsorption of calcium over strontium is a higher observed ratio (OR) in the urine than in the plasma. The OR of plasma and diet is .25; the OR of urine to diet is roughly four times as great. This biological discrimination has been outlined in numerous studies of strontium metabolism in a variety of organisms, and the pathways for distribution of strontium in nature have been described (38, 39).

Plants, however, discriminate against strontium relatively little compared to mammals. Such consistent, though variable discrimination against strontium will enable its concentration to be used to indicate an organism's level in the food chain. Herbivores will have the highest strontium levels, and carnivores will have the lowest. Other organisms will occupy intermediate positions depending on the composition of their diet. Mixed feeders of grasses or succulents will be higher than grazing herbivores, and omnivores will range rather broadly between herbivores and carnivores. Toots and Voorhis (40) and Parker and Toots (9) made use of this distribution of strontium in the food chain to offer a reconstruction of the dietary specializations of extinct fossil species. Toots and Voorhis (40) reported that the mean strontium content could be used to distinguish between Pliocene carnivores and herbivores, but also a difference was seen between browsers and grazers because of the concentration of strontium in leaves versus stems. But they warned that such distinctions could be made only if the abudance of strontium was maintained at a constant level and there was no significant postmortem change in the mineral phase. This caution has frequently not been heeded, however.

Archaeological Evidence for the Paleodiet

Brown (41) was the first to use the Sr/Ca ratio of archaeological bone to compare diets of several prehistoric cultures. She compared samples taken from sites in the Mississippi Valley (Woodland cultures) with samples from four sites in Mexico and a collection from Iran. The results were used to distinguish between cultures on the basis of the proportions of the diet from animal or plant sources. The changes in proportions gave evidence of dietary shifts through time—that is, a greater consumption of plant foods. A distinction between sexes was also reported; females averaged a higher strontium concentration. Brown explained this by postulating that females had a lower status in the prehistoric society and thus subsisted on a diet consisting of less meat than the higher-status males. Factors of physiological differences due to increased bone turnover because of pregnancy and lactation were not considered. However, since Brown's pioneering study, there have been many improvements in the collection and analysis of samples together with the wider recognition of the variables that influence Sr/Ca ratios.

One of the next applications of bone strontium was an attempt to distinguish between fossil fauna from East African hominid sites (ca. 1–2 million years B.P.). Boaz and Hemple (42) examined a variety of taxa from baboon (major food sources, grasses and seeds) and colobine monkey (mainly leaf eaters) to giraffes (browsers) and lions (carnivores). The investigators carefully recorded the Sr/Ca ratios of bone fragments and dental enamel by microprobe and X-ray fluorescence methods. The initial results of bone strontium analysis showed no correlation between strontium and the diets of the fossils that were presumed to be analogous to the diets of closely related modern species. Further tests of enamel by X-ray fluorescence failed to distinguish between herbivores and carnivores. Boaz and Hemple concluded that the fossils must have been affected by postmortem changes in the strontium content. They likened the increases in strontium to the uptake of fluorides. This paper raised questions about the likelihood of the retention of "life values" of strontium in fossil bones, a question considered later in "diagenic changes."

Schoeninger (43) published one of the first comprehensive attempts to use strontium analysis as an aid to archaeological studies. She examined a large number of skeletons from an advanced agricultural society in Chalcatzingo, Mexico (1150–550 B.C.). The overall size of the archaeological site, the distribution of artifacts, and the mortuary items accompanying certain burials suggested a highly stratified society, probably at the "chiefdom" level. Relying on extensive archaeological and ethnographic studies, Schoeninger assumed that the presence of grave goods (mortuary items) and their quality were a measure of status held by the individual. She reasoned, from ethnographic studies of recent peoples, that diet would be correlated with status, that the higher-status individual would have proportionately more of the desirable food, probably meat, in his diet. A cluster analysis of grave goods was compared to the distribution of bone strontium values, and, as predicted, the mean value of strontium for those burials of high status individuals was the lowest, indicating a higher meat-to-plant ratio.

Schoeninger's study was carefuly conceived and executed with measurements of bone strontium made by two methods—neutron activation and atomic absorption spectrometry of 58 and 91 bone samples, respectively. The results of the absolute values were not identical owing to "matrix interaction" of trace elements. However, results from both methods ranked the samples in similar positions relative to their strontium values. Also, she recognized that individual metabolic variation would result in differing strontium levels, an insight gained from the measure of a high coefficient of variation (20%) of strontium in a controlled study of 35 mink raised on an identical diet. She assumed that the strontium ion in bone mineral is very stable and that diagenesis should not have affected bone strontium levels. Her confidence in the use of strontium values to establish status hierachy has not always been shared, and interpretation of status was criticized for being on shaky ground (23). A major cultural problem is the concept of what constitutes a "high-status" diet. Dietary preferences vary widely among the world's cultures today and are further confounded by the favored use of grubs, insects, seeds, and roots by some societies. The strontium content of these substances is not known. Also, the lack of sexual identification of each bone sample raises further questions about these interpretations of status.

Comparisons of human and faunal remains from different time periods were made by Sillen (44) in order to test the strontium method for paleodiet reconstruction. Unlike the previous archaeological studies, Sillen dealt with older human and associated faunal materials. He sampled bone fragments from human, carnivore, and herbivore remains that were excavated from Hayonim Cave, Israel. The carnivores and herbivores came from two distinct temporal sequences, the Natufian (9970 B.C.) and the Aurignacian (16,000–20,000 B.P.). The human bone samples were from the Natufian layer only, a time of incipient agriculture when, according to other archaeological evidence, the people had a mixed omnivorous diet containing quantities of grain, ancestor to modern domesticated varieties. Samples were taken from cortical bone only and analyzed by atomic absorption spectroscopy. Sillen's results showed a large difference between herbivore and carnivore samples from the Natufian level, as would be expected from their diets. The adult human bone samples fell midway between carnivore and herbivore ranges. However, the fauna from the Aurignacian level of the cave showed no significant differences. There was complete overlap in the strontium values of all herbivore and carnivore samples. In fact, the carnivore strontium values were higher than those from the more recent Natufian. On the other hand, the strontium values of some of the herbivores (gazelles) were lower than those of their more recent descendants.

Postmortem chemical changes of the bone were considered by Sillen to be the most plausible explanation, since the high Sr/Ca ratio of a carnivorous genus like *Felis* could not be explained by diet changes between Natufian and Aurignacian levels. Because of postmortem chemical changes, this study raised serious questions about the time range of applicability of Sr/Ca ratios to dietary reconstructions. Sillen did note, however, that it was a useful method for differentiating between human and faunal remains at the most recent levels.

Another study that brought into question paleodiet reconstruction was the analysis of teeth from modern human vegeterians and nonvegeterians from Calcutta, India (45). Atomic absorption spectroscopy was used to determine the strontium content of sound tooth enamel. The results showed no difference between the samples; the method could not differentiate between dental enamel of people on a purely vegetable diet and those on a partly vegetable diet. Since it is unlikely that any of the fossil hominids were other than omnivores, the analysis of dental strontium is unlikely to be a useful method given these data. The factors of mixed diets and the lack of synchrony of the fossils further confound the problem of paleodiet analysis. Elias (45) adds that strontium levels may also differ because of species-specific physiological differences.

Schoeninger (46) continued to apply the comparisons of Sr/Ca ratios found in faunal and human remains in a paleolithic context but this time with an internal control. The ratios found in human bone were taken in relation to the accompanying fauna. The human bone strontium was divided by the mean strontium values of the herbivores. Additionally, she examined specimens by X-ray diffraction to determine the degree of postmortem deposition of carbonate. Secondary carbonate deposits were seen in the earlier materials (ca. 70,000–30,000 B.P.), but the later levels (5,000–10,000 B.P.) showed little change in the mineral phase.

The results of these diffraction patterns together with those of the reference herbivores aided the comparison of dietary components between time periods. Schoeninger reasoned that since human or animal bones have undergone the same diagenesis as determined by their similar apatite patterns, the relative strontium amounts would be the same, though their absolute value may have increased. The results showed that there was a fairly consistent proportion of meat to vegetable material consumed from 70,000 to 35,000 years ago. The Sr/Ca ratio of the human diet was about 70 percent of the ratio of the herbivores. A marked change was seen in the materials from later time levels (ca. 10,000 B.P.), when a dietary shift occurred boosting the Sr/Ca ratio to 90 percent of the related herbivores. These results, though necessarily based on small samples of scarce and valuable hominid fragments, correlated well with the other archaeological evidence, which indicated a greater reliance on the harvesting of grains.

An interesting application of this study is made to answer the perplexing question of what influence food production had on the reduction of human robusticity mentioned earlier. The study showed that diet changes (i.e., a reduction in animal protein) occurred about 20,000 years later than the appearance of the first skeletally modern humans. That is, the human skeletal form became gracile long before the introduction of food production.

After this study investigators became more cautious in their conclusions, and more recognition was given to possible diagenic changes. More attention was paid to faunal bone from species of known dietary habits. At times, such investigations have helped, but new questions have been raised. Bumsted (34), in a review of bone chemical analysis applied to questions of human diet, noted that samples of antelopes and bison are distinct in their strontium levels, with a higher concentration in the antelope. The bison, however, could not be distinguished from the human in terms of its bone strontium level. This similarity between human and grazing herbivore still awaits explanation, and at this time there is no ready answer. It is merely another oddity in the search for dietary evidence from bone composition. Considering such faunal differences, a clue may be found in the report by Price (47) that demonstrated significant strontium variation among modern deer. It may be, as Bumsted observed, that animal foods do not provide a single class of chemical input. The soils, water, and vegetation differ between regions, sometimes to a significant degree.

Klepinger (48) noted unusually high strontium levels in bones in an Iron Age site in Sicily which she attributed to the concentrations in the surrounding soil of the burials and in the nearby spring water. Regional differences of strontium concentration were also noted as a significant factor by Sillen and Kavanagh (49). In their extensive review of strontium and paleodiet research, they emphasized that the content of strontium in skeletons from Arizona will not be comparable to remains recovered in Illinois, for example. This regional factor was further illustrated by Schoeninger (31) in a recent paper comparing herbivores and carnivores from the Lake Turkana region in Kenya with several Pleistocene fauna from Los Angeles. The fauna consisted of a variety of herbivore and carnivore genera, including several carnivorous birds. The distribution of strontium values of the world sample overlapped so completely that no predictions about diet could be made. However, those bones collected from the Lake Turkana area showed a separation between carnivores and herbivores that suggests that only fauna inhabiting a single drainage basin should be compared. Human nomads covering wide environmental ranges can be another problem.

Waterborne solutes can confound trace element analysis in other ways in addition to diagenic changes. Aquatic and marine resources can significantly increase strontium in the food chain and influence its concentration in the bone. Prehistoric peoples supplementing their diet with mussels from rivers or streams will increase their strontium intake, and their bone strontium will thus suggest a lower meat diet than was actually the case (50). Marine waters have 100 times the concentration of strontium of fresh water, and this is also reflected in the bones of prehistoric Eskimos (35). Their diet was heavily dependent on sea mammals, which resulted in some of the highest levels of bone strontium reported. More recent populations showed a decline in strontium that the authors interpret as increased dependence on terrestrial resources like caribou. The average caribou strontium was 235.5 ppm versus 619.5 ppm for polar bear, a carnivore preying on marine mammals like seals.

Associated fauna are often used as a check of regional environmental influences on strontium concentration variability. The extensive study of late Archaic (3000–700 BC) remains from the Ohio River Valley relied on examination of bones of white-tailed deer. Since this animal was a frequently used food source, skeletal remains are found at a majority of the archaeological sites. The strontium concentration ranged from 250 to 1021 ppm, and there were significant differences between the collections found at three major sites (47). Even when corrected with reference to deer bones, the human bone strontium averages showed different concentrations, reflecting a variation in subsistence base. Certain groups had relied more heavily on freshwater mussels, and other populations, represented at the more recent occupation sites, had replaced hickory, oak, and hazel nuts with more seeds. This shift in subsistence base was also reflected by a change in carbon isotope ratios.

Age and Metabolic Factors and Strontium Values

The use of associated fauna as baseline references is not without its problems. Studies of modern deer bones show an increase of strontium from 4 months to 88 months (51). Accumulation of strontium with age has also been described in humans by Benfer (52), who reasoned that the high intake of strontium, because of the quantity of shellfish consumed, would cause increased levels with age. He also noted that Sr/Ca ratios were less variable among females, for whatever reason. Whether this is due to dietary differences or biological discrimination variation is not known. Studies of other populations both human and faunal have described sexual dimorphism for Sr/Ca ratios (35,53). One possible explanation, frequently offered, is the more rapid bone remodeling rate among pregnant and lactating females. Since in prehistoric times, females were either pregnant or lactating most of their adult lives, this is a possibility to consider.

In young mammals age plays an equally important role, but in the reverse of the above. Infant mammals have lessened capability to discriminate. The OR of strontium reaches a peak at 1 year in humans and then declines by up to 50 percent over the next two decades (36). The initial diet, milk, or formula in modern or breast milk in prehistoric populations is low in Sr/Ca ratios, and even though infant tissue discrimination is low, the buildup of bone strontium is slow until solid food is added. This leads to considerably higher Sr/Ca values until the age of 10 years. Anthropologists have made use of the discrimination of placenta and mammary glands and the higher Sr/Ca in solid foods to try to compare variations in childhood diets (49).

Compared to human milk, other diet sources are high in Sr/Ca; most plant foods and even meat contain more strontium. The strontium intake would increase in proportion to the foods added to supplement breast milk. Sillen and Smith (54) used this reasoning to examine the variation of strontium in child and infant skeletons recovered from an eastern Mediterranean Arab cemetery (A.D. 800–1300). The skeletons varied in age from newborn to 7 years. X-ray diffraction showed no crystallographic changes in the apatite and presumably no diagenesis. Sr/Ca ratios were calculated, and the lowest were found in those bones under 1 year and the highest between 1.5 and 2 years. The level declines slowly after this peak to an adult range.

The fitted curve conformed closely to those curves describing data for numerous contemporary populations and is interpreted by the authors as a reflection of the introduction of solid foods during the weaning period. The time, 1.5–2 years of age, conforms to the practice of the duration of breast feeding among modern Arab communities. Though the sample sizes at each age are small (3–6), the highest Sr/Ca in the child skeletons and the distribution of values conform very close to the expected, given the modern experiences with strontium discrimination.

Associated with the question of Sr/Ca ratios in bones of the growing child is a problem of bone remodeling rates. Ribs have a rate of 10–19 percent per year compared to 0.9 percent for the tibia (55). These differences can lead to conflicting results if bone samples are mixed, especially if there is a variation of strontium intake, as could occur in a migratory population using alternate water sources. This variation can appear in the rib before the denser, more compact bones. If adult dietary strontium were held constant, then some workers reason that Sr/Ca would be evenly distributed throughout the skeleton. However, this is probably not the case. In addition to the rib differences, long-bone epiphyses have been reported to have different Sr/Ca levels from the midshafts (56).

Tanaka (57) also reported higher Sr/Ca ratios in bone diaphysis than epiphysis. He recorded values for most of the skeleton gained from autopsy samples, aged birth to 79 years. The values ranged from .661 for the skull to .367 in vertebrae. There was a slight increase with age, as expected from other studies. In addition, archaeological bone has shown variation between ribs and femurs for several of the major trace elements, including strontium (5). This, plus the factor of a reduction in remodeling rates with age, raises a question about assumptions of even strontium distribution and the conclusion that any portion of the body has the same ratio.

Interpretative problems are further emphasized by excavated skeletons of more recent dates that show a wide range of values for trace elements. Grupe (58) examined samples of human skeletons from northern Germany of Eleventh and Twelfth Century dates and found low correlations of trace elements in trabecular and compact bone. Differences between samples from the same individuals varied as much as 100 percent, even when the samples were taken only a few centimeters apart from the same bone fragment. Over the entire skeleton, trace element concentrations of both compact and trabecular bone sometimes showed intra-individual variability that exceeded the inter-individual variability (59).

PALEODIET COMPLEXES AND TRACE ELEMENT CONCENTRATIONS

The diversity of plant and animal resources used for food, the different preparation techniques, and environmental factors contribute a high level of complexity to paleodietary interpretation. Some foods are unusually high or low in major bone-seeking elements, or they may be bound to insoluble complexes. Other food may contain compounds that bind and inhibit absorption through the intestinal mucosa. Cooking may add or subtract elements, such as the absorption of strontium from boiling water. Given the wide range of foraging techniques employed by prehistoric peoples, together with food preparation choices, any analysis of trace element content of bone to determine paleodiet is open to broad interpretation and subject to a wide range of error. Because of these problems, investigators are more frequently considering a complex of trace elements together as evidence of diet composition.

Typically, nine trace elements are considered. Strontium, magnesium, and manganese are considered to be representative of a vegetable diet. Copper and zinc concentrations are indicative of a higher proportion of meat. Since nuts, hickory, hazel, and oak, typically found in abundance at woodland sites in the Midwest, will provide high levels of most elements, an unwanted complication arises. Hatch (60) proposed that vanadium would offer a way to assess the relative contribution of nuts to dietary zinc and copper. The extraordinarily high strontium content in nuts should have caused a high bone strontium in the late Archaic populations of the middle Mississippi Valley. But this was not the case, as described earlier. These bone samples from the midwestern Archaic had less strontium than the later populations, which were becoming dependent on more seed collecting and domesticated plants like maize.

A possible explanation may be the presence of a binding agent in the nut meat itself that prevented or at least reduced the absorption of strontium. This substance may be similar to the pectin compounds naturally occurring in fruit and plant gums that have been experimentally shown to reduce absorption of alkaline earth metals (see later). Hickory nuts were cracked and placed in boiling water; the nut meat and oils rose to the top and were scooped off. It is likely that this substance was congealed into a kind of nut butter similar to that used by early French settlers, according to P. J. Watson (personal communication), a specialist in Midwestern archaeology. This method of food preparation, together with the use of plant gums, could have added pectin compounds to the digestive tract. There is ample ethnographic evidence to support this interpretation; aboriginal peoples in recent times, and even today, used plant exudates to add a tasty sweetener to their diet. Unfortunately, the significance of these observations are only now becoming realized since so few chemical composition data are available. The use of such supplements may be another confounding factor, however.

Despite these problems, taken as a group, several bone trace elements do show shifts through time and may be indicative of major dietary components. In addition to strontium, zinc is the one most frequently used. Examination of prehistoric populations from Illinois showed a significant reduction of zinc levels in those skeletons from the period when the subsistence base shifted to a heavy dependence on maize cultivation. The reasoning was that, since zinc is present in high quantities in animal protein, a shift away from animal food sources to a limited number of cultivated plants would result in lowered zinc intake over a lifetime (61).

Zinc concentrations have also revealed sexual and status differences among populations from these same time periods. As more plants are cultivated, the population diet shifted toward less animal protein, but the most significant change occurred in the female diet, since females received even less animal protein. This is reflected in their relatively lower zinc levels as agricultural development proceeded. The same relationship has been reported for other archaeological populations (53). Such observations are supported by a study of modern-day Papuans in Oriomo, New Guinea, that showed significantly lower zinc levels in the hair of females. This was explained by the lower consumption of meat by women confirmed during an ethnographic field study (62).

The dietary factor that will complicate zinc absorption as well as calcium, iron, manganese, and copper is the presence of phytate in many grains and seeds. Studies of the influence of high-bran diets on trace elements have demonstrated the formation of insoluble phytate chelates (63). This prevents absorption and leads to deficiency states that can have serious growth consequences, especially in the case of zinc. In areas of the world where populations are dependent on grains high in phytate as their major food source, this chelation of zinc has caused serious growth defects (6, 64). Similar influences could have occurred in prehistoric times as many populations began to gather wild grains and later to cultivate them. The ingestion of the trace element binding phytate would have increased markedly under these dietary conditions. A particular consideration would be the well-reported dietary shifts that occurred in parts of North America when more seed plants were added to the diet. The probability that the lowered zinc levels might be due to this phenomenon should not be overlooked.

Iron and magnesium deficiencies are other conditions noted by anthropologists studying prehistoric bone. Since many of the skeletal remains are frequently those of young children whose bones bear pathological lesions, causes are often sought. A frequent pathology is one of the thinning and even the perforation of the cortical bone of the skull, especially the parietal and occipital bones. Another feature is the deposition of spongy bone on the superior surfaces of the orbits or its perforation (criba orbitalia). The causes of these conditions have been variously described as vitamin deficiencies or anemias, especially in the case of iron deficiency anemia.

Some studies have reported correlations between these lesions and iron and magnesium deficiencies. Samples taken of bone and hair from a well-preserved prehistoric population in Nubia (A.D. 550–1450) who suffered a high frequency of criba orbitalia showed a close correspondence between the pathology and iron and magnesium deficiencies (65). However, these pathological lesions are of complex etiology, which cannot easily be interpreted from the prehistoric bone. Zaino (66) pointed this out when he examined bone iron in a collection of skeletons from an Arizona Pueblo (A.D. 900–1100) There was a frequent occurrence of criba orbitalia and porotic hyperostosis, but bone iron concentrations were measured within normal ranges, which suggested a diet adequate in iron. The surrounding soils had a lower iron level, so Zaino ruled out any postmortem losses of the element.

In a study of a tropical population, the prehistoric Mayan, Saul (2) made a convincing case for iron deficiency anemia and attendant bone lesions, however. The form and location of the cranial lesions of spongy hyperostosis are consistent with those associated with anemia, he argued. Further, of the lesions found in 32 individuals, seven were children with the active variety, and the 25 adults showed a healed variety. Saul explained that a greater number of iron absorption problems are suffered by tropical populations, with diets high in plant and low in animal sources, parasitic loads, and increased sweat losses. Since these factors apply to other trace elements as well, special consideration must be given trace elements of bone when the remains of prehistoric populations from different climatic zones are used for paleodiet reconstruction.

Lead is another trace element that may usefully be applied in studies of past populations. Measurements of lead ingested are generally very small, and because the minute quantities distributed in the food chain are within the excretory capacity of the body, this element does not normally accumulate in the skeleton to a great degree. However, with the introduction of technologies dependent upon large amounts of lead for utensils, solders, or pipes, skeletal-borne lead increased materially, especially as discovered in Roman and Greek remains (67). A good example of skeletal lead burdens in recent populations was given by a historical archaeological study of Colonial households in the Chesapeake Bay area (A.D. 1670–1730). Excavations not only turned up evidence of numerous pewter vessels but also showed a distinct class difference in their usage. The wealthier families used these plates and drinking vessels exclusively, but the laborers were excluded from the risk of this source of lead ingestion. Because of their lower status, they were limited to the use of ceramic and wood containers. This class difference is reflected in bone lead content recovered from two groups distinguished on the basis of their burial locations, which were spatially segregated according to social class (68).

INTERFERENCE WITH INTESTINAL TRACT ABSORPTION

One of the more interesting factors that can complicate paleodiet interpretations is the mix of component food particles and their elemental constituents. Phytate as an inhibitor has already been mentioned, so this section will consider the various influences on strontium and calcium absorption. The studies of ^{90}Sr fallout and its movement in the food change have given ample experimental evidence of Sr/Ca ratios in the whole animal (37). A result of major significance for paleodiet evolution was the report that calcium intake strongly influenced strontium absorption and excretion. Strontium is regulated by total calcium ion concentration (69) and human plasma strontium levels varied with calcium in the diet. Higher calcium intakes contributed to a greater strontium discrimination, whereas lower calcium conditions led to higher strontium (70). Phosphorus added to either low- or high-calcium diets decreased strontium levels.

In attempts to find an inhibitor for ^{90}Sr absorptions, several food substances were tried in addition to phosphorus and calcium compounds. The alginates and other natural polymers of plant gums and muculages were tried (71). Sodium alginate inhibited strontium uptake in the rats at several dietary levels from 24 percent alginate to a low of 1.4 percent. Calcium absorption was only slightly affected, and calcium metabolism was not sufficiently disturbed to influence normal growth. A most interesting observation for the anthropologist, as noted above, are the similarity of other natural substances, such as the pectins, which have equally good strontium-binding capacity. The use of gums, fruits, and berries could introduce a quantity of pectins into the digestive tract. Though only slight effects on calcium are reported, the pectins may bind with other trace elements, though no observations have yet been offered.

It is a matter for further investigation to aid bone trace element research. It is likely that the food supplements used by a prehistoric or a contemporary aboriginal people have a greater influence on growth and health and hence bone composition then has been recognized to date. Also, the casual addition of the occasionally collected grub, insect, fruit, or berry may have important affects on dietary absorption. Few of these items, by the way, have been analyzed for their trace element components.

The influence of waterborne trace elements is another important consideration. Here epidemiology data have been most helpful in understanding the effects of water sources. Studies of calcium content of drinking water have shown that persons using low-calcium sources had a significantly higher (16%) ^{90}Sr in their bone than persons who received additional calcium in their drinking water. Higher fluoride ingestion also made a significant difference, as studies of enamel from thousands of adult and deciduous teeth have demonstrated (72). The contributor of water to trace element intake may lead to a wide variation among communities. These differences are probably responsible for variation in hard-tissue levels (73). In addition, Losee and Adkins (74) reported the high rate of strontium absorbed by cooked vegetables. These studies of water involvement and trace element uptake make soils and water sources an important factor to contend with both in the living organism and after interment of the skeleton.

FOSSILIZATION AND DIAGENESIS: CONTRIBUTIONS TO TRACE ELEMENT AND PROTEIN VARIATION

The study of the skeletal evidence for dietary information assumes that the bone chemical composition of either organic or mineral phases is representative of life values. Unfortunately, this is seldom wholly true. Once a body has been deposited in lake sediments, grave, open site, or cave floor, numerous features of the environment begin to act. The state of the body's preservation, including its skeleton, depends on these features. Archaeologists have recovered remains in various stages of preservation that range from intact mummified bodies to fragile, fragmentary bones, and any skeletal analysis must take account of the environmental conditions. For the sake of simplicity in this discussion, I shall consider only those conditions that relate to the skeletal integrity, since most of the published dietary analyses have dealt only with the preserved bone. Valuable information, however, has been obtained from mummified or frozen tissues as well as from intact bodies preserved in marshes or peat bogs. These types of preserved remains require special methods not unlike those of forensic pathology, and these methods are ably described by Cockburn and Cockburn (75). In a majority of burials, though, once the soft tissue has been removed through decay, the skeleton is more or less well preserved, depending on a variety of circumstances.

Trace Element Variation

The composition of the soils and water in contact with the bone play major roles, but temperature, especially seasonal alteration, influences preservation as well. The first vital consideration is soil pH. Even under only slightly acidic conditions, rapid bone loss will occur; the lighter bones of young children and infants are quickly reduced in mass and are frequently destroyed (76). The repeated wetting–drying or freezing–thawing will contribute to bone loss. This "weathering" of bone will cause a decrease in density, beginning with the trabeculae (77). Soil chemical composition also influences bone. The quantities of carbonates or silicates may contribute to preservation, but the greatest influence, from the perspective of trace element analysis, is the ion exchange due to soil and water.

For example, the discussion of bone iron as representative of living values can be assumed only for dry, arid regions, not for humid areas (66). The state of preservation for Anazasi Pueblo burials in Arizona will be vastly different from the majority of the sites in the Mississippi Valley. As Parker and Toots (9) emphasized, the variety of chemical changes of the skeleton is a function of the chemical environment of the burial. Many studies have considered the quantities of groundwater as an important factor because of the erosive, leaching effects and because of the addition of trace elements to bone. The longer a bone has been buried, the more concentrated certain substances may become. The most famous of examples is the absorption of fluorides by buried bone, a phenomenon that has proved useful for the relative dating of some archaeological and paleontological sites. However, bones from different locales cannot be compared because of varying water fluoride concentrations (78).

The variations of soil trace element influences were further illustrated by St. Hoyme and Koritzer (79), who compared enamel of prehistoric North American teeth from the Midwest and the East Coast, dating from about A.D. 600. They recorded 11 trace elements, including strontium, commonly found in dental enamel surfaces. The wide range of recorded values was explained by reference to soil compositions in different drainage systems. The assumption was that little or no postmortem enamel change occurred, a point that could be debated if the studies of enamel trace element exchange are considered. Curzon and Cutress (37) described decreasing gradients of trace elements, especially strontium, from the enamel surface inward, which they considered strong evidence of posteruptive deposition from saliva-borne elements. This observation, together with the findings of Boaz and Hemple (42), suggests, possible postmortem exchanges with waterborne ions, as well.

In the study of early Hellenistic Greek burials, mentioned earlier, considerable attention was given to the state of preservation of isotope integrity in the bones examined (5). Concentrations of most elements were probably the result of soil contamination due to groundwater filtering through the bones, an event more influential in the porous ribs than the long bones. Edward and his co-workers argued that, despite this postmortem influence on chemical integrity, the elements considered most useful for dietary studies remained unchanged; these were calcium, strontium, and zinc. Comparison of these elements in surrounding soil showed a lower concentration than that of bone, so contamination through leaching was unlikely, though the process had occurred for other elements.

A more complete analysis of bone diagenesis was attempted by Lambert and co-workers (80). They reasoned that the leaching process would distribute elements in irregular gradient patterns from bone to burial soil. Samples of soil were taken at 5-cm increments above, below, and beside the burials. Strontium and zinc showed the same concentration in all directions and did not vary with the distance from the bone. However, calcium, iron, aluminum, potassium, and copper varied with distance; the pattern of distribution was uneven as well. Calcium, for example, showed higher than normal concentrations next to the bone and decreased with distance. The soil concentrations of iron, aluminum, and potassium decreased nearest the bone, which suggested a contamination of the bone by these elements, according to the authors. Strontium and zinc are probably the most resistant to the leaching process, so bone contamination should be least, while calcium and sodium are subject to a greater loss.

Since the bones studied dated to A.D. 400–600, the authors concluded with a cautious note, there may be a decrease in reliability of bone mineral measurement with duration of burial. However, archaeologically older bones and bones in advanced stages of decomposition have been less thoroughly studied.

Another extensive examination of bone trace elements and diagenesis was made of historic burials from three different periods—the late Iron Age (750–650 B.C.), Archaic Greek (550–500 B.C.), and Hellenistic Greek (330–211 B.C.) (48). Cortical bone samples were taken from tibia, femur, or humerus, and 10 elements were recorded plus the Sr/Ca ratios. Six of the 10 elements did not show a predictable trend with length of burial time, so the authors were unable to predict direction of diagenesis. Only four of the elements (Mn, Ca, Cd, Mg) showed a undirectional change with time; manganese and cadmium increased, and magnesium and calcium decreased. These burials, from a semiarid site in the mountains of Sicily, provide little help for those who wish evidence of predictable diagenesis trends. The changes that occurred over the approximately 500 years between the earliest and most recent burials were not great, perhaps because of rainfall variations during the intervening 2,200 years since the more recent of the burials. Whatever the reason, the answer to bone diagenesis will not be an easy one. There is likely a time limit that restricts trace element analysis, as suggested earlier (44, 46).

The degree of diagenesis in buried bone continues to be a focus of much investigation, especially the concentration of stable strontium. The results of several recent studies have not been encouraging for the use of Sr/Ca ratios for dietary reconstruction. Archaeological bone may offer a wide variation in the concentration of strontium due to the state of preservation and the burial environment. Specific differences of locality are important considerations as is the duration of burial, described above.

Williams (81) examined samples of fossilized mammal bone taken from several sites of paleoanthropological importance in East Africa. He recorded the trace elements of dietary and chronological interest with special attention to strontium. The distribution profiles in the fossil bone measured from the cortical surface to the medullary cavity were relatively flat and the strontium/calcium ratio was exceptionally high (up to 47.0). Williams, at first, thought this high ratio was due to a Sr-rich diet. However, examination of a bone recently deposited on the surface (about one year) showed that there was a rapid postmortem uptake of strontium by faunal remains in the area. This uptake was most likely due to a high concentration in the ground water and soil surrounding the covered portion of the bone. Comparisons with the fossil bones of the area suggested that the high strontium concentrations were likely due to diagenesis. These results caused Williams to conclude with a cautionary note about the use of "dietary tracers in the inorganic phases of bone." Each archaeological site must be evaluated individually to evaluate the degree of postmortem change.

In another study of Sr/Ca ratios of buried bone, Sealy and Sillen (82) also noted significant differences due to the burial environment. Animal and human bone recovered from shell middens in the Cape region of South Africa showed high levels of strontium, for example. Repeated washings of the archaeological samples lowered the Sr/Ca because, compared to fresh bone, strontium was released from a "highly soluble, diagenic mineral compartment." They concluded that this was due to the presence of high levels of strontium circulating in the shell middens. This has further added to the evidence for the need to identify the burial medium, especially the influences of the accumulated debris that have high concentrations of those elements of dietary interest.

Different bones of the skeleton may be more or less subject to diagenesis. Ribs, for example, are frequently used in analysis, because they have little value for morphological studies, so one is often willing to use ribs for methods that require destruction of the sample. Ribs, though, have a higher rate of contamination by the groundwater (5,53); calcium and sodium are among the elements frequently recorded at lower levels in the rib fragments. However, three elements—Sr, Zn, and Mg—showed statistically identical levels in rib and femur (80).

Some workers claim that the choice of bone samples is not critical for strontium, zinc, or magnesium analysis (53). However, given the reports for variation of trace elements in autopsied material and the differing remodeling rates, it would be best to be cautious in sample selection. In fact, at least one study points out the possibility that even cortical bone may not be as homogeneous as has been assumed (48). As a further check on possible diagenesis contamination, femur cross sections were made of bones recovered from Midwestern woodland sites (83). The authors reasoned that an element entering bone from the soil would be distributed unevenly throughout the section. They examined each cross section with an electron microprobe and mapped the distributions of those elements in question. The density of Fe, Al, K, Mn, and Mg near the periosteal surfaces ruled out their usefulness for paleodiet reconstruction. The distribution of Zn, Sr, and Pb throughout the samples appeared not to be altered and would probably be useful as dietary indicators. This study was of a small sample (eight individuals) and did not account for the possible exchanges of elements like calcium or sodium. Also, the penetration of the marrow spaces by waterborne soil particles and contact with trabecula bone were not considered. However, the study represents one more concern with diagenesis of the mineral phase.

Bacterial and Fungal Contamination

Bacterial residues in bone are a major contaminating source to be considered. In addition, the presence of rhizones and fungi may add to changes of isotopic ratios or trace element diagenesis, a factor little appreciated. Mycelia of fungus can penetrate the smallest of spaces in dense, compact, mineralized tissues and even the tubules within the dentin of teeth. What residues they deposit or remove have yet to be determined, but a few experiments have demonstrated fungi influence on bone composition. Grupe and Piepenbrink (84), using fresh pig bone inoculated with two types of fungi and kept in a simulated soil medium enriched with the several elements of dietary interest, showed changes influenced by fungi growth. Comparisons of the control and fungi-infected samples showed changes of the elements in the infected samples that varied over a wide range, depending upon the type of fungi and the concentration of the element in the surrounding medium. One fungi species (*P. brevicompactum*) caused near-depletion of all elements of dietary interest and radically increased the Ca/P ratio to 18, while in other fungal media (*Cladosporium sp.*), the bone retained ratios of about 2.3 to 3. In like manner the elements strontium, boron, magnesium, and zinc underwent marked changes and were reduced to low levels.

Fungi may also cause considerable microstructural changes in bone. A careful histologic and electron microscopic study of the palatine torus of the Neanderthal from Mt. Circeo I, Italy showed areas of irregular bone (85), woven bone with many irregular canniculi. These features were very similar to those that were experimentally produced in fresh bone. Fragments of human vertebra, obtained at autopsy, were placed in flower pots containing garden soil and moistened and kept at room temperature. After the 45th day, the bone had been penetrated by extensive mycellium growth.

The bone was viewed by optical and electron microscopes, and the mold specimens were identified. The mold had caused resorption pits and notching on the bone surfaces, which had deep, punched-out-looking pits that resembled Howship's lacunae. This fungus genus, *Mucor,* produced bony channels, which appeared to be one of its characteristic actions (85). Resorption seems to be produced by the fungal membrane in contact with the bone, though mechanisms of the osteoclastic-like activity are not completely clear. The authors believe that the fungi produce enzymes that attack both mineral and organic phases of the bone. Such fungal action would explain the appearance of the Neanderthal palatine torus described by Sergi and co-workers (86). They postulated that, during fossilization, bone mineral actually decreased in parts of the skull. Their microradiographic studies of the exostotic bone regions showed such a decrease in calcium content. If such observations can be confirmed in other specimens, then the factors of change due to microorganisms must be carefully considered. Such clues have been provided by Wyckoff (87), who noted that bacteria can be an agent that may add protein like material to fossils, either from ancient or from recent contamination.

More recently, Hanson and Buikstra (88) observed microorganism-caused changes in prehistoric bone from the lower Illinois Valley. The growth of bacteria and/or fungi into the vascular spaces led to a resorption of the surrounding tissue and created broader tunnels and destroyed the histological identity of the bone. The authors noted that 23% of the 119 histological sections they examined showed microfocal destruction and were not suitable for histomorphometric evaluation. Likewise, bones so altered by microorganism action were suspect for use in dietary reconstruction because of the likely contamination of the mineral concentrations. Soil composition and pH influences microbe growth as well as the state of bone preservation which emphasized the need for analysis of the burial environment when archaeological bone is used as a source of data for dietary reconstruction.

Changes in the Organic Phases of Bone

The studies of carbon isotope ratios to determine dietary carbon sources, either C3 or C4 plants, depend on the stability of the bone carbon-bearing fractions. Calcium carbonates bound to bone mineral are a poor source because of their ready exchange with the environmental sources of carbonates. Therefore, estimates of ^{13}C values are not considered useful when derived from the carbonates (89). Even the attempts to remove postmortem deposits with acetic acid have not helped. Land (11) compared Pleistocene and Holocene deer bones with fresh-killed samples and found that the carbon isotope ratios were too inconsistent to be of use. This problem of diagenesis requires that only collagen be used, since the assumption is that there is little diagenesis of this protein. However, alterations and degeneration of collagen are known to occur.

Bone collagen is subject to change over time, and to some degree its products are released into the environment. Decomposition may or may not selectively release certain amino acids while retaining others. Some authors have argued that diagenic degredation of collagen is linear, with no preferential retention of specific amino acids (90), while others have reported changes in certain amino acid concentrations compared to fresh bone (91). Whatever the relative changes of amino acids in archaeological bone, several authors have described the duration of burial by comparing concentrations with that of fresh bone. Knight and Lauder (92) examined bone samples of various archaeological ages and, by chromatography, identified the amino acids of the hydrolysate. Bones containing both proline and hydroxyproline were likely less than 50 years old. A nitrogen content of greater than 3.5 mg percent was considered good evidence of bone less than 100 years old, while 2.5 mg percent suggested an origin of 350 years or less. In his extensive study of animal fossils, Wyckoff (87) noted that amino acid changes varied with age and environmental conditions. Slow hydrolysis of peptide bonds occur, which increases protein solubility (93).

In general, even in a constant environment, the older the fossil bone, the less organic matrix, and there is an extreme variation in amino acid composition. The quantity of water plays a essential role, but even the endogenous water in bone is usually sufficient for hydrolysis to occur. Laboratory experiments have established that water distribution was as important as temperature in the diagenesis process, which is to be expected from the numerous studies that have shown mineral exchanges. What is not as obvious, however, is the extent of diagenesis on human bone collagen.

Most bones in natural environments, according to Hare (93), show diminished amounts of protein presumably due to the leaching process. Bones so leached often lack mechanical strength, as samples from many archaeological sites have demonstrated. Von Endt and Ortner (94) also showed protein changes through controlled experiments. The more easily water is diffused, the more readily the protein is altered. Size is an important factor, as shown by the experiments that kept bone fragments at a constant temperature in a water bath. Hare and his coworkers (93) showed that the quantity of nitrogen released was proportionate to bone size. These conditions of collagen diagenesis have been recognized as a problem for the analysis of ^{13}C ratios in archaeologically derived bone. Bones from Tehuacan, Mexico, over the past 7,000 years have undergone some collagen diagenesis, but DeNiro and Epstein argued that, though collagen concentrations varied from 12 percent to 5.4 percent, diagenesis did not alter isotope ratios (13). A similar conclusion was reached earlier, by DeNiro and Epstein (89) in their study of feeding patterns of African hyrax. They stated that the collagen fraction is not subject to carbon exchange with the environment. They added the caution that a rigorous analysis of diagenesis effects on isotope ratios is still needed (13). The implication is that, though collagen may be degraded and amino acids lost, carbon and nitrogen isotope ratios will remain the same. This is further highlighted by DeNiro's 1985 (95) study in which he qualified his original conclusion. He noted that any postmortem process that adds or subtracts a collagen component will affect isotope ratios if a large enough quantity is involved. Therefore, any prehistoric collagen samples with carbon and nitrogen ratios outside the observed range for fresh collagen should be suspect.

Further comparisons of collagen were made to describe several kinds of diagenic changes and to confirm these earlier results. De Niro and Weiner (97) took samples of prehistoric and modern terrestrial herbivores and marine carnivores for analysis by chemical, enzymatic and spectrascopic methods. They were able to distinguish between the altered organic components of the prehistoric bone by comparisons with modern samples. The "good" samples—prehistoric bone without diagenic change—yielded the same results as did modern bone obtained by all three methods. The "bad" prehistoric samples gave widely divergent values because of postmortem changes in the organic fraction that rendered them useless for stable isotope analysis as suggested in De Niro's earlier study.

Finally, the state of bone preservation varies so widely that in some environments fossilization may preserve much of the collagen intact. In well-preserved Pleistocene species from arid regions like Arizona, striated fibers of collagen indistinguishable from that in fresh bone were observed by Matter (96). In other samples, recognizable collagen was not found, but degradation products were occasionally seen. Several samples contained undecomposed protein in quantities sufficient for amino acid analysis (87). Care must be taken not to confuse fossil protein with proteinaceous material residues from microbial action, as noted above. Ultimately the filling of every fine crevice, crack, or void in bone or tooth brings many ions and compounds into intimate contact with the structural elements; at times some products are removed. Therefore, after a vertebrate organism dies and the decay process begins, the numerous and complex changes of diagenesis will contribute to alterations of the life values of those isotopes or trace elements of dietary interest.

ARCHAEOLOGICAL DIETS: SOME CONCLUSIONS

Interpreting the past is never easy. Even if one is provided most of the remains of ancient human activity in an archaeological site, the task of reconstruction may still be monumental. A major and much disputed question is, and has always been, the ways in which people exploited their environment to gain a subsistence. Much time has been spent analyzing plant and animal remains, their distribution, and their identity in order to shed light on the survival of prehistoric humans. An equal challenge is the explanation of why the human species began to grow in numbers about the time it discovered new methods of food procurement. To examine these issues more thoroughly, precise data on food composition and consumption are needed. Human skeletal remains have been viewed as an essential source of information about diet only over the past two decades. Previously, with few exceptions, human skeletons were examined only for the data they might provide about race, body size, and disease. Even then, unless the skeletons were from an earlier era, the Neanderthals, for example, they did not attract much attention. But now, with new tools at hand, precise chemical and histological analysis may be made. But there are several cautions and guidelines that must be followed if the data are to be meaningful.

The first and most crucial question is how representative of life values are the isotope ratios and trace element concentrations. Work on this question is in its early stages, and more attention is being paid to comparisons between fossil, recent, and fresh bone. Additionally, faunal remains are used for references of postmortem changes. It is the recombination or rearrangement of mineral and organic components that cause a shift from life values, and this "diagenesis" will continue to require the utmost attention through experimentation and comparison. The features of the soils surrounding the bones and the quantities of water as well as temperature cause each burial or archaeological site to be unique. Investigators, intent on determining paleodiet from the skeletal evidence must keep this in mind. The slow diagenic processes over time have shifted sets of values at more than one site, as described above. The values may even approach an equilibrium between human and faunal bone, even though in life the differences in isotope and trace element concentration are far apart.

A major requirement of any dietary analysis based on studies of bone is that the samples be of the same provenience. They must be from the same time period to be comparable, not widely separated by hundreds or thousands of years. Even relatively small differences of a few hundred years may cause large value shifts for certain elements, as described by Klepinger (48). The bone should be from burials within the same drainage system, an important requirement noted by Schoeninger (31). In addition, the bones selected from different individuals or different species must be comparable; rib to rib or tibia to tibia. This will reduce the error that can result from comparison of bones of varying densities.

The use of trace elements for dietary reconstruction has come a long way since the first tentative statements by Toots and Voorhies (40). But there is still a long way to go before the skeleton can be used fully for the vital environmental record it contains. Too many workers, however, have continued to make assumptions about hard tissue integrity. Not enough attention has been paid to the dental tissues, whose state of preservation and longevity in the fossil record far exceeds that of bone. Bone strontium is useful for determining trophic levels, but dental enamel may be even better. Strontium in enamel apatite crystals correlates with concentrations in food and water and its main uptake is during tooth formation. There is little change with age or from diagenesis in contrast to bone or to other dental tissues: cementum and dentin (98). The work by Curzon and Cutress (37) on dental trace elements provides many examples. Also, they offer illustrations of nonbiological exchanges of trace elements between the mineralized tissues and the environment. Far from being inappropriate as a data source, as some would suggest, the enamel may provide a significant data reference.

The organic components of bone may be as important as the mineral phases in providing dietary evidence. Collagen composition of the archaelogical bone gives a measure of the state of preservation and provides evidence of dietary composition and disease influences. Amino acid composition of collagen of archaeological bone from recent times (200 to 400 years ago) shows considerable variation which may be relevant to diet, disease or preservation. Dennison and Houghton (99) compared samples taken from four burial sites, two in New Guinea and two in New Zealand. Significant differences were described for several amino acid concentrations especially threonine, serine, tyrosine, and glutamic acid. Differences were found between the two New Zealand collections; the temperate zone burials on the South Island had a higher leucine, lysine, and arginine concentration

370 ARCHAEOLOGICAL DIETARY CONSIDERATIONS

than the tropical site on the North Island. The samples taken from the two New Guinea localities also showed significant differences for threonine, serine, tyrosine, phenyalanine, and glutamic acid. Diagenesis differences likely played a major role in the New Zealand materials because of preservation differences. However, the two New Guinea sites were within 12 km of each other and the authors consider that the burial environments were similar. They suggest that the amino acid differences are due to diet and disease. Those individuals with skeletal pathologies had significantly different amino acid combinations; higher glycine, and lower serine, glutamic acid, and aspartic acid levels suggestive of low protein diet and anemia typical of chronic malaria. Such conclusions are supported by observations of contemporary populations living in these areas of New Guinea.

To conclude a broad summary like the preceding, one might be tempted to add a lengthy list of variables that influence the ultimate interpretation, the nature of the samples, and the environmental conditions, to say nothing of the analytical methods. However, it is sufficient to note that the state-of-the-art of dietary interpretation from archaeologically derived bone is at the beginning stages, but the method holds much potential. At this time the analyses of paleodiet from bone are useful, but only in the context of dietary information gained from other sources. As more careful controls are exerted and additional faunal and plant data are collected, the trace element concentrations and isotope ratios of bone will become increasingly valuable.

REFERENCES

1. Angel, J. L. (1975) In: Polgar S. (ed) *Population, Ecology and Social Evolution.* The Hague: Mouton p. 167.
2. Saul, F. P. (1972) Papers Peabody Mus. Archaeol. Ethnol. 63.
3. Armelagos, G. J. Van Gerven, D. P., Martin, D. L., Huss-Ashmore R. (1984) In: Clark, J. D., Brandt, S. A. (eds), *Hunters to Farmers.* Berkeley: Univ. of Calif. Press, p. 132.
4. Von Endt, D. W. Ortner, D. J. (1982) Am. J. Phys. Anthropol. 59:377–385.
5. Edward, J., Fossey, J. M., Yaffe, L. (1984) J. Field Archaeol. 11:37–46.
6. Prasad, A. S. (1985) Nutr. Research suppl. 1, p. 295.
7. Goodman, A. H., Martin, D. L., Armelagos, G. J. (1984) In: Cohen, M. N., Armelagos, G. J. (eds), *Paleopathology at the Origins of Agriculture.* Orlando: Academic Press, p. 13.
8. Robson, J. R. K., Wadsworth, G. R. (1977) Ecol. Food Nutr. 6:187–202.
9. Parker, R. B., Toots H. (1980) In: Behrensmeyer, A. K., Hill, A. P. (eds) *Fossils in the Making.* Chicago: Univ. of Chicago Press, p. 197.
10. Tauber H. (1981) Nature 292:332–333.
11. Land, L. S., Lundelius, Jr., E. L., Valastro, S. (1980) Paleogeogr. Paleoclimatol. Paleoecol. 32:143–151.
12. Tieszen, L. L., Boutton, T. W. Tesdahl, K. G., Slade, N. A. (1983) Oecologia 57:32–37.
13. DeNiro, M. J., Epstein, S. (1981) Geochim. Cosmochim. Acta. 45:341–351.
14. Ambrose, S. H., DeNiro, M. J. (1986) Nature 319:321–324.
15. Craig, H. (1957) Geochim. Cosmochim. Acta. 12:133–149.
16. Calvin, M., Benson A. A. (1948) Science 107:476–480.

17. Kortshack, H. P., Hart, C. E., Butt, C. O. (1965) Plant Physiol. 40:209–213.

18. van der Merwe, N. (1982) Am. Sci. 70:596–606.

19. Vogel, J. C. (1978) South Afr. J. Sci. 74:298–301.

20. Jones, R. J., Ludlow, M. M., Troughton, J. H., Blunt, C. G. (1979) J. Agr. Sci. 92:91–100.

21. Minson, D. J., Ludlow, M. M., Troughton, J. H. (1975) Nature 256:602.

22. Jones, R. J., Ludlow, M. M., Troughton, J. H., Blunt, C. G. (1981) Search 12:85–87.

23. Klepinger, L. L. (1984) Ann. Rev. Anthropol. 13:75–96.

24. Matthews, D. R., Bier, D. M. (1983) Ann. Rev. Nutr. 3:309–339.

25. Buikstra, J. E., Cook, D. C. (1980) Ann. Rev. Anthropol. 9:433–470.

26. Vogel, J. C., van der Merwe, N. J. (1977) Am. Antiq. 42:238–242.

27. Chisholm, B. S., Nelson, D. E., Schwarcz, H. P. (1983) Curr. Anthropol. 24:396–398.

28. Sullivan, C. H., Kruger, H. W. (1983) Nature 301:177.

29. Schoeninger, M. J., DeNiro, M. J. (1982) Nature 29:577–578.

30. Gaebler, O. H., Vitti, T. G., Vukmirovich, R. (1966) Can. J. Biochem. Physiol. 44:1249–1257.

31. Schoeninger, M. J. (1985) J. Hum. Evol. 14:515–525.

32. Keegan, W. F., DeNiro, M. J. (1988) Am. Antiq. 53:320–336.

33. Price, T. D., Schoeninger, M. J., Armelagos, G. J. (1985) J. Hum. Evol. 14:419–447.

34. Bumsted, M. P. (1985) J. Hum. Evol. 14:539–551.

35. Connor, M., Slaughter, D. (1984) Arctic Anthrop. 21:123–134.

36. Gran, F. S., Nicolaysen, R. (1964) *A Theoretical Analysis of Ratio-Strontium Metabolism and Deposition in Humans.* Copenhagen: Scandinavian Univ. Books.

37. Curzon, M. E. J., Cutress, T. W. (1983) *Trace Elements and Dental Disease.* Boston: John Wright.

38. Comar, C. L., Russell, L., Wasserman, R. H. (1957) Science 126:485–492.

39. Lenihan, J. M. A., Loutit, J. F., Martin, J. H. (eds) (1967) *Strontium Metabolism.* London, NY: Academic Press.

40. Toots, H., Voorhies, M. R. (1965) Science 149:854–855.

41. Brown, A. (1973) Bone Strontium Content as a Dietary Indicator in Human Skeletal Populations. Ph.D. dissertation. Ann Arbor, Univ. of Michigan.

42. Boaz, N. T., Hample, J. (1978) J. Paleontol 52:928–933.

43. Schoeninger, M. J. (1979) Am. J. Phys. Anthropol. 51:295–310.

44. Sillen, A. (1981) Am. J. Phys. Anthropol. 56:131–137.

45. Elias, M. (1980) Am. J. Phys. Anthropol. 53:1–4.

46. Schoeninger, M. J. (1982) Am. J. Phys. Anthropol. 58:37–52.

47. Price, T. D. (1985) J. Hum. Evol. 14:449–459.

48. Klepinger, L. L., Kuhn, J. K., Williams, W. S. (1986) Am. J. Phys. Anthropol. 325–331.

49. Sillen, A., Kavanagh, M. (1982) Yearbook of Phys. Anthropol. 25:67–90.

50. Schoeninger, M. J., Peebles, C. S. (1981) J. Archaeol. Science 8:391–397.

51. Farris, G. S. (1967) Factors Influencing the Accumulation of Strontium-90, Stable Strontium and Calcium in Mule Deer. Ph.D. thesis, Dept. of Radiology, Colorado State Univ., Fort Collins.

52. Benfer, R. A. (1984) In: Cohen, M. N., Armelagos, G. J. (eds) *Paleopathology At the Origins of Agriculture.* NY: Academic Press, p. 531.

53. Lambert, J. B., Valasak, S. M., Thometz, A. C., Buikstra, J. E. (1982) Am. J. Phys. Anthropol. 59:289–294.

54. Sillen, A., Smith, P. (1984) J. Archaeol. Sci. 11:237–245.

55. Stout, S. D., Simmons, D. J. (1979) Yearbook Phys. Anthropol. 22:228–249.

56. Martin, A. (1969) Brit. J. Rad. 42:295–298.

57. Tanaka, G., Kawamura, H., Nomura, E. (1981) Health Physics 40:601–614.

58. Grupe, G. (1988) J. Archaeol. Sci. 15:123–129.

59. Grupe, G., Herrmann, B. (eds) (1988) *Trace Elements in Environmental History.* Berlin, Heidelberg, New York: Springer-Verlag.

60. Hatch, J. W., Geidel, R. A. (1985) J. Hum. Evol. 14:469–476.

61. Huss-Ashmore, R., Goodman, R., Armelagos, G. J. (1982) In: Schiffer M. B. (ed) *Advances in Archaeological Method and Theory.* New York: Academic Press, p. 395.

62. Ohtsuka, R., Suzuki, T. (1978) Ecol. Food Nutr. 6:243–249.

63. Renan, M. J., van Rensburg, S. J. (1980) Phys. Med. Biol. 25:433–444.

64. Berlyne, G. M., Ben Ari, J., Nort, E., Shainkin, R. (1973) Am. J. Phys. Anthropol. 29:910–911.

65. Hummart, J. R. (1983) Am. J. Phys. Anthropol. 62:167–176.

66. Zaino, E. C. (1968) Am. J. Phys. Anthropol. 29:433–436.

67. Waldron, H. A. (1973) Med. Hist. 17:391–399.

68. Aufderheide, A. C., Neiman, F. D., Wittmers, Jr., L. E., Rapp, G. (1981) Am. J. Phys. Anthropol. 55:285–291.

69. Comar, C. L., Bronner, F. (1964) *Mineral Metabolism, An Advanced Treatise.* New York: Academic Press.

70. Spencer, H., Lewin, I., Samachson, J. (1967) In: Lenihan, J. M. A., Loutit, J. F., Martin, J. H. (eds) *Strontium Metabolism.* London New York: Academic Press, p. 111.

71. Waldron-Edward, D., Paul, T. M., Skoryna, S. C. (1967) In: Lenihan, J. M. A., Loutit, J. F., Martin, J. H. (eds) *Strontium Metabolism.* London/New York: Academic Press, p. 329.

72. Knizhnikov, V. A., Marei, A. N. (1967) In: Lenihan, J. M. A., Loutit, J. E., Martin, J. H. (eds) *Strontium Metabolism.* London/New York: Academic Press, p. 71.

73. Wolf, N., Gedalial, I., Yariv, S. (1973) Arch. Oral Biol. 18:497–499.

74. Losee, F. L., Adkins, B. L. (1968) Nature 219:630–631.

75. Cockburn, A., Cockburn, E. (eds) (1980) *Mummies, Disease, and Ancient Cultures.* Cambridge: Cambridge Univ. Press.

76. Wing, E. S., Brown, A. B. (1979) *Paleonutrition. Method and Theory in Prehistoric Foodways.* New York: Academic Press.

77. Stout, S. (1978) Curr. Anthropol. 19:601–604.

78. Oakley, K. P. (1969) *Framework for Dating Fossil Man.* 3rd Edition. London: Weidenfeld and Nicolson.

79. St. Hoyme, L. E., Koritzer, R. T. (1976) Am. J. Phys. Anthropol. 45:673–686.

80. Lambert, J. B., Simpson, S. V., Szpunar, C. B., Buikstra, J. E. (1985) J. Hum. Evol. 14:477–482.

81. Williams, C. T. (1988) In: Grupe G. & Herrmann B. (eds) *Trace Elements in Environmental History.* Berlin, Heidelberg, New York: Springer-Verlag, pp. 27–40.

82. Sealy, J. C., Sillen, A. (1988) J. Archaeol. Science 15:425–438.

83. Lambert, J. B., Simpson, S. V., Buikstra, J. E., Hanson D. (1983) Am. J. Phys. Anthropol. 62:409–423.

84. Grupe, G., Piepenbrink, H. (1988) In: Grupe G. & Herrmann, B. (eds.) *Trace Elements in Environmental History.* Berlin, Heidelberg, New York: Springer-Verlag, pp. 103–112.

85. Marchiafava, V., Bonucci, E., Ascenzi, A. (1974) Cal. Tis. Res. 14:195–210.

86. Sergi, S., Ascenzi, A., Bonucci, E. (1972) Am. J. Phys. Anthropol. 36:189–198.

87. Wyckoff, R. W. G. (1972) *The Biochemistry of Animal Fossils*. Bristol: Scientechnica (Publishers) Ltd.

88. Hanson, D. B., Buikstra, J. E. (1987) J. of Archaeol. Science 14:549–563.

89. DeNiro, M. J., Epstein, S. (1978) Geochim. Cosmochim. Acta. 42:495–506.

90. Dennison, K. J. (1980) J. of Archaeol. Science 7:81–86.

91. DeNiro, M. J. (1987) Am. Scientist 75:182–191.

92. Knight, B., Lauder I. (1969) Human Biol. 41:322–341.

93. Hare, P. E. (1980) In: Behrensmeyer A. K., Hill, A. P. (eds) *Fossils in The Making*. Chicago: Univ. of Chicago Press, p. 208.

94. Von Endt, D. W., Ortner, D. J. (1984) J. Archaeol. Sci. 11:247–253.

95. DeNiro, M. J. (1985) Nature 317:806–809.

96. Matter, P., Davidson, F. D., Wyckoff, R. W. G. (1970) Comp. Biochem. Physiology 35:291–298.

97. DeNiro, M. J., Weiner, S. (1988) Geochimica Acta 52:2197–2206.

98. Molleson, T. (1988) In: Grupe G. & Herrmann B. (eds) *Trace Elements in Environmental History*. Berlin, Heidelberg, New York: Springer-Verlag, pp. 67–82.

99. Dennison, K. J., Houghton, P. (1986) J. Archaeol. Science 13:393–401.

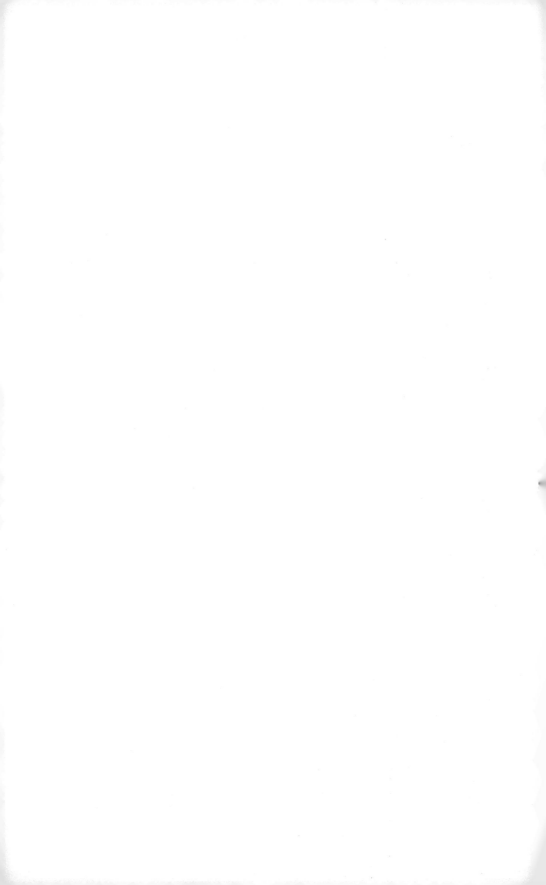